THE HISTORY OF
Occupational Therapy

THE FIRST CENTURY

THE HISTORY OF
Occupational Therapy

THE FIRST CENTURY

Lori T. Andersen, EdD, OTR/L, FAOTA

Kathlyn L. Reed, PhD, OTR, FAOTA, MLIS

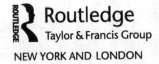

Routledge
Taylor & Francis Group

NEW YORK AND LONDON

The History of Occupational Therapy: The First Century includes ancillary materials specifically available for faculty use. Included are PowerPoint slides and *Instructor's Manual*. Please visit http://www.routledge.com/9781617119972 to obtain access.

First published 2017 by SLACK Incorporated

Published 2024 by Routledge
605 Third Avenue, New York, NY 10158

and by Routledge
4 Park Square, Milton Park, Abingdon, Oxon OX14 4RN

Routledge is an imprint of the Taylor & Francis Group, an informa business

Library of Congress Cataloging-in-Publication Data

Names: Andersen, Lori T., 1954- author. | Reed, Kathlyn L., author.
Title: The history of occupational therapy : the first century / Lori T.
   Andersen, Kathlyn L. Reed.
Description: Thorofare, NJ : SLACK Incorporated, [2017] | Includes
   bibliographical references and index.
Identifiers: LCCN 2016053330| ISBN 9781617119972 (hardback : alk. paper)
Subjects: | MESH: Occupational Therapy--history | History, 20th Century |
   Occupational Therapy--trends
Classification: LCC RM735 | NLM WB 555 | DDC 615.8/515--dc23 LC record available at
https://lccn.loc.gov/2016053330

ISBN: 9781617119972 (hbk)
ISBN: 9781003524571 (ebk)

DOI: 10.4324/9781003524571

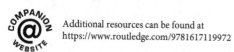

Additional resources can be found at
https://www.routledge.com/9781617119972

DEDICATION

This book is dedicated to all the history makers—past, present, and future.

CONTENTS

The History of Occupational Therapy: The First Century includes ancillary materials specifically available for faculty use. Included are PowerPoint slides and *Instructor's Manual*. Please visit http://www.routledge.com/9781617119972 to obtain access.

ACKNOWLEDGMENTS

Special acknowledgement is given to the chairs and co-chairs of the AOTA History Committee over the years, who repeatedly started the task of getting a book written on the history of occupational therapy but could not finish the task for one reason or another. These former chairs include Mary Merritt, Myra McDaniel, Robert K. Bing, Marianne Catterton, Helen Hopkins, Ruth Griffin, Carolyn Baum, and Ruth Levine Schemm.

Special acknowledgement is also given to the Junior Leagues of America, who provided the funds to buy equipment and supplies needed to start and maintain occupational therapy programs throughout the United States, provided countless volunteer hours in the clinics, and sometimes paid the salary of early occupational therapy practitioners. Without the help of the Junior Leagues, fewer occupational therapy service programs would have been started and survived. Many thanks are due to the members of Junior Leagues over the past 100 years for their interest, service, and support.

The authors also express their appreciation to the AOTF/AOTA for their willingness to share archival materials from the Wilma L. West Library. A special thank you is extended to Mindy Hecker and Helene Ross for their hospitality during our visits to the Wilma L. West Library and assistance in obtaining resource materials and artifacts.

ABOUT THE AUTHORS

Lori T. Andersen, EdD, OTR/L, FAOTA, received her Bachelor of Science degree in Rehabilitation Services from Springfield College, her Master of Science degree in Occupational Therapy from the Medical College of Virginia, and her Doctorate in Education from Nova Southeastern University. She has more than 15 years of experience in clinical practice and more than 20 years in academia. Her academic positions in occupational therapy have included the following: Associate Professor at Florida Gulf Coast University, Professor at Nova Southeastern University, Visiting Clinical Associate Professor at Florida International University, and Professor at Brenau University. She is now enjoying retirement, pursuing such passions as traveling and researching the history of occupational therapy.

Kathlyn (Kitty) L. Reed, PhD, OTR, FAOTA, MLIS, is Associate Professor Emeritus, School of Occupational Therapy, Texas Woman's University, Houston, Texas. She completed her basic education in occupational therapy at the University of Kansas, received a master's degree in occupational therapy from Western Michigan University, obtained a doctorate in special education from the University of Washington, and was awarded a second master's in information and library studies from the University of Oklahoma. She has been active in occupational therapy for over 50 years as a practitioner, educator, and consultant. Reed has authored several textbooks in occupational therapy and co-authored textbooks in physical therapy and speech-language pathology. She was named a fellow of the American Occupational Therapy Association (AOTA) in 1975, received the AOTA Award of Merit in 1983 and presented the Eleanor Clarke Slagle lectureship at the AOTA annual conference in 1986. She has served in the AOTA Delegate and Representative Assemblies representing three different state associations and was chair of the AOTA Ethics Commission. She is a member of the Texas Occupational Therapy Association, the World Federation of Occupational Therapists and the Society for the Study of Occupation. Her interests include tracking assessments developed by occupational therapists, analyzing models of practice in occupational therapy, and studying the philosophy and history of the profession.

FOREWORD

The past is never dead. It's not even past.
—William Faulkner (1953, p. 73)

In this quote, William Faulkner calls forth a haunting truth about how history waits for us around the next corner; how it reminds us that its lessons should be heeded if we are wise. But too often it seems humans fall prey to the naïve and impatient conceit of youth and are fooled by the illusion that there is nothing from the past that is worth knowing.

Of course, ideas and events from the past do live on, often lurking in the shadows of the familiar or the taken-for-granted. The poet/philosopher David Whyte makes the keen observation that "alertness is the hidden discipline of familiarity" (2003). He suggests that the familiar (established habits and ideas) can teach us if we let them, since they too were informed by earlier conversations —the dialogues that take place with ourselves or with others as we make sense of the world.

Fortunately, life provides occasions that remind people (as individuals or groups) to acknowledge the important lessons of the past. In the present case, it is the timely publication of this fascinating and important book, inspired by the 100th anniversary of occupational therapy. Centennial celebrations are like family reunions in that they naturally invite useful reflections and memories, calling forth reminders that everything we know, sense, and understand is ultimately the result of someone or some group whose footprints once graced the paths we now tread.

Awareness of history enables us to recognize the story lines of our past, to appreciate the genius, inspiration, persistence and work of our forebears, and to understand the importance of context, since progress often results from the alignment of ideas, opportunities, individuals, and chance.

Yet, simply being alert to a profession's history may be insufficient to provide useful guidance for the paths ahead. Unwary professions can fail to recognize the distinctions between the past and present and the potential implications of planned changes on current and future practice. Care is needed to avoid the assumption that innovations necessarily equate with improvements or progress. Similarly, in the global environment of the 21st century, it is useful to make distinctions between the developments of a profession in one country in contrast to that of others. Although occupational therapy began in the United States, it has evolved quite differently in other countries with different social and political contexts. Some might argue, with justification, that progress in some other countries has equaled or surpassed that made in the United States.

This well documented historical volume is a monumental and timely contribution to the literature of occupational therapy. It carefully describes changes in the profession that have been influenced by events such as wars, legislation, economics, reimbursement practices, regulatory changes, and educational standards. It also deftly describes the evolution of concepts influencing practice, drawing upon the well-regarded expertise of Kathlyn Reed in this area.

The editors have been careful to avoid extraneous commentary about the personalities of key figures and the stories of conflict and character that provide the color (and often the explanations) for why some things happened and others did not. While group living is imperative to human survival, it is imperfect to be sure, and the inevitable conflict that occurs within groups often causes distractions from the tasks at hand. This can sometimes lead to inattention in important areas, prolonged disagreement, delayed decision-making, or misdirected and uninspired leadership.

Perhaps also, it is useful to devote attention to the values that guide decisions and actions of a profession over time. Questions have and can be made with legitimacy about the profession's inconsistencies when it comes to values and actions—that is, what is said versus what is actually done (Hammel, 2009; Kielhofner, 2005). Or, why new practice concepts may be insufficiently debated or challenged (e.g., Mocellin, 1995, 1996)?

In the United States, Peloquin (1994, 2005, 2007) and Yerxa (1994) have been notable among those who been courageous and thoughtful contributors to an important conversation about the core values, aspirations, and beliefs that influenced occupational therapy's founding and how these remain relevant over time. Questions about values, ethics, and professional responsibilities serve importantly as a profession's moral compass. Current questions might include: Why does a relative lack of diversity persist among the profession's practitioners in the United States (Abreu & Peloquin, 2004; US Department of Health and Human Services, 2013)? And, since mental health is such a compelling national issue, how did organized occupational therapy in the United States ever allow itself to abandon its rich traditions in this area (Bonder, 1987)? More important, perhaps, are observations by the late Maralynne Mitcham (2014) regarding the lack of clarity and focus in the structure and pedagogies of educational curricula around occupation as the central concept of occupational therapy.

As suggested earlier, a profession's inattention to its founding ideas can result in navigational errors, eroding its heritage and compromising it ethics and responsibility to the public. Thoughtful leaders should be alert to potential implications of changes on core values such as therapeutic use of self, or client-centered care based on a full appreciation of the everyday lives of clients and their personal narratives. Even the use of the term *client* to identify recipients of care has been seen as an erosion of the field's ethos (Sharrot & Yerxa, 1985).

This volume also notes the increased attention to research that has been ushered in by managed care and the calls for evidence-based practice (e.g., Tickle-Degnen, 1999). To be sure, it is understandable and necessary for a health profession to improve its practices as research validates or disproves theories and techniques that were previously based only on clinical traditions. While the evolution of evidence-based practice in occupational therapy during the 21st century is generally seen as a positive development, it is not without its critics. Some argue that studies focusing only on things that can be readily measured too often overlook qualitative dimensions of care that are not easily reduced to numbers (e.g., Hammell, 2001). For example, failure to study dimensions of personal meaning for the client could ultimately diminish occupational therapy's claims to authenticity, relevance, and distinct value (Engelhardt, 1977, 1983; Kielhofner, 2005; Yerxa, 1967).

Toward the end of his life, American poet William Carlos Williams, who worked as a physician to support his passion for writing, penned a beautiful poem to his wife. Two lines in that composition, called "Asphodel, That Greeny Flower" (1994) seem relevant here:

> *It is difficult to get the news from poems*
> *yet men die miserably every day for lack of what is found there.*

In a world currently torn by violence, ideological conflict, and social injustices, there is a manifest need for health care that embraces the World Health Organization's definition of health, unconstrained as it is by economic motives and myopic distinctions between body, mind, and soul. Many years ago, I wrote that I welcomed the 21st century as an era where occupational therapy's promise would be fully realized by embracing the inspiring ideas of its founders, grounded as they were in the healing potential of human occupation (Christiansen, 1999). The AOTA Centennial Vision effort, which I had the privilege of helping to lead, took care to include goals intended to advance the profession while preserving its ethos (AOTA, 2007; Moyers, 2007). As occupational therapy moves ahead, one hopes that future leaders in the United States and elsewhere will be alert and courageous in protecting occupational therapy's rich heritage.

One day perhaps, ages hence, there will be a sequel to this important book, in whatever mediated form exists at that time. My earnest hope is that it documents that the territory inhabited by the profession has become as large as its language; inspired as it has been by ideas and people borne of courage, imagination, practicality, compassion, and a deeply rooted sense of social justice.

Charles H. Christiansen, EdD, OTR, FAOTA
Retired CEO, American Occupational Therapy Foundation
Clinical Professor, The University of Texas Medical Branch at Galveston
Principal and Founder, StoryCrafting, LLC
Rochester, Minnesota

References

Abreu, B. C., & Peloquin, S. M. (2004). The issue is-embracing diversity in our profession. *American Journal of Occupational Therapy, 58*(3), 353-358.

American Occupational Therapy Association. (2007). AOTA's Centennial Vision and executive summary. *American Journal of Occupational Therapy, 61*(6), 613-614.

Bonder, B. R. (1987). Occupational therapy in mental health: Crisis or opportunity? *American Journal of Occupational Therapy, 41*(8), 495-499.

Christiansen, C. H. (1999). Defining lives: Occupation as identity: An essay on competence, coherence, and the creation of meaning, 1999 Eleanor Clarke Slagle lecture. *American Journal of Occupational Therapy, 53,* 547-558.

Engelhardt, H. T. (1977). Defining occupational therapy: The meaning of therapy and the virtues of occupation. *American Journal of Occupational Therapy, 31*(10), 666-672.

Engelhardt, H. T. (1983). Occupational therapists as technologists and custodians of meaning. In G. Kielhofner (Ed.), *Health Through Occupation: Theory and Practice in Occupational Therapy* (pp. 139-145). Philadelpha, PA: F.A. Davis.

Faulkner, W. (1953). *Requiem for a nun.* New York, NY: Random House.

Hammell, K. W. (2001). Using qualitative research to inform the client-centred evidence-based practice of occupational therapy. *The British Journal of Occupational Therapy, 64*(5), 228-234.

Hammell, K. W. (2009). Sacred texts: A sceptical exploration of the assumptions underpinning theories of occupation. *Canadian Journal of Occupational Therapy, 76*(1), 6-13.

Kielhofner, G. (2005). Scholarship and practice: Bridging the divide. *American Journal of Occupational Therapy, 59*(2), 231-239.

Mitcham, M. D. (2014). Education as Engine. *American Journal of Occupational Therapy, 68*(6), 636-648.

Mocellin, G. (1995). Occupational therapy: a critical overview, part 1. *The British Journal of Occupational Therapy, 58*(12), 502-506.

Mocellin, G. (1996). Occupational therapy: a critical overview, part 2. *The British Journal of Occupational Therapy, 59*(1), 11-16.

Moyers, P. A. (2007). A legacy of leadership: Achieving our centennial vision. *The American Journal of Occupational Therapy, 61*(6), 622.

Peloquin, S. M. (1994). Moral treatment: How a caring practice lost its rationale. *American Journal of Occupational Therapy, 48*(2), 167-173.

Peloquin, S.M. (2005). Embracing our ethos, reclaiming our heart. *American Journal of Occupational Therapy, 59,* 611-625.

Peloquin, S. M. (2007). A reconsideration of occupational therapy's core values. *American Journal of Occupational Therapy, 61*(4), 474.

Sharrott, G. W., & Yerxa, E. J. (1985). Promises to keep: Implications of the referent "patient" versus "client" for those served by occupational therapy. *American Journal of Occupational Therapy, 39*(6), 401-405.

Tickle-Degnen, L. (1999). Organizing, evaluating, and using evidence in occupational therapy practice. *American Journal of Occupational Therapy, 53*(5), 537-539.

US Department of Health and Human Services. (2013). The US Health Workforce Chartbook. *National Center for Health Workforce Analysis.* Rockville, MD: Health Resources and Services Administration.

Whyte, D. (2003). *Everything is waiting for you.* Langley, WA: Many Rivers Press.

Williams, W. C. (1994). *Asphodel, That Greeny Flower and Other Love Poems.* New York, NY: New Directions Publishing Corporation.

Yerxa, E. J. (1967). 1966 Eleanor Clarke Slagle lecture. Authentic occupational therapy. *American Journal of Occupational Therapy, 21*(1), 1.

Yerxa, E. J. (1994). Dreams, dilemmas, and decisions for occupational therapy practice in a new millennium: An American perspective. *American Journal of Occupational Therapy, 48*(7), 586-589.

INTRODUCTION

To understand who we are and where we are going,
we first need to understand who we were and where we came from.

In studying the history of occupational therapy, one may see first, only interesting events, second, a series of records left by medical authorities of the past which help to establish the value of this treatment for the sick today, and finally, we may, through these events, examine the forces which contributed to development in the past and may affect progress in the future. (Haas, 1944, p. 3)

This quote underscores the importance of understanding history to appreciate the efforts of those who came before to foster the development of occupational therapy and to learn from the lessons of the past to effectively plan for the future. We are reminded by Bob Bing (1961, pp. 296-297) that "the names, the pictures, the thoughts of those who came before us are indeed a profound reminder of the possibility that someday, someone may be looking back and may be wondering who we were and what we did." The eve of the Centennial Celebration, the commemoration of the first 100 years of occupational therapy, calls for a historical review and reflection and a renewed effort to set the direction for the next 100 years.

This book was written for all occupational therapy practitioners and occupational therapy students who want to learn more about the history of occupational therapy, especially about the people, activities, and influences that shaped the development of the profession. The objective of this scholarly book is to provide these readers with the historical context of the profession, from the formative stages in the 18th century to the eve of the Centennial Celebration in 2017, as well as a glimpse into the future. Extensive use of photographs of pioneers, leaders, and advocates of occupational therapy; pictures of occupational therapy artifacts, including newspaper clippings and historical documents; maps showing historical locations in occupational therapy practice and education; and sidebars that give glimpses into personalities and events add visually stimulating and educational perspective to the contextual history.

The chapters follow a chronological timeline, providing discussions and reflections on the influence of highlighted personalities, key places and times, sociocultural events and issues, political events and legislation, economic and technological issues, educational factors that led to the progressive maturation of the profession, changes in practice over the years, and development of the national association and related organizations. In the early chapters, the prominent personalities of the profession—including the backgrounds and experiences they brought to the table, the foundations they laid, and the crises and battles they faced—are the central focus of the discussion. In later chapters, the issues and problems that faced the profession in the modern world become more central to the discussion.

All history must be viewed from the perspective of the present and is thus a changing target. What was important to our founders may seem trivial to us today. What seems important to us today may seem unimportant to future generations of occupational therapy practitioners. We have tried to present a fair and unbiased approach to writing the history but recognize that our eyes and minds are rooted in today and that tomorrow may bring a different set of eyes and minds that analyze the same issues from a different angle. Nevertheless, we hope our efforts provide readers with a better understanding of their professional roots and stimulate further study and research into the historical details of occupational therapy.

Lori T. Andersen, EdD, OTR/L, FAOTA
Kathlyn L. Reed, PhD, OTR, FAOTA, MLIS

References

Bing, R. K. (1961). *William Rush Dunton, Junior—American psychiatrist, a study in self* (Doctoral dissertation). College Park, MD: University of Maryland. Available from ProQuest Dissertations and Theses database. UMI no. 6305931.

Haas, L. (1944). *Practical occupational therapy for the mentally and nervously ill*. Milwaukee, WI: The Bruce Publishing Company.

1

The Formative Stages
Ancient Times to 1900s

Key Points

- The health benefits of activity and occupation were first recognized in ancient times.
- Shifting paradigms of scientific knowledge, sociocultural beliefs, and religious beliefs influenced medical treatment through the years.
- The Industrial Revolution was a significant milepost in the history of civilization, affecting the daily life of communities, families, and individuals.
- A number of social and political movements and reforms, including the Progressive Era, the Arts and Crafts Movement, and the establishment of settlement houses, were precursors to the development of the profession of occupational therapy.
- Occupational therapy developed from a confluence of established ideas and influences that developed over hundreds of years, not new knowledge or technology.

Highlighted Personalities

- Phillipe Pinel
- William Tuke and Henry Tuke
- Benjamin Rush
- Amariah Brigham
- Thomas Story Kirkbride
- Dorothea Dix
- John Ruskin and William Morris
- Jane Addams

Key Places

- Bicêtre Asylum and Salpêtrière Hospital in France
- York Retreat in England
- Pennsylvania Hospital in the United States
- Hull House in Chicago

Andersen, L. T., & Reed, K. L.
The History of Occupational Therapy: The First Century (pp. 1-13).
© 2017 Taylor & Francis Group.

Key Times/Events

- Medieval times
- Age of Enlightenment
- Industrialization Revolution
- Progressive Era

Political Events/Issues

- Progressive Movement

Economic Events/Issues

- Industrialization Revolution

Sociocultural Events/Issues

- Moral treatment
- Change from an agrarian to a manufacturing society
- Move from rural to urban areas
- Wave of immigration
- Progressive Movement
- Arts and Crafts Movement
- Settlement houses

Technological Events/Issues

- Shifting medical paradigms with advances in scientific knowledge
- Industrialization

INTRODUCTION

Credo:
That occupation is as necessary to life as food and drink.
That every human being should have both physical and mental occupation.
That sick minds, sick bodies, sick souls, may be healed thru occupation.
—Dr. William Rush Dunton, Jr., 1919

The year 1917 stands as a historic year in the establishment of occupational therapy in the United States; however, the seeds for the development of occupational therapy were planted hundreds of years ago. With strong roots in psychiatry, the philosophy of occupational therapy is entrenched in the beliefs and values of the treatment of individuals with mental illness.

From ancient times, the treatment of those with mental illness was influenced by changes in sociocultural and religious beliefs, advances in scientific knowledge, current political issues, and current economic concerns. In more modern times, several social and political reform movements contributed directly or indirectly to the evolution of occupational therapy, including the use of moral treatment, which began in the Age of Enlightenment, the Arts and Crafts Movement, the Settlement House Movement, the Progressive Movement, and the Mental Hygiene Movement, all of which began in the late 19th and early 20th centuries.

THE RISE OF MORAL TREATMENT

Strongly rooted in psychiatry, occupational therapy emerged from the successful use of occupation in the treatment of mental illness hundreds of years ago. In ancient times, as early as 2000 B.C., the therapeutic benefit of occupation was recognized when music and dance were used to soothe troubled minds and lift one from depressed states and morbid moods (Haas, 1944, p. 3). During the first century, Galen, a prominent Greek physician, also promoted the benefit of occupation, stating, "employment is nature's best physician and is essential to human happiness" (Dunton, 1947, p. 1; Haas, 1944, p. 3).

In medieval times, physical and mental illnesses were thought to be caused by disturbances in body fluids and humors, including blood, phlegm, and yellow and black bile. Physicians of the time believed that restoration of balance in the body humors through bloodletting, purging, and enemas would help to alleviate symptoms of physical and mental disorders. Additionally, people with mental illness were said to be possessed by demons and were being punished for their heretical religious beliefs (Pinel, 1806, p. xxi). Not of rational mind, these people were deemed to be a danger to themselves and others. They were placed in asylums to separate them from society and were forced to live in conditions that were overcrowded and unsanitary. Inhumane care was typical of the lunatic asylums in medieval times. Often constrained in shackles, the mentally ill were frequently tortured to excise the demons and punish them for their sins. One of the worst asylums of the day was the Hospital of Saint Mary of Bethlem in London, also known as Bethlem Royal Hospital. The nickname of the asylum, Bedlam, an antiquated term for a lunatic asylum, became synonymous with the chaos, confusion, and irrational nature of asylums ("Bedlam," n.d.) (Figure 1-1).

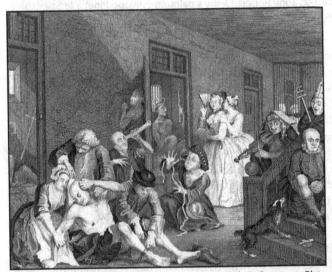

Figure 1-1. William Hogarth's painting of the Rake's Progress, Plate VIII, The Madhouse, depicts a man in Bedlam asylum in London being laughed at by aristocratic visitors who paid for the opportunity to see the lunatics.

The Age of Enlightenment, or Age of Reason, began at the end of the 17th century and continued through the 18th century. This new age brought cultural and intellectual movements with contemporary beliefs and perspectives. Society embraced individualism, reason, and advanced knowledge through science rather than relying on tradition and religious beliefs. Intellectuals turned to science as a way to understand human behavior and mental illness. Although many physicians continued to believe in a physical cause of mental illness, a belief in a psychological basis or moral cause for mental illness was emerging. Society and the medical community gradually shifted their view of mental illness toward a more humanistic view, in which all people, even those with mental illness, were perceived to be capable of rational thought. The new theory stated that the stresses of life caused people with mental illness to lose their ability to reason. These people, having no control over these stresses, the moral causes of lunacy, were not to blame for their illness. This belief in a moral reason or moral cause of mental illness gave rise to moral treatment. The shifts in sociocultural, religious, and political beliefs that emphasized the value and worth of an individual and the equality of individuals supported the rise of moral treatment and compassionate care (Bockoven, 1963, p. 11).

In late 18th century Europe, a number of institutions for the mentally ill began to incorporate the principles of moral treatment, improving the treatment of people with mental illness. Most prominent of these were the York Retreat in England and the Bicêtre Asylum and Salpêtrière Hospital in Paris. Dr. Philippe Pinel served as superintendent of Bicêtre Asylum and Salpêtrière Hospital. In his essay, "Treatise on Insanity," Pinel provides a historical discussion on the causes and treatments of mental illness.

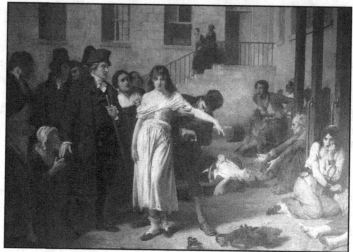

Figure 1-2. Tony Robert-Fleury's painting Philippe Pinel à la Salpêtrière shows Pinel unshackling a patient.

He included some of his observations on treating people with kindness and firmness, and on the beneficial effects of participation in "laborious or amusing occupations" (Pinel, 1806, p. 193). During his time as superintendent at Bicêtre Asylum and Salpêtrière Hospital, Pinel unshackled patients from chains, provided more sanitary living conditions, and encouraged participation in activities (Paterson, 2002) (Figure 1-2).

William Tuke and Henry Tuke, father and son, founded York Retreat in 1796 following the sudden death of a family friend. The friend, Hannah Mills, had been placed in an asylum, isolated from family and friends. The Tukes expressed concern that the substandard treatment in the asylum might have caused her death. The Tukes, who were Quakers, social reformers, and humanitarians, believed that those with mental illness were spiritual beings still capable of rationale thought if provided with kind yet firm treatment. All patients at the York Retreat were called Friends according to the Quaker tradition. Consistent with religious and political beliefs of the time, the Quakers considered those afflicted with mental disorders as valued individuals and equals entitled to humane treatment and not as people possessed by demons deserving of torture and punishment for their sins (Charland, 2007). Although the Tukes embraced moral treatment at York Retreat, traditional medical treatment of balancing body humors with purging and bloodletting were also used. Located on a country estate, York Retreat provided a healthy, peaceful environment to minimize the stresses of daily life (Figure 1-3). A structured regime of exercise, work, and leisure shaped daily routines. Patients were expected to display socially appropriate behavior in their dress, at meals, and in interactions with others. The Quaker influence of York Retreat also encouraged spiritual reflection as part of treatment (Charland, 2007).

Samuel Tuke, William's grandson, touted the benefits of participation in activities to occupy minds with healthy thoughts in a book about the York Retreat.

> Every means is taken to seduce the mind from its favourite but unhappy musings, by bodily exercise, walks, conversations, reading, and other innocent recreations. The good effect of exercise, and of variety of object, has been very striking in several instances at this Institution. (Tuke, 1813, p. 98)

York Retreat's census was small, just 30 patients. The high staff-to-patient ratio allowed for more individualized care to facilitate recovery from mental illness. Systematic clinical observations supported the fact that the conditions of patients at the Retreat improved with moral

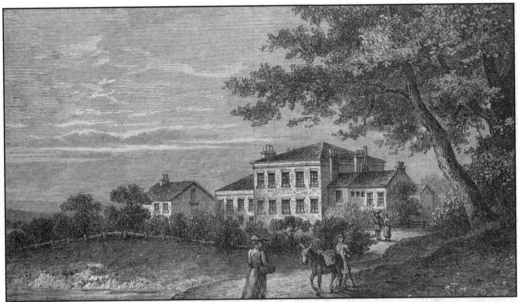

Figure 1-3. Drawing showing the estate and original building of York Retreat.

treatment (Charland, 2007). The reputation of York Retreat spread, and many from as far away as the United States came to see this model of practice first hand (Quiroga, 1995, p. 21).

Dr. Benjamin Rush of Philadelphia, a noted physician and signer of the Declaration of Independence, was a proponent of moral treatment in the United States in the late 18th century. Many considered Dr. Rush, a politician, reformer, educator, and physician, to be the father of American psychiatry (Figure 1-4). As an intellectual and a man of science, he attempted to find explanations for the causes of diseases and to categorize diseases of the mind rather than relying on tradition and religious beliefs. He sought evidence to support the effectiveness of treatments for diseases of the mind. As the superintendent of Pennsylvania Hospital in Philadelphia, one of the first hospitals in the United States to embrace moral treatment for individuals with mental illness, he took immense pride in eliminating shackles and cruel treatments in favor of more humane care. Pennsylvania Hospital's philosophy provided kind yet firm treatment that expected patients to adhere to social norms in a comfortable environment with fresh air and light. Patients were encouraged to participate in such activities as reading, listening to stories, exercise, games, and work activities to divert their minds from the deranged ideas and thoughts that were thought to cause their mental illness. Although he implemented moral treatment at Pennsylvania Hospital, Dr. Rush also continued to use physical interventions focused on balancing the body humors and fluids (Reed & Sanderson, 1999, pp. 20-21; Rush, 1812, pp. 174-180, pp. 241-244).

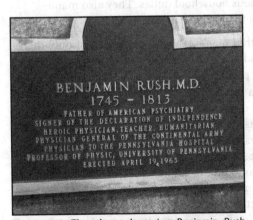

Figure 1-4. The plaque honoring Benjamin Rush at his gravesite at Christ Church Burial Ground in Philadelphia. At the Fourth Annual Meeting of the National Society for the Promotion of Occupational Therapy in Philadelphia, President Eleanor Clarke Slagle credited Benjamin Rush with starting the first occupational therapy work in America. (Copyright © Dr. Lori T. Andersen. Reprinted with permission.)

A number of other mental institutions that embraced the philosophy of moral treatment opened their doors in the early 19th century, including McLean Asylum (Hospital) in Massachusetts,

Frankford Insane Asylum in Pennsylvania, Bloomingdale Asylum in New York, Hartford Retreat for the Insane in Connecticut, Kentucky Lunatic Asylum in Kentucky, Worcester Insane Asylum (State Hospital) in Massachusetts, and Vermont Asylum for the Insane (Brattleboro Retreat) in Vermont. Others, such as New York State Lunatic Asylum at Utica, followed in the 1840s.

Dr. Amariah Brigham became superintendent of New York State Lunatic Asylum in 1843 (Hunt, 1858) (Figure 1-5). He was among a number of asylum superintendents at that time who championed moral treatment as an

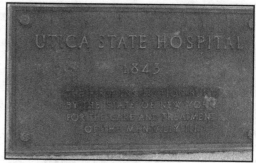

Figure 1-5. Plaque indicating the year Utica State Hospital opened. The hospital was originally known as New York State Lunatic Asylum at Utica.

effective cure for mental disorders. Many of these superintendents collaborated to establish the Association of Medical Superintendents of American Institutions for the Insane, the forerunner to the American Psychiatric Association (Luchins, 1988). The official journal of the association, the *Journal of Insanity*, was edited by Dr. Brigham. Also a frequent contributor to the journal, Dr. Brigham often wrote about moral treatment. According to Dr. Brigham, moral treatment involved:

> Removal of the insane from home and former association, with respectful and kind treatment, under all circumstances, and in most cases manual labor, attendance on [sic] religious worship on Sunday, the establishment of regular habits and of self-control, diversion of the mind from morbid trains of thought... (Brigham, 1847, p. 1)

In a description of New York State Lunatic Asylum and activities, Brigham indicated:

> Attached to the Asylum, is an excellent farm, of above one hundred and forty acres, affording pasturage and hay for the cows and horses that will be necessary, and good land for raising all the vegetables required by the household. The patients, in good weather, perform much labor on the farm, and in the garden, by which they are gratified and improved. Some also work in the joiners' shop, some make and repair mattresses, and several work at making and mending shoes. The women make clothing, bedding, and do the ironing, and assist in various household duties. They also manufacture many useful and fancy articles for sale. (Brigham, 1844, pp. 5-6)

Many of these activities, such as farming and other manual labors, provided not only therapeutic activities for the patients but also income and support to enable asylums to become self-sufficient, self-sustaining communities (Haas, 1944, p. 10).

The superintendents of the asylums believed that a person's environment, with social and moral problems and other stresses of life, contributed to his or her mental illness. Therefore, a move from a stressful environment to a peaceful environment was hypothesized to facilitate recovery. Asylums were located on rural estates away from urban centers to provide a stress-free environment. In the 1840s, the Association of Medical Superintendents of American Institutions for the Insane considered the structural design of a building to be of paramount importance (Luchins, 1988). Thomas Kirkbride, superintendent of Pennsylvania Hospital in the 1840s, developed the Kirkbride Plan, an architectural plan for asylum buildings. The architectural design of Kirkbride buildings generally consisted of a center building with long wings, allowing for a pleasant environment with plenty of fresh air and light (Figure 1-6). The Kirkbride Plan was used to build asylums all over the country. The first one built, New Jersey State Hospital at Trenton, formerly known as New Jersey State Lunatic Asylum, was built in 1848. Other Kirkbride hospitals include the following:

- Pennsylvania State Lunatic Asylum at Harrisburg
- Taunton State Hospital at Taunton, Massachusetts

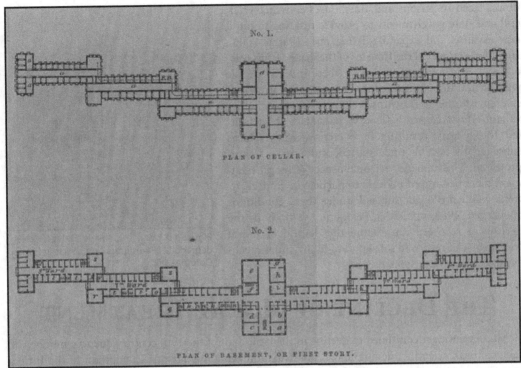

Figure 1-6. Drawing showing the layout of a typical Kirkbride building.

- Northampton State Lunatic Asylum at Northampton, Massachusetts
- Institute of Pennsylvania Hospital at Philadelphia (Kirkbride's Hospital)
- Hudson River State Hospital for the Insane at Poughkeepsie, New York
- St. Joseph State Hospital at St. Joseph, Missouri (formerly known as Missouri State Hospital for the Insane)
- Athens State Hospital for the Insane at Athens, Ohio
- Clarinda State Hospital at Clarinda, Iowa
- Independence State Hospital at Independence, Iowa
- Fergus Falls Regional Treatment Center State Hospital at Fergus Falls, Minnesota
- Broughton State Hospital at Morganton, North Carolina (formerly known as the Western Carolina Insane Asylum)
- Oregon State Hospital at Portland, Oregon
- Northern Michigan Asylum for the Insane at Traverse City, Michigan
- St. Elizabeth's Hospital at Washington, D.C. (formerly known as Government Hospital for the Insane)
- Kankakee State Hospital in Kankakee, Illinois
- Sheppard Pratt Hospital at Towson, Maryland

Some Kirkbride hospitals are still in existence today (Geller & Morrissey, 2004; McElroy, n.d.).

In spite of efforts to improve treatment for those with mental illness, problems continued. Dorothea Dix, a mid-19th century reformer, was intent on securing the protection of people with mental illness (Figure 1-7). A person of strong opinions, critical nature, and bold, imperious manner, she exposed the fact that many of the insane were housed inappropriately in prisons and almshouses. Dix's graphic first-hand accounts of the horrific conditions that people with mental illness faced in prisons and almshouses convinced federal and state governments to provide funding to build new asylums and expand existing ones (Parry, 2006). Her efforts triggered the transfer of the insane from prisons and almshouses to asylums, where initially people with mental illness received more humane treatment in safe environments (Luchins, 1988). Unfortunately, her valiant efforts caused a flood of patients to be admitted to asylums, resulting in overcrowding. Asylums subsequently became understaffed, and care was compromised. The humane, personal aspect of moral treatment that encouraged patients to participate in occupations could no longer succeed under these conditions (Bockoven, 1963, pp. 38-39; Peloquin, 1994). With the decline in recovery rates came the demise of moral treatment and return to substandard living situations in asylums (Bockoven, 1963, p. 31).

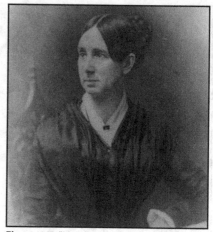

Figure 1-7. "Man is not made better by being degraded." Photograph of social reformer Dorothea Dix.

THE DECLINE OF MORAL TREATMENT

Moral treatment continued to decline in the latter half of the 19th century due to a number of sociocultural, scientific, demographic, political, and economic factors. In addition to the influx of patients from prisons and almshouses, families who no longer wanted to care for aging family members with dementia had them admitted to asylums. The wave of immigration in the mid-19th century also had an effect. With limited ability to speak English, immigrants often had difficulty adjusting to life in America. Society viewed immigrants with suspicion because of their differing sociocultural values, political beliefs, and habits. Many thought that foreign countries were encouraging emigration of their undesirables. Immigrants were often deemed to be mentally ill because of their different habits, routines, and traditions. Placed in asylums, immigrants began to make up an increasingly higher percentage of the patient populations. As these immigrants were not raised with the traditions and habits of Americans, many doubted that moral treatment, which encouraged good habits, hygiene, and routines, would benefit these immigrants (Bockoven, 1963, p. 24; Luchins, 1988).

In the latter half of the 19th century, advances in scientific and medical knowledge and the growth of neurology, a new medical specialty, prompted a paradigm shift. Neurologists believed that mental illness was organic—caused by a brain lesion—and as such could not be cured. Moral treatment, no longer based on current science, became obsolete. Asylum superintendents faced criticism because they were out of touch with current knowledge (Luchins, 1988; Peloquin, 1994). This shift came at a time when many of the early proponents, such as Dr. Amariah Brigham, had either left their posts or passed away, leaving few to advocate for the benefits of moral treatment (Bockoven, 1963, pp. 20-21). In 1854, Dr. John Gray, who was appointed superintendent of Utica State Hospital, also became editor of the American Journal of Insanity, positions previously held by Dr. Brigham (Bockoven, 1963, p. 41). Brigham's and Gray's philosophies on mental illness differed drastically. Dr. Brigham believed mental illness was inorganic—a disease of the mind. Dr. Gray believed mental illness was organic—a disease of the brain (Bockoven, 1963, p. 41; Lidz, 1985, p. 36). The shift in thinking became evident in the premier psychiatric journal of the day, as well as in the treatment philosophies of institutions.

The effectiveness of moral treatment was no longer supported by the annual reports of asylums, which had previously touted a high cure and discharge rates. Additionally, politicians recognized that asylums built according to Kirkbride's architectural requirements were very expensive. As a result, legislators no longer wanted to provide funding to build additional asylums (Bockoven, 1963, pp. 20-21; Luchins, 1988).

ARTS AND CRAFTS MOVEMENT

The Industrial Revolution, a significant turning point in history, began in England in the 18th century and slowly expanded to other countries. It was a time of great progress, with technological innovations such as the printing press, the steam engine, powered machine tools, improved processes to make iron, and manufacturing processes for mass production. The ripple effect of these innovations included advances in transportation systems, agriculture, and knowledge through distribution of print materials. A number of sociocultural and economic changes occurred, including an increase in the population, an increase in per capita income, a shift from rural to urban areas as people moved to work in factories, and a shift from an agricultural society to an industrial society. Mass production enabled more people to purchase goods as prices decreased.

The Industrial Revolution made great strides in advancing civilization, but it also brought some drawbacks. Prior to the Industrial Revolution, most goods, clothing, furniture, and foods were produced by individuals in their homes. There was a pride of workmanship in making handcrafted goods and a satisfaction in creating a well-made product that contributed to quality of life. Most viewed manufactured goods as being of a lesser quality than handmade goods in both design and construction. Factory workers had little to no control over the design or outcome of a finished product and therefore could not gain any personal satisfaction from a machine-made product (Levine, 1986, 1987; Schemm, 1994). The move to an industrial society caused a major concern that it would cause a decline in standards and moral values when people began to value materialism more than quality work (Schemm, 1994).

John Ruskin and William Morris, both social reformers, started the Arts and Crafts Movement in England as a reaction to the problems caused by the Industrial Revolution. The Arts and Crafts Movement embraced the belief that the action of making handmade goods integrated the mind and body, providing intrinsic satisfaction to the craftsman. As such, the Arts and Crafts Movement embraced a return to an appreciation of traditional design and craftsmanship (Schemm, 1994). Arts and crafts societies formed in various cities as part of the Arts and Crafts Movement in the United States. The aim of these societies was to ensure that artistic ability and technical ability to make handcrafted goods was not lost. Societies sponsored exhibitions to display handcrafted utilitarian objects of art and competitions to encourage higher standards. Societies also sponsored lectures, craft books, and other publications to educate people on making various crafts.

One of these societies, the Chicago Arts and Crafts Society, was incorporated at Hull House, a settlement house in Chicago, on October 22, 1897. The objectives of this society included:

> To recognize and encourage handicraft among its members, and through them in others, in order that the stimulation derived from this means may be a helpful factor in the development of those new ideals which present conditions, to-wit, industrial organization and the machine render necessary.

> To consider the present state of the factories and the workmen therein, and to devise lines of development which shall retain the machine in so far as it relieves the workman from drudgery, and tends to perfect his product; but which shall insist that the machine no longer be allowed to dominate the workman and reduce his production to a mechanical distortion. (Chicago Arts and Crafts Society, 1897)

The Society of Arts and Crafts (Boston) was formally incorporated on June 28, 1897 (Eaton, 1949). The mission of the Society, in concert with the Arts and Crafts Movement, was to "develop and encourage higher standards in the handicrafts" (Society of Arts and Crafts, 2014). This society still exists today. Architect George Edward Barton, one of the incorporators, later became one of the founders and incorporators of the National Society for the Promotion of Occupational Therapy (NSPOT), the precursor to the American Occupational Therapy Association (AOTA) (Eaton, 1949).

PROGRESSIVE MOVEMENT

The last decade of the 19th century guided in the Progressive Era, a time of tremendous social, economic, political, and technological change. Driven in part by the Industrial Revolution, the Progressive Era began as a social movement but evolved into a political movement to address some of the negative consequences brought on by the Industrial Revolution, including a lack of concern for worker safety, poor work conditions, poor wages, and the onslaught of child labor in factories (Figure 1-8). This era also witnessed corruption in government and industry, political scandals, and corporate monopolies that sacrificed the public good for profits.

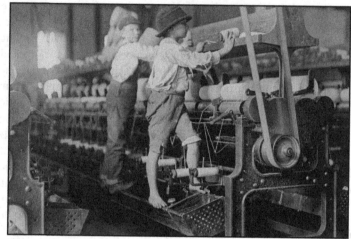

Figure 1-8. Photograph of children laboring in a textile factory in Macon, Georgia.

Progressives, the name given to the social and political reformers of this era, wanted to institute reforms to make the United States a better place to live. Their goal was to promote social justice and improved quality of life for all. Progressives firmly believed in the value of science, technology, and education. They set out to improve the environment and conditions of life for all people, pushing a series of reforms in the areas of medicine, public health, education, business, and banking by setting standards and regulating certain professions and industries. One reform of the Progressive Era, the setting of standards for medical education, resulted from the Flexner Report of 1910. With the objective of improving medical care, a committee of the American Medical Association (AMA) asked Abraham Flexner to study the state of medical education in the United States. Flexner surveyed 155 medical schools' admissions requirements, curricula, facilities, methods of assessment, and graduation requirements. Based on these findings, the Flexner Report of 1910 made recommendations to reform medical education, setting standards strongly based in science (Kunitz, 1974). This emphasis on standard setting had future implications for a number of medical professions, including occupational therapy.

SETTLEMENT HOUSE MOVEMENT

The elite middle class of this era, especially women, felt a sense of duty and obligation to work for social reform, and they did so through various types of philanthropic activities. Jane Addams, a well-known reformer representative of these philanthropic women, worked hands-on to improve the condition of the working class. Born to privilege, Jane, a very charismatic woman with a strong sense of duty, worked and led others to improve the living and working conditions of citizens. Like others, including Eleanor Roosevelt, wife of President Franklin Roosevelt, Jane Addams participated in establishing and running settlement houses to promote social and political reform.

In the United States, settlement houses were modeled after Toynbee Hall in England, one of the first settlement houses established in the world. Settlement houses served as neighborhood centers that provided living arrangements and a place for people of different social classes and cultures to gather to learn from organized educational programs and from each other. Discussions to foster the understanding of differing sociocultural backgrounds were encouraged at these gatherings (Reed & Sanderson, 1999, p. 23). Settlement houses also served as research centers that scientifically examined social, economic, and educational problems (Stritt,

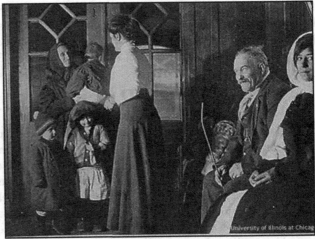

Figure 1-9. Front door at Hull House, Chicago, Illinois. (Hull-House Photograph Collection, Special Collections and University Archives, University of Illinois at Chicago.)

2014). The founders of settlement houses intended to use this information to identify issues and influence social policy.

In the United States, settlement houses were established in urban neighborhoods where the working poor and newly arrived immigrants lived. To help immigrants assimilate into American society and adjust to their new country's language, customs, and values, settlement houses provided classes in language, social, and work skills (Quiroga, 1995, pp. 37-38).

Women like Lillian Wald and Jane Addams were well known for the settlement houses they established. Wald established Henry Street Settlement in New York City and Jane Addams established Hull House in Chicago, one of the most famous settlement houses (Figure 1-9). The Chicago Arts and Crafts Society was established at Hull House, which was a good match because Hull House and the proponents of the Arts and Crafts Movement had a similar focus on social reform. The Chicago Arts and Crafts Society sought to counteract the worker alienation that resulted from the mass production of goods. At the same time, Hull House offered demonstrations and classes in making crafts so people could understand the processes and experience the pride and satisfaction in using one's hands to create beautiful, functional objects (Quiroga, 1995, pp. 41-42) (Figure 1-10).

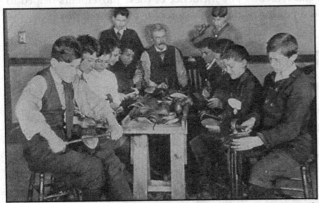

Figure 1-10. Boy's cobbling class at Hull House. (Hull-House Photograph Collection, Special Collections and University Archives, University of Illinois at Chicago.)

Lillian Wald, Jane Addams, and others associated with the Settlement House Movement gradually became politically active to further their goals. They recognized the need to influence government to solve social problems facing the poor, workers, and immigrants. Jane Addams and her colleagues quickly became political forces in Chicago, advocating for social justice and influencing public policy. Lillian Wald and Florence Kelley became political forces in New York City and Philadelphia, respectively. Concerned with children's welfare, they were instrumental in getting federal legislation passed in 1912 to establish the Children's Bureau. This federal bureau was estab-lished to safeguard the welfare of children and dealt with such social issues as infant mortality, juvenile delinquency, and child labor. A friend and colleague of Jane Addams at Hull House, Julia Lathrop, became the first director of this federal program (Brown, 2001, pp. 14-22).

REFLECTION

The origin and development of occupational therapy, rooted in psychiatry, was influenced by sociocultural values, religious beliefs, political attitudes, economic issues, and scientific knowledge that shaped the treatment of those with mental illness. As society emerged from medieval times, religious beliefs and sociocultural values changed. There was a renewed willingness to accept sci-ence and knowledge instead of holding fast to traditional beliefs. During the Renaissance, society adopted a humanistic view of man, recognizing all people as individuals with moral worth and deserving of respect. Mental illness, once thought to be caused by demons, was now believed to be caused by the ills and stresses of living in certain unhealthy environments. From the Renaissance to the 19th century, many of the principles of occupational therapy began to form through the work of reformers such as Philippe Pinel, William and Henry Tuke, Benjamin Rush, Amariah Brigham, Dorothea Dix, and Jane Addams. Through sheer force of desire and persistence, these advocates of change worked tirelessly to improve the social welfare of people with mental illness.

In the mid-19th century, moral treatment was derailed due to political and economic issues. Asylums were overcrowded with society's castoffs, including a significant percentage of immi-grants coming to the United States in the late 19th century. Asylums became more expensive to build and operate. In a change in scientific beliefs, mental illness was thought to be organic with no cure. Additionally, lack of evidence supporting the benefit of moral treatment contributed to its demise.

In the late 19th century, the Industrial Revolution, a major turning point in the history of civi-lization, triggered numerous sociocultural, technological, economic, and political changes, some good and some bad. The Arts and Crafts Movement, the Progressive Movement, and the Settlement House Movement, reactions to the ills of the Industrial Revolution, endeavored to improve quality of life for all. Occupational therapy emerged in this early 20th century environment, embracing many of the values of these movements. The Arts and Crafts Movement originated out of the desire to restore the worth of individuals by promoting the value of handmade goods. The Progressive Movement embraced science, social justice, political reform, and the sharing of knowledge. Finally, settlement houses served as research centers to study social, economic, and educational problems and advocated for social justice and social reforms. The influence of these movements helped to shape the values, beliefs, principles, and direction of the profession of occupational therapy.

REFERENCES

Bedlam. (n.d.). Merriam-Webster's online dictionary. Retrieved from http://www.merriam-webster.com/dictionary/bedlam

Bockoven, J. S. (1963). *Moral treatment in American psychiatry.* New York, NY: Springer Publishing Company, Inc.

Brigham, A. (1844). Article I: Brief notice of the New York State Lunatic Asylum at Utica. *American Journal of Insanity, 1,* 5-6. Retrieved from http://archive.org/details/psyamericanjourno1ameruoft

Brigham, A. (1847). Article I: The moral treatment of insanity. *American Journal of Insanity, 4,* 1. Retrieved from https://archive.org/details/americanjournal04184amer

Brown, V. B. (2001). Addams, Jane. In R. L. Schultz & A. Hast (Eds.), *Women building Chicago 1790-1990: A biographi-cal dictionary* (pp. 14-22). Bloomington, IN: Indiana University Press.

Charland, L. C. (2007). Benevolent theory: Moral treatment at the York Retreat. *History of Psychiatry, 18*(1), 61-80. doi:10.1177/0957154X07070320

Chicago Arts and Crafts Society. (1897). *Chicago Arts and Crafts Society constitution.* Chicago, IL: Author.

Dunton, W. R. (1947). History and development of occupational therapy. In H. S. Willard & C. S. Spackman (Eds.), *Principles of occupational therapy* (pp. 1-9). Philadelphia, PA: J. B. Lippincott Company.

Eaton, A. H. (1949). *Handicrafts of New England* (pp. 281-294). New York, NY: Harper Brothers.

Geller, J. L., & Morrissey, J. P. (2004). Asylum within and without asylums. *Psychiatric Services, 55*(10), 1128-1130.

Haas, L. (1944). *Practical occupational therapy for the mentally and nervously ill.* Milwaukee, WI: The Bruce Publishing Company.

Hunt, E. (1858). *Biographical sketch of Amariah Brigham, late superintendent of the New York State Lunatic Asylum, Utica, N.Y.* Utica, NY: W. O. McClure.

Kunitz, S. J. (1974). Professionalism and social control in the Progressive Era: The case of the Flexner Report. *Social Problems, 22*(1), 16-27.

Levine, R. E. (1986). Historical research: Ordering the past to chart our future. *Occupational Therapy Journal of Research, 6*(5), 259-269.

Levine, R. E. (1987). The influence of the arts-and-crafts movement on the professional status of occupational therapy. *American Journal of Occupational Therapy, 41*(4), 249-254.

Lidz, T. (1985). Adolf Meyer and the development of American psychiatry. *Occupational Therapy in Mental Health, 5*(3), 33-53.

Luchins, A. S. (1988). The rise and decline of the American asylum movement in the 19th century. *Journal of Psychology: Interdisciplinary and Applied, 122*(5), 471-486.

McElroy, E. (n.d.). Kirkbride buildings. Retrieved from http://www.kirkbridebuildings.com/

Parry, M. S. (2006, April). Dorothea Dix (1802-1887). *American Journal of Public Health, 96*(4), 624-625. doi:10.2105/AJPH.2005.079152

Paterson, C. F. (2002). A short history of occupational therapy in psychiatry. In J. Creek (Ed.), *Occupational therapy and mental health* (3rd ed., pp. 3-14). London, UK: Churchill Livingstone.

Peloquin, S. M. (1994). Looking back: Moral treatment: How a caring practice lost its rationale. *American Journal of Occupational Therapy, 48*(2), 167-173.

Pinel, P. H. (1806). *A treatise on insanity.* Sheffield, UK: W. Todd. Retrieved from http://archive.org/details/treatiseoninsanioopine

Quiroga, V. A. M. (1995). *Occupational therapy: The first 30 years: 1900 to 1930.* Bethesda, MD: American Occupational Therapy Association.

Reed, K. L., & Sanderson, S. N. (1999). *Concepts of occupational therapy* (4th ed.). Philadelphia, PA: Lippincott Williams & Wilkins.

Rush, B. (1812). *Medical inquiries and observations, upon the diseases of the mind.* Philadelphia, PA: Kimber & Richardson. Retrieved from http://archive.org/details/medicalinquiries1812rush

Schemm, R. L. (1994). Bridging conflicting ideologies: The origins of American and British occupational therapy. *American Journal of Occupational Therapy, 48*(11), 1082-1088.

Society of Arts and Crafts. (2014). The Society of Arts and Crafts: Background and history. Retrieved from http://www.societyofcrafts.org/about/about.asp

Stritt, S. (2014). The first faith-based movement: The religious roots of social progressivism in America (1880-1912) in historical perspective. *Journal of Sociology and Social Welfare, 41*(4), 77-105.

Tuke, S. (1813). *Description of the retreat, an institution near York for insane persons.* Philadelphia, PA: Isaac Peirce. Retrieved from http://collections.nlm.nih.gov/muradora/objectView.action?pid=nlm:nlmuid-2575045R-bk

2

Conception and Formal Birth
1900s to 1917

Key Points

- Functional and pragmatic psychology viewpoints influenced the thinking of Adolf Meyer and his new science of psychobiology—the inseparable mind-body connection—one of the principles of occupational therapy today.
- The Arts and Crafts Movement, moral treatment, the Progressive Movement, and the Mental Hygiene Movement influenced the formal birth of occupational therapy.
- The Progressive Era of the early 20th century, with its sharing of ideas, progressive thought, and emphasis on science, brought the early proponents of occupation together.
- The early founders brought different skills, abilities, and values to the table.
- Occupational therapy was born of a confluence of ideas, not one paradigm.
- Key events and people shaped the profession of occupational therapy.

Highlighted Personalities

- William James
- Thomas Dewey
- Adolf Meyer
- Julia Lathrop
- George Edward Barton
- William Rush Dunton, Jr.

- Herbert Hall
- Susan Cox Johnson
- Thomas Bessell Kidner
- Isabel Gladwin Newton
- Eleanor Clarke Slagle
- Susan E. Tracy

Andersen, L. T., & Reed, K. L.
The History of Occupational Therapy: The First Century (pp. 15-49).
© 2017 Taylor & Francis Group.

Key Places

- Devereux Mansion in Massachusetts
- Adams Nervine Hospital in Jamaica Plains, Massachusetts
- Sheppard and Enoch Pratt Hospital in Towson, Maryland
- Occupational Experiment Station in Chicago, Illinois
- Chicago School of Civics and Philanthropy in Chicago, Illinois
- Hull House in Chicago, Illinois
- Henry B. Favill School of Occupations in Chicago, Illinois
- Consolation House in Clifton Springs, New York
- Industrial Room, Clifton Springs Sanitarium
- Experiment Station for the Study of Invalid Occupations in Jamaica Plains, Massachusetts

Political Events/Issues

- Progressive Movement
- Government regulation
- Consumer protection (anti-trust legislation)

Association Issues

- Founding of the profession
- Initial Contemplation of Educational Standards

Key Times/Events

- Progressive Era
- Founding meeting of National Society of the Promotion of Occupational Therapy

Sociocultural Events/Issues

- Moral treatment
- Pragmatism
- Functional psychology
- Progressive Movement
- Arts and Crafts Movement
- Settlement House Movement
- Mental Hygiene Movement
- Manual training

Economic Events/Issues

- Industrialization

Technological Events/Issues

- Medical technology: x-ray, electrocardiogram
- Communication technology: telegraph, radio, telephone
- Transportation technology: railroad, automobile, airplane

INTRODUCTION

"Never doubt that a small group of thoughtful, committed citizens can change the world. Indeed, it is the only thing that ever has."
–Margaret Mead

At the turn of the century, the Progressive Movement was in full swing, led by Presidents Theodore Roosevelt, William Howard Taft, and Woodrow Wilson. Consumer protection, regulation of commerce, anti-trust legislation, workers' rights movements, the women's suffrage movement, and development of the national park system were all initiatives and movements intended to improve quality of life for citizens. Advances in science and new inventions furthered development of the railroad transportation system, the telephone system, and the use of radios. Electricity was now lighting cities. Henry Ford implemented the assembly line. As a result, his Ford automobiles become more affordable. The Panama Canal, an engineering marvel, was built. The United States assembled a powerful navy, including powered submarines. Renewed interest in science initiated reforms in intellectual thinking and education. Within the context of these advances and reforms, the opportunity and desire to develop the new profession of occupational therapy took shape. The productive 3-day inaugural meeting of the National Society for the Promotion of Occupational Therapy (NSPOT) was the beginning of the founders' and leaders' vision and work to establish a strong foundation for the Society and profession.

INTELLECTUAL THINKING

A renewed interest in science and systematic investigation was ushered in by the Progressive Era in the late 19th and early 20th centuries. The economic, political, and social reform of the Progressive Movement of the early 20th century also brought educational reform and, along with it, the gradual emergence of research universities and a new group of intellectual thinkers. These intellectuals challenged traditional thinking and focused their efforts on advancing knowledge in various fields and professions, including the social sciences, which sought to answer social problems.

William James and John Dewey were two of the leading thinkers of the late 19th and early 20th centuries. William James is considered the father of American psychology, and John Dewey is best known as an educational reformer with a belief in learning by doing. Both James and Dewey were psychologists and philosophers. Both were proponents of philosophy of pragmatism, which provided the underpinnings for functional psychology.

In the early 20th century, there were two opposing philosophical schools of thought shaping philosopher's view of the world: structuralism (the primary school of thought) and pragmatism. According to the structuralism school of thought, everything, including human behavior, could be broken into parts and analyzed, and the mind (psychology) and the body (physical) were separate entities. In contrast, pragmatism described human behavior in terms of a system approach wherein human thought or action was influenced by life experiences and the environment. Pragmatism viewed the mind, body, and context as inextricably intertwined and emphasized the importance of context in human behavior. These differing viewpoints had implications for research on human behavior. Structuralism searched for universal laws and principles of human behavior through introspection of a person in controlled laboratory studies, whereas the hallmark of pragmatism was naturalistic study because context and individual differences were considered to be of prime importance (Serrett, 1985).

In concert with the pragmatism school of thought, the central tenet of functional psychology is that mental processes are used to adjust to environmental demands and are needed to think, learn, and live. Mind and body form an inseparable system that give humanity purpose, function, and life. Dewey saw the importance of the mind-body connection and strongly believed that a man's mind and his hands were crucial for successful adaptation to life (Serrett, 1985).

Best known as an educational reformer, Dewey's doctrine, learning by doing, is emblematic of this philosophical viewpoint and was a shift away from learning by rote. This way of learning was not focused on learning a specific trade or skill, but rather on developing problem-solving ability, "which reproduces, or runs parallel to, some form of work carried on in social life" (Dewey, 1915, p. 131). Dewey saw this as a means to develop skills to survive in life. A person facing a problem or difficulty must determine the best way to solve the problem. This requires the ability to plan, to "project mentally the result to be reached," and to determine strategies and steps to be taken (Dewey, 1915, pp. 133-134). Learning takes place through this process. This pragmatic and functional psychology view was also addressed by Burnham (1924) when he wrote: "In the individual, integration and the power of adjustment may be developed, physically, by coordinating activity, and mentally, in the doing of purposeful tasks" (p. 677). This doing of tasks helps develop attitudes and influence behavior; in other words, through the doing of tasks, one learns.

The work of James and Dewey greatly influenced the work of their friend and colleague, Adolf Meyer, a psychiatrist. Meyer in turn greatly influenced the central tenets of occupational therapy (Hooper & Wood, 2002; Serrett, 1985). With the philosophical viewpoint that melded the mind and body, Meyer began a new scientific discipline called psychobiology. The premise of psychobiology is seen in Meyer's Philosophy of Occupation Therapy (Meyer, 1922/1977), in which he provides an example of the mind-body connection. He recognized this connection when observing patients participating in activities in an asylum:

> A pleasure in achievement, a real pleasure in the use and activity of one's hands and muscles and a happy appreciation of time began to be used as incentives in management of our patients instead of abstract exhortations to cheer up and to behave according to abstract or repressive rules. (Meyer, 1922/1977, p. 640)

He further explained that man is not of separate physical or psychological structures, but that man is a live organism whose function cannot be analyzed by looking at its structural parts:

> Our body is not merely so many pounds of flesh and bone figuring as a machine, with an abstract mind or soul added to it. It is throughout a live organism pulsating with its rhythm of rest and activity, beating time (as we might say) in ever so many ways, most readily intelligible and in full bloom of its nature when it feels itself as one of those great self-guiding energy-transformers which constitute the real world of living beings. (Meyer, 1922/1977, p. 641)

William James was also known for his philosophy of habit. He believed that there was a physical basis for habits and promoted the viewpoint that "an acquired habit, from the physiological point of view, is nothing but a new pathway of discharge formed in the brain, by which the certain incoming currents ever after tend to escape" (James, 1892/1985, p. 55). James described the practical effect of habits as simplifying movements and requiring less conscious attention, thereby reducing fatigue from cognitive exertion. People perform many tasks automatically without much conscious effort. James believed that the plasticity of the brain allows for the eventual shaping of habits and changing of habits. He believed that the nervous system could be an ally in education, especially in early life, through repetition of activities and a daily regime to form good habits. He also believed that, based on the plasticity of the brain, there was an opportunity to change habits through continual repetition (James, 1892/1985). This philosophy became the basis for habit training used by Adolf Meyer and Eleanor Clarke Slagle at the Phipps Psychiatric Clinic at Johns Hopkins.

RESURGENCE OF MORAL TREATMENT

> "It should be remembered that the term applied to this form of therapy was in those days moral treatment or labor. The term occupation came in somewhat later." (Dunton, 1917, p. 382)

Based on moral treatment's principles of individuality and the need to participate in occupation, "the history of moral treatment in the United States...is the history of occupational therapy before it acquired its 20th century name" (Bockoven, 1971, p. 223). These principles were rooted in the political, cultural, and religious beliefs of the early 19th century, when moral treatment flourished. After its demise in the late 19th century, there was a renaissance of the concept of moral treatment in the first decades of the 20th century. This renaissance gave momentum to the development of occupational therapy.

Although moral treatment had lost its footing just a quarter century before, many men and women still living had personal contact with or knowledge of moral treatment proponents of the past (Bockoven, 1971). Benjamin Rush, who implemented humane care for the mentally ill in Pennsylvania Hospital, was a second cousin to William Rush Dunton Jr.'s grandmother. Dunton attended university with Thomas Kirkbride's son, Franklin. It is possible that connections such as these helped transmit knowledge and the values of moral treatment to Dunton in the next generation. At the founding meeting of the NSPOT, William Rush Dunton Jr. spoke about such notables as Benjamin Rush and Thomas Kirkbride advocating for engaging patients in work for therapeutic purposes (Dunton, 1917). His extensive reading of the literature on moral treatment was the basis of his paper, but it is likely that his interest in moral treatment was sparked by his personal connection to Benjamin Rush and Thomas Kirkbride.

MENTAL HYGIENE MOVEMENT

In 1900, Clifford W. Beers, a graduate of Yale University, suffered a mental breakdown. He was shuttled around to various insane asylums for treatment of his manic-depressive episodes. He was subjected to horrendous conditions and ill treatment in these asylums. In 1907, Beers decided to write an autobiographical book to expose the deplorable state of affairs in insane asylums. While writing the book, he sought the advice of William James and Adolf Meyer. Meyer was supportive, editing the book for Beers and suggesting that Beers use this opportunity to promote social change by increasing awareness and understanding of mental illness. Taking this suggestion, Beers began to organize supporters to work toward social reforms to improve the care for those with mental illness. It was Meyer who suggested the term *mental hygiene* as a name for Beers' movement.

Beer's book, *A Mind That Found Itself*, was published in 1908. It was a huge success and galvanized the public for reform. A heightened awareness of social problems and a belief that the government should be responsible for the care and safety of the mentally ill set the stage for the development of the Mental Hygiene Movement. The National Committee for Mental Hygiene was formally established on February 19, 1909 (Lief, 1948, pp. 280-281). William James and Julia Lathrop of Hull House, who had taken an interest in mental health after reading Beers' book, were among those attending the founding meeting at the old Hotel Manhattan in New York City (Meyer, 1935/1948, p. 313).

The Connecticut Society for Mental Hygiene was founded May 6, 1908, by the National Committee founders, and it served as a model for other state societies. The second and third state societies to organize were the Illinois Society for Mental Hygiene, which formed in July 1909, and the New York State Society for Mental Hygiene, which formed in May 1910 (National Committee for Mental Hygiene, 1912, pp. 6-7). The Mental Hygiene Movement facilitated change through education of physicians and the public, as well as implementation of public health initiatives that focused on the prevention of mental illness. Additionally, the Mental Hygiene Movement prompted improved care for patients in asylums, including use of occupations, individualized care, and better living environments (Peloquin, 1991a).

CONCEPTION AND BIRTH
OF THE NEW PROFESSION

In the early years of the 20th century, many people became involved in the science, practice, and promotion of the therapeutic use of occupation. Occupational therapy was beginning to be practiced in parts of the United States. Consistent with the values of the Progressive Movement and the development of various professions, many began to share ideas on the therapeutic use of occupation.

Prominent psychiatrist Adolf Meyer was a major proponent of the therapeutic use of occupation. Although not active in the formation of a professional society, he was a strong supporter and advocate. A group of six professionals—including physician William Rush Dunton Jr., architects George Edward Barton and Thomas Bessell Kidner, social worker Eleanor Clarke Slagle, arts and crafts instructor Susan Cox Johnson, and secretary Isabel Newton—were responsible for the formal birth of the professional society to promote the therapeutic use of occupation. They gathered together from March 15 to 17, 1917, in Clifton Springs, New York, for the inaugural meeting of the NSPOT. Susan E. Tracy, a nurse, and Herbert James Hall, a physician, were not at the founding meeting but were instrumental in the early development of the Society. As such, both are considered by many to be near founders. The founders and near founders each brought different skills, values, beliefs, and experiences to shape the new profession of occupational therapy. Many others throughout the country worked on behalf of the new profession, sharing the common belief that meaningful work and occupation could facilitate restoration of health.

Adolf Meyer

Adolf Meyer, an alienist (an early term for psychiatrist), was a lifelong proponent of occupational therapy. His paper, "Philosophy of Occupation Therapy," describes his introduction to the therapeutic use of occupation and his own experiences with using occupation in psychiatric facilities (Meyer, 1922/1977) (Figure 2-1). Many of the principles he espoused—including the need for man to adapt to his environment; the need to develop habits through training; and the need to understand the effect of life history on health, time use, and balance—still form the basis for the principles of occupational therapy.

Born on September 13, 1866, in Switzerland, Meyer studied neurology and psychiatry. After graduating in 1892, he immigrated to the United States because he believed he would have better professional opportunities there. He moved to Chicago, where he opened a neurology practice and taught at the University of Chicago. While in Chicago, he met John Dewey and Julia Lathrop, both of whom had a profound effect on his thinking and professional life. Meyer and Lathrop became close colleagues after she arranged a meeting with him to learn about social services in Europe. Their close relationship was evident in some of their actions. When Meyer was recovering from a fall, Lathrop invited him to stay for a week at Hull House (Lief, 1948, p. 49). Later, Meyer named his daughter, born in 1916, Julia Lathrop Meyer. John Dewey also had a close professional relationship with Adolf Meyer while in Chicago. They reconnected at the turn of the century when both moved to New York City, dining together on a weekly basis to continue their intellectual discourse.

In 1893, Meyer took a job as a neuropathologist at the Eastern State Hospital for the Insane in Kankakee, Illinois. There he performed autopsies on patients to determine whether there was a correlation between brain lesions and mental illness. Frustrated by the lack of record keeping documenting patients' symptoms and behaviors while alive, Meyer instituted processes to record physical, mental, and developmental life histories and living environments of patients to further his research. As a result, at Meyer's insistence,

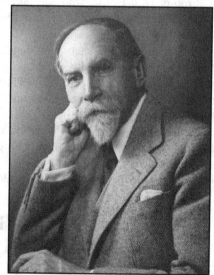

Figure 2-1. Adolf Meyer, psychiatrist. (Printed with permission from the Archive of the American Occupational Therapy Association, Inc.)

documentation of life histories became an important part of a patient's evaluation. To ensure he had adequate information for his research, Meyer established a method for standardized documentation for case records. Believing that mental illness was not just a disease of the brain, Meyer began to develop his theories of psychobiology and to investigate how life experiences and ability to adapt were factors in mental illness (Lidz, 1966/1985; Scull & Schulkin, 2009). Dr. Meyer's research provided the theoretical basis for the therapeutic effects of occupation.

Meyer moved to Worcester State Hospital for the Insane in Worcester, Massachusetts, in 1895 to become the director of research and then moved on to the Pathological Institute of the New York State Hospitals in 1902, where he met and married Mary Potter Brooks (Lidz, 1966/1985; Scull & Schulkin, 2009). Meyer's wife helped to ignite her husband's interest in the therapeutic use of occupation. She successfully implemented a program using occupations to facilitate recovery of patients housed in the psychiatric hospital on Ward's Island in New York City. Considered the first psychiatric social worker, Mrs. Meyer visited patients in their homes to learn about their living environments. Examination of the living environments of patients as a potential factor contributing to their illness was furthered by Mrs. Meyer's home visits. By working with patients in the community, Mrs. Meyer could better understand the cultural and social environments of individual patients. She used this information to assist patients adapt to the different circumstances in their environments.

Meyer moved to Baltimore in 1910 to serve as Chair of the Psychiatry Department at Johns Hopkins Medical School and as the director of the newly established Henry Phipps Psychiatric Clinic. Endowed by philanthropist Henry Phipps, the clinic officially opened on April 16, 1913. Phipps was inspired to provide funding for the clinic after reading Clifford W. Beers' book, *A Mind That Found Itself*, an autobiographical exposé on life and abuses in an insane asylum. Meyer was able to entice Eleanor Clarke Slagle, a social worker from Chicago, to move to Baltimore to work at the Phipps Psychiatric Clinic (Baum, 2002; Peloquin, 1991a).

Meyer believed that mental problems were problems of living and disorganized habits (Meyer, 1922/1977). With Slagle's help, he instituted a program of habit training at the clinic. As part of this program, patients followed prescribed daily routines and were encouraged to use time appropriately to organize and balance daily activities of work, play, rest, and sleep (Meyer, 1922/1977; Peloquin, 1991b; Reed, 1993, p. 36). Meyer's conviction in the importance of time use and balance is emphasized in this statement from his well-known address, "The Philosophy of Occupation Therapy":

> Our conception of man is that of an organism that maintains and balances itself in the world of reality and actuality by being in active life and active use, i.e. using and living and acting its time in harmony with its own nature and the nature about it. It is the use that we make of ourselves that gives the ultimate stamp to our every organ. (Meyer, 1922/1977, p. 641)

George Edward Barton

George Edward Barton was a major force in the organization of the inaugural meeting of the NSPOT. He was elected the first President of the Society at the founding meeting. Born on March 7, 1871, in Brookline, Massachusetts, Barton studied to be an architect. A man of many talents and interests, Barton spent time in Great Britain near the end of the 19th century. There he met William Morris, one of the leaders of the Arts and Crafts Movement. Morris' influence sparked Barton's interest in studying social problems brought on by industrialization. In 1897, Barton became an incorporator and secretary the Boston Arts and Crafts Society, one of the many formed in the United States as an outgrowth of the Arts and Crafts Movement (Figures 2-2 and 2-3).

Barton was diagnosed with tuberculosis in 1901. He suffered recurring attacks from that time until the end of his life in 1923. He eventually moved to Denver, a place deemed to have a healthy climate that helped people recover from tuberculosis. Rest, a good diet, fresh air, and sunshine

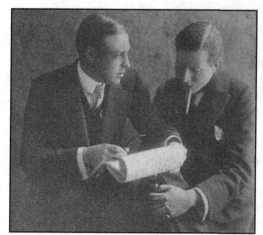

Figure 2-2. George Edward Barton (left) and the famous English actor George Arliss (right). (Printed with permission from the Archive of the American Occupational Therapy Association, Inc.)

were the conventional treatments of many tuberculosis sanitariums at that time. While residing in Colorado, George Barton married Agatha Farrington, a divorcee with two children, on November 25, 1911. They divorced in 1915 (Colorado State Archives, 1911, 1915; Engagement, 1911).

Once Barton recovered his health, he continued his architectural practice in Colorado. One of his major projects was developing plans for the Myron Stratton Home in Colorado Springs. The Myron Stratton Home was not a single building, but rather a small village with a number of cottages and dormitories to house poor children and older adults who were physically unable to earn a living. The buildings and grounds were carefully planned to ensure ample space and facilities for living, learning, and working. The complex included playgrounds, a swimming pool, a gymnasium, a farm, a dairy, recreation and reading rooms, and school rooms. The intent was to provide employment to all residents, young and old. The young boys would learn trades such as carpentry, brick laying, metal work, plumbing, farming, and typesetting. The young girls would receive instruction in sewing, cooking, and other domestic trades (Barton, 1911, pp. 22-34; "Homes for Unfortunates," 1914, pp. 698-700).

In 1912, the Governor of Colorado asked Barton to examine the effects of famine on Kansas farmers. It was during this mission that his left foot froze. He developed gangrene in his foot, requiring amputation of two toes. While recovering from the surgery, Barton developed hysterical paralysis on his left side. In 1913, Barton was referred to Dr. James G. Mumford, Superintendent at Clifton Springs Sanitarium in upstate New York, for help. He spent a year resting and regaining his health at the sanitarium. Unable to participate in simple tasks and frustrated with the lack of encouragement from physicians to regain his functional ability, Barton turned to Dr. Elwood Worcester of the Emmanuel Church and founder of the Emmanuel Movement in Boston for consultation. Dr. Worcester started the Emmanuel Movement in response to the perceived inadequacies of medical care, a perception shared by many at the time. Scientific advances had prompted the medical profession to focus primarily on the physical aspect of illness. Seeing a need to treat the whole person, Dr. Worcester believed religion could treat the mental and emotional aspects of illness. A clinic was established at the Emmanuel Church that offered both medical and psychological services, including individual and group counseling. The clinic offered moral, educational, and

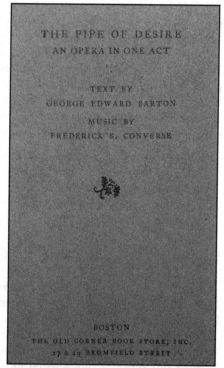

Figure 2-3. George Edward Barton wrote the play "The Pipe of Desire" in 1905. It became the libretto for an opera written by Frank Converse and was the first opera to be presented at the Metropolitan Opera House that was written by Americans and given in English. (Copyright © Dr. Lori T. Andersen. Reprinted with permission.)

psychological treatments, which were provided by both religious and medical professionals (Green, 1934).

Barton, disappointed in the lack of support or assistance provided by physicians to restore him to a productive life, was grateful for Dr. Worcester's guidance. Dr. Worcester encouraged Barton to prove that people could overcome disabilities, first by overcoming his own disabilities and then by teaching others how to do so. In effect, Dr. Worcester was encouraging Barton to regain his health by helping the other fellow regain his health.

Barton wanted to change the hospital system to not only restore health to people, but to return them to independence and productive work. He purchased a house next to Clifton Springs Sanitarium and renovated it to make it more accessible and comfortable for him. He also built facilities on the property for the purpose of rehabilitating other people who lacked independence. An adjacent lot was converted into a garden, and the barn was converted into a workshop with numerous tools that could be carefully selected for use by patients, grading activities, and a choice of tools appropriate to each patient's ability. Barton continued to learn about the medical aspects of dis-

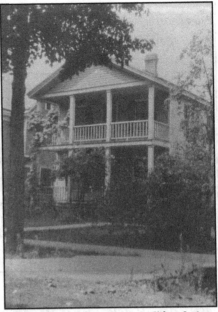

Figure 2-4. Consolation House in Clifton Springs, New York. (Printed with permission from the Archive of the American Occupational Therapy Association, Inc.)

ability through self-study and by taking classes with the nurses at Clifton Springs Sanitarium. To further his understanding of human movement, he studied the work of Frank and Lillian Gilbreth, both motion efficiency experts. Barton saw the need to analyze motions required for a patient to perform a task, the motions the patient was able to perform, and the motions that needed to be encouraged to select an appropriate occupation for a patient. Barton also thought it important to choose an occupation that stimulated the patient's interest and to analyze the environment in which a task was to be performed (Newton, 1917a, p. 325).

Barton's house, known as Consolation House, officially opened on March 7, 1914 (Figure 2-4). Physicians began to refer patients to Barton once they saw how he had regained his physical abilities (Barton, 1968; Reed & Sanderson, 1999, pp. 423-425). He accepted patients only through a physician referral (Newton, 1917a). It is likely that Barton experienced the magic of occupational therapy through his efforts to help the other fellow, an effort that was also therapeutic for him.

Interested in the therapeutic value of occupation, Barton began to look into the work of Dr. Herbert Hall and Susan Tracy, who were also using occupation to heal (Barton, 1914). In November 1914, Barton corresponded with Susan Tracy and William Rush Dunton, Jr., about their occupation work and their desire to organize those with similar interests (Dunton, 1926). Dunton, eager to promote occupation work, wrote a letter requesting Barton to submit a paper

---

SIDEBAR 2-1

Early Use of the Term *Occupational Therapy*

In his book *Teaching the Sick*, George Edward Barton states that he first used the term *occupational therapy* on December 28, 1914, at a conference of hospital workers called by the Massachusetts State Board of Insanity (p. 17).

---

on his work for publication in the *Maryland Psychiatric Quarterly* (Dunton, 1914). Their correspondence continued through the founding of the professional association (Sidebars 2-1 and 2-2).

SIDEBAR 2-2

Curious Companions

In a newspaper article published in the *Geneva Times* on Friday, May 9, 1958, Bill de Lancey recounts a story about George Edward Barton's travels in England as a young architect. Barton was bicycling through the English countryside to visit and make sketches of a number of lesser-known churches designed by a well-established architect. Barton, known to be quirky, had purchased a pair of gaudy trousers for his trip. While bicycling, he encountered an English gentleman on a bicycle who joined him for several hours. The gentleman commented on Barton's garish outfit and was admonished by Barton for this slight. The gentleman did join in when Barton began to whistle operatic arias, followed by singing. At the end of their time together, the gentleman declared, "I've enjoyed this very much, but I hope we never meet again." Barton did see the Englishman again. The Englishman was King Edward VII.

William Rush Dunton, Jr.

William Rush Dunton Jr., a physician and psychiatrist, is considered the father of occupational therapy. Born on July 24, 1868, he lived a long, productive life, passing away at the age of 98 on December 23, 1966 (Figures 2-5 and 2-6). Through the years, Dunton, with his level head and steady hand, was the glue that held the association together. Dunton was known to be kind, full of wisdom, and possessed of a sparkling wit (American Occupational Therapy Association [AOTA], 1967).

In 1895, 2 years after earning his medical degree, Dunton began his 29-year tenure at newly established Sheppard Asylum in Towson, Maryland. It was here that Dunton learned about moral treatment and the therapeutic use of occupation. In 1857, businessman Moses Sheppard's will provided $600,000 for the construction of Sheppard Asylum. After learning of the poor treatment of the daughter of an employee received in an asylum, Sheppard hoped to remedy this by constructing an asylum in which "courteous treatment and the comfort of all patients" was given priority in the construction of buildings, the designing of grounds, and the provision of medical care. The asylum's purpose was to provide treatment that would cure, "combining science and experience" to this end (Forbush & Forbush, 1986, p. 15). All patient residences were to have "privacy, sunlight, and fresh air" (Forbush & Forbush, 1986, p. 15). The Civil War and financial constraints of the endowment (only the interest from the endowment was to be used for construction

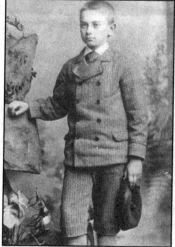

Figure 2-5. William Rush Dunton, Jr., at age 12. (Printed with permission from the Archive of the American Occupational Therapy Association, Inc.)

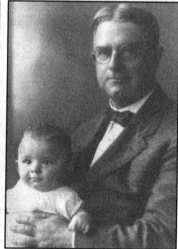

Figure 2-6. William Rush Dunton, Jr., with his grandson William Dunton Furst in 1925. (Printed with permission from the Archive of the American Occupational Therapy Association, Inc.)

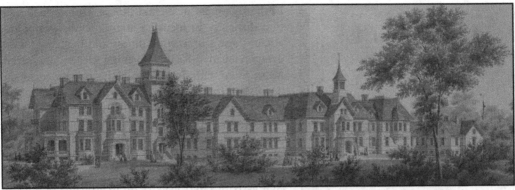

Figure 2-7. Calvert Vaux's architectural design proposal showing the front elevation of the Sheppard Asylum.

and operation) delayed construction for several decades. The asylum finally opened in 1891 under the direction of Edward N. Brush, MD, previously the Assistant Superintendent of the Pennsylvania Hospital for the Insane. The financial stability and future of asylum was secured in 1896 when a second benefactor, businessman Enoch Pratt, bequeathed $2 million to the facility. His only stipulation was that the name be changed to the Sheppard and Enoch Pratt Hospital (Figure 2-7).

Dr. Dunton was hired by Dr. Brush to head the clinical and pathology laboratory at Sheppard Asylum. Frustrated that his research was not producing significant results, Dr. Brush suggested that full-scale efforts may not be warranted at that time. He recommended that Dunton become involved in clinical work with patients. Following this advice, Dunton divided his time between patient care and his research on the topic of dementia praecox (Bing, 1961, pp. 128-129). He began to publish his findings and present his research at professional conferences, gaining professional recognition in the field of psychiatry. In 1905, Johns Hopkins University Medical School gave him a part-time clinical appointment to teach psychiatry and neurology (Bing, 1961, p. 149).

In 1912, having established his reputation as a psychiatrist and researcher of dementia praecox, Dunton's interests turned to use of occupations as a therapeutic measure for those with mentally illness. The Casino Building, built in 1902 on the grounds of Sheppard and Enoch Pratt Hospital, was a center for occupations and recreation (Figure 2-8). Dunton had minimal involvement in these activities from 1902 to 1912 but had always been drawn to Dr. Brush's belief in the "judicious regimen of activity" for patients (Bing, 1961, p. 130). While previously occupation had been used for occupation's sake without concern for the best therapeutic choice for the individual, Dr. Brush believed that, for the best outcome, the careful selection of activities and implementation of a regimen of activities should be based on the individual needs of each patient (Bing, 1961, p. 131).

Dr. Dunton was put in charge of the occupations program at Sheppard and Enoch Pratt Hospital in 1912. He set his research agenda to study the therapeutic benefits of occupation, beginning with a review of the literature. He used the medical library of Dr. Edward Brush, the Superintendent of Sheppard Asylum, to research the history of psychiatry, moral treatment, and the use of occupation

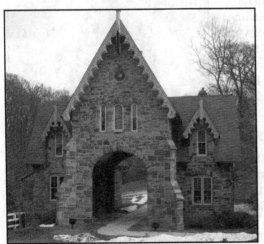

Figure 2-8. The Gatehouse was the primary entrance to the Sheppard and Enoch Pratt Hospital until 2001.

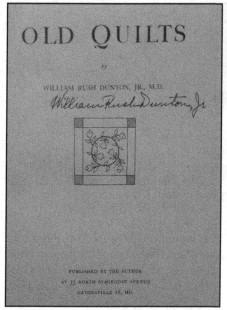

Figure 2-9. In 1946, William Rush Dunton self-published a book on quilts titled *Old Quilts*. The book is now a collector's item, prized by occupational therapists and quilters. (Copyright © Dr. Lori T. Andersen. Reprinted with permission.)

in the treatment of mental illness. Dunton believed that difficulty in focusing attention was symptomatic of those with mental illness and that those with dementia had difficulty forming clearly organized ideas, those with depression had a narrow focus on depressive thoughts, and those in an excited stage had difficulty organizing the rapid-fire thoughts entering the mind. Participation in occupation would help them refocus attention and facilitate recovery by substituting healthy thoughts in place of delusions, hallucinations, and/or depressive thoughts. New activities were also useful in arousing new ideas and interests to take one's mind off of problems (Bing, 1961, p. 167; Dunton, 1921, pp. 27-28).

Dunton understood the importance of history. It is because of his efforts that we have a wealth of documents and artifacts from the early years of National Society for the Promotion of Occupational Therapy and American Occupational Therapy Association. He saved his correspondence with other founders and was the editor of the first official journals association. *The Maryland Psychiatric Quarterly*, the *Archives of Occupational Therapy*, and *Occupational Therapy and Rehabilitation* published many of the early occupational therapy papers, as well as many of the proceedings of the association meetings. Preferring to work quietly in the background, he used his persistent yet gracious manner to gently press George Edward Barton to organize the inaugural meeting of NSPOT.

Recognizing the importance of having trained personnel to direct activity programs, Dunton read Susan E. Tracy's book, *Studies in Invalid Occupations*, a textbook for training nurses and aides in therapeutic use of occupations. Dr. Brush encouraged Dunton to develop training classes for the nurses at Sheppard and Enoch Pratt Hospital. Nurses learned a number of handicrafts, including leatherwork, reed basketry, book binding, embroidery, and metal work. His course materials were published in his book, *Occupation Therapy: A Manual for Nurses*, in 1915 (Bing, 1961, p. 170). Dunton, a prolific writer, published a number of journal articles and books, including a self-published book on quilts (Figure 2-9).

Eleanor Clarke Slagle

Eleanor Clarke Slagle is known as the mother of occupational therapy and has the most recognizable name of all the founders (Figure 2-10). The prestigious American occupational therapy lectureship, the Eleanor Clarke Slagle lecture, was named after her. Born Ella May Clarke in Hobart, New York, in 1870 (1875 New York State Census; 1880 U.S. Federal Census), she

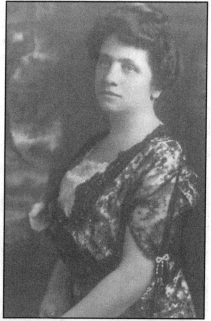

Figure 2-10. Young Eleanor Clarke Slagle. (Printed with permission from the Archive of the American Occupational Therapy Association, Inc.)

married Robert E. Slagle in 1894. Robert and Eleanor moved to Chicago after the wedding. They also lived in St. Louis and Kansas City, Missouri, during their marriage. Robert and Eleanor separated around 1910, about the same time Robert Slagle moved to Nampa, Idaho (1910 U.S. Federal Census). They divorced around 1914 or 1915 (United States Corporation Bureau, 1914, p. 819). The circumstances surrounding the separation and divorce are not known. Robert Slagle remarried in 1915 (1920 U.S. Census; *Idaho Press-Tribune*, 1986).

Slagle is described as "a woman with a strong personality [who] possessed broad vision, charm, dignity, and a presence which commanded admiration and respect" (AOTA, 1967, p. 292). While in Chicago, she became interested in social service work with the mentally and physically handicapped. She enrolled as a social work student in 1908 at the Chicago School of Civics and Philanthropy, a forerunner of the University of Chicago School of Social Service Administration (Dobschuetz, 2001). The Chicago School of Civics and Philanthropy was established in 1908 as an outgrowth of the Settlement House Movement. Graham Taylor, head of Chicago Commons, a settlement house, was the first president, and Julia Lathrop of Hull House was the first vice president. Part of the Progressive Movement, the aim of the school was "to promote through instruction, training, investigation and publication the efficiency of civic, philanthropic and social work, and the improvement of living and working conditions" (Chicago School of Civics and Philanthropy, 1909, p. 9). The belief was that humanitarian work was skilled professional service that required specialized training, including education in research methods to help determine solutions for social ills (Chicago School of Civics and Philanthropy, 1909, p. 9). It heralded the start of new professions such as social work.

Site visits to public and private facilities were part of each educational program. During observational visits to Kankakee State Hospital, Slagle was struck by the poor conditions and lack of meaningful activities for patients (Loomis, 1992). This had a profound influence on her. In view of Slagle's newfound interest in care of institutionalized patients with mental illness, Julia Lathrop suggested she enroll in a special course in occupations and educational methods at the Chicago School of Civics and Philanthropy. This 6-week course, started by Julia Lathrop in the summer of 1908 (Loomis, 1992), taught crafts to hospital attendants working with the mentally ill. Lathrop had been inspired to start the course by Adolf Meyer, her friend and colleague, and was assisted by Rabbi Emil Hirsch and artisans from the Chicago Arts and Crafts Society. The course applied the philosophy of the Arts and Crafts movement to the treatment of the mentally ill (Levine, 1987).

Slagle completed this special course in occupations for attendants in institutions for the insane in the summer of 1911. She assisted in teaching the course the next year during the summer of 1912 (Chicago School of Civics and Philanthropy, 1912, p. 39). After completing this course, Slagle spent 6 months at Upper Peninsula State Hospital in Newberry, Michigan, and 6 months at Central Islip State Hospital in Long Island organizing and conducting occupational therapy classes for nurses, attendants, and patients at those institutions. The course Slagle took at the Chicago School of Civics and Philanthropy served as a model for the courses she developed (Dobschuetz, 2001).

In 1912, Adolf Meyer recruited Slagle to move to Baltimore to work at the newly established Phipps Psychiatric Clinic at Johns Hopkins University. From 1912 to 1914, she organized and directed the department of occupational therapy. She also offered a 3-week course to nurses in training at Johns Hopkins, a course that oriented student nurses to the therapeutic use of occupations (Peloquin, 1991b). Soon after Slagle's arrival in Baltimore, William Rush Dunton, hearing of Slagle's expertise in occupation work, arranged to meet her. They became close friends and colleagues, frequently dining together and sharing knowledge and ideas, including the idea to form a society for sharing experiences in using occupation for therapeutic purposes.

In 1915, Slagle was recruited by the Illinois Society for Mental Hygiene to conduct a workshop for patients with mental and physical disabilities. She was appointed as the Director of Occupations for the Illinois Society for Mental Hygiene. In this role, she established and ran the Occupational Experiment Station in Chicago. During this time, Slagle also lectured at the Chicago School of Civics and Philanthropy.

The purpose of the Occupational Experiment Station was two-fold: it provided a community-sheltered workshop for discharged patients who needed supportive employment in work rooms for the handicapped, and it provided classes for training teachers of occupations (Thomson, 1914, 1917; Slagle, 1919b, p. 121). The patients referred to this workshop included borderline "mental cases" and orthopedic "cripples" (Slagle, n.d.). The workshop was a success. More space was needed, so a second location was opened. Additionally, during the summer of 1915, Hull House granted use of their workshops to provide even more space to accommodate the work being done. From October 1, 1915, to October 1, 1916, the Occupational Experiment Station was successful in returning 31% of patients to gainful employment. Of the 77 individuals treated at the workshop, 24 returned to wage-earning positions outside the department. Only 16 were not helped at all (Thomson, 1917).

In 1917, Slagle was appointed as General Superintendent of Occupational Therapy by the Illinois Department of Public Welfare

CHICAGO SCHOOL OF CIVICS AND PHILANTHROPY

Fifteenth year opened October 1, 1917
Winter term begins January 2, 1918

GENERAL TRAINING COURSE FOR SOCIAL WORKERS
One-year course for college graduates. Two-year course for other qualified students.

SPECIAL PLAYGROUND COURSE
With technical classes, at Hull-House Gymnasium, in folk dancing games, story-telling, dramatics, preparation of pageants and gymnastics.

SPECIAL COURSE FOR PUBLIC HEALTH NURSES
March 4 to June 25

SPECIAL COURSE IN CURATIVE OCCUPATIONS AND RECREATION
(In co-operation with the Illinois Society for Mental Hygiene)
Dealing with the problem of re-education of the physically sick, the mentally disturbed, and the wounded and handicapped soldier. January 2nd to June 7th.

For further information address the Dean, 2559 Michigan Ave., Chicago

Figure 2-11. Chicago School of Civics and Philanthropy Announcement of Special Courses in Curative Occupations and Recreation.

(Slagle, n.d.). She also continued her role with the Illinois Society of Mental Hygiene as director of the workshop and school for occupation workers (Slagle, n.d.). On October 24, 1917, the Illinois Society for Mental Hygiene named the society's occupational department the Henry B. Favill School of Occupations in honor of Dr. Henry B. Favill, the highly respected physician. Dr. Favill, who died in 1916, was instrumental in organizing the Illinois Society of Mental Hygiene and served as the first vice president (Favill, 1917, p. 87). In January 1918, the Illinois Department of Public Welfare, in collaboration with the Henry B. Favill School, the Illinois Society of Mental Hygiene, and the Chicago School of Civics and Philanthropy, established a training school for occupational therapists (Chicago School of Civics and Philanthropy, 1917; "Training school," 1918, p. 635) (Figure 2-11). This 5-month special course in curative occupations and recreation in cooperation was designed to teach students how to care for those with physical and mental disabilities, including disabled soldiers. Classes were held at Hull House and at the Chicago School for Civics and Philanthropy. Many of the students completed their practice training work at Elgin State Hospital and Chicago State Hospital to help fulfill the mission of the State of Illinois to provide services to those in state mental institutions (Slagle, 1919a, pp. 29-32). The Henry B. Favill School is considered to be the first training school for occupational therapists in the United States.

Susan Cox Johnson

Susan Cox Johnson was born in Corsicana, Texas, on December 29, 1875. Johnson is described as a woman with an "attractive personality and a charming, gracious manner which won her many friends" (Occupational Therapy Notes, 1932, p. 152). Although she is the founder who is least known, she was very involved in moving the profession forward through the setting of educational standards. A designer and arts and crafts teacher, Johnson wrote a textbook titled Textile Studies, published in 1912. She worked as a high school teacher in Berkeley, California, and then moved

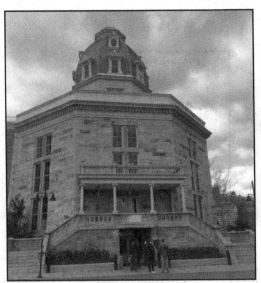

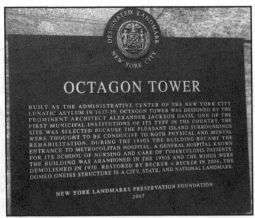

Figure 2-13. The Octagon Tower Plaque designating the tower as a city, state, and national landmark. (Reprinted with permission from Dr. Carol A. Lambdin-Pattavina.)

Figure 2-12. The Octagon Tower, former entrance to Metropolitan Hospital on Blackwell's Island, still stands as the entrance to luxury waterfront residences on Roosevelt Island. (Reprinted with permission from Dr. Carol A. Lambdin-Pattavina.)

to the Philippines in 1912 to teach arts and crafts (Quiroga, 1995, p. 129). Johnson returned to the United States 2 years later.

In August 1916, Johnson accepted a position in New York City as Director of Occupations for the Department of Public Charities. The Commissioner of Public Charities had established this committee on occupations to demonstrate the benefit of providing occupations to patients and inmates of public hospitals and almshouses. Once in her position, Johnson hired two teachers and began a program teaching handicrafts to patients with nervous disorders at the Central and Neurological Hospital on Blackwell's Island and to patients with tuberculosis at the Metropolitan Hospital, also on Blackwell's Island. In the early 1900s, asylums, sanitariums, and penitentiaries were often built on islands or other areas away from the rest of society. Blackwell's Island, located in the East River on the east side of Manhattan, housed an asylum, sanitarium, and penitentiary at various times in history. Blackwell's Island was renamed Welfare Island in 1921 and again renamed Roosevelt Island in 1973. Part of the old asylum, the Octagon Building was renovated in 2006 and is now the entrance to luxury waterfront residences (Figures 2-12 to 2-14).

At the hospitals on Blackwell's Island, patients participated in rug making, basket weaving, knitting, crocheting, and toy making. Johnson observed that depressed patients participating in occupations became cheerful and more social. Important to patient success was the "thoughtful selection of materials and designs and … careful supervision of the patient's efforts" (Johnson, 1917, p. 414). The products created were made available for sale, adding to patient satisfaction and self-esteem knowing they were more self-sufficient. Tennis nets, one of the main products manufactured by the patients, were commercially available (Johnson, 1917; Public Welfare Committee, 1917, pp. 51, 68). Johnson also taught occupations courses for the Department of Nursing and Health at Teachers College, Columbia University. The courses taught a number of crafts such as basketry, leather work, and chair caning to nurses and social workers. The courses provided medical, psychological, and economic perspectives of therapeutic use of occupations to help patients become self-sufficient (Quiroga, 1995, p. 130).

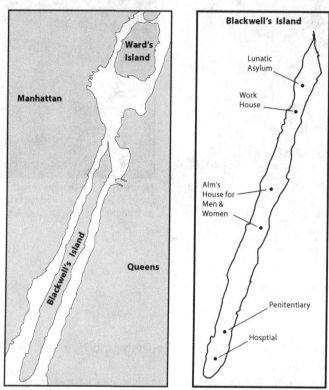

Figure 2-14. Map of New York City area showing the location of Blackwell's Island and Wards Island. Susan Cox Johnson worked on Blackwell's Island. Adolf Meyer's wife, Mary Potter Brooks Meyer, worked on Wards Island.

Thomas Bessell Kidner

Thomas Bessell Kidner was born in Bristol, England, in 1866. He was educated as an architect. As part of his training, Kidner took classes in building construction and manual arts such as carpentry and joinery. This was consistent with the beliefs of the Arts and Crafts Movement, which deemed it was important to learning these skills to fully appreciate the artistic quality of the materials (Friedland, 2007; Friedland & Davids-Brumer, 2007). After graduating, he accepted a technical education teaching position at a high school in Bristol. Kidner was "a man of fine presence, rather formal in dress, clear and concise in his way of speech" (AOTA, 1967, p. 292).

As the world's economy slowly moved from agriculture to industry, Sir William MacDonald, a Canadian and wealthy owner of the MacDonald Tobacco Company, saw the need to develop a workforce with practical skills for industry. He offered to pay the salaries of selected manual training teachers to develop technical education programs in Canadian elementary schools. Kidner, with his teaching experience in technical education, was selected by the MacDonald Manual Training Fund to go to Canada and develop these programs. In 1900, he moved his family to Nova Scotia. There he worked for the province as Director of Technical Education. He stayed in Canada past the 3-year commitment, holding similar positions in New Brunswick and Calgary.

Kidner embraced the philosophy of learning by doing championed by John Dewey. Manual training, a new progressive aspect of general education, consisted of participation in handwork

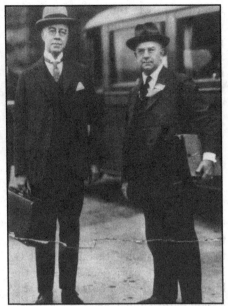

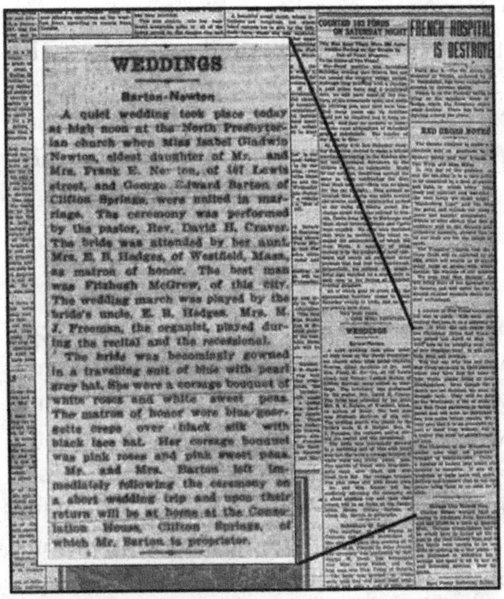

Figure 2-15. Thomas Bessell Kidner (left) and William Rush Dunton (right) at the train station. (Printed with permission from the Archive of the American Occupational Therapy Association, Inc.)

or crafts, which was believed to develop brain centers as well as physical skills (Kidner, 1910, p. 10). Kidner believed that manual training (elementary level) prepared one for technical education (secondary level) and a vocation. Kidner became a noted expert in the area of manual training and technical education. His book, *Educational Handwork*, provides graded craft activities for schoolchildren. In his book, he wrote:

> The acquisition of dexterity and skill of hand; the training of the eye to a sense of form and beauty; the formation of habits of accuracy, order, and neatness; the inculcation of a love of industry and habits of patience, perseverance and self-reliance, are some of the results which may be claimed as peculiarly belonging to work with the hands as a means of education. (Kidner, 1910, p. 9)

World War I began in Europe in the summer of 1914. Although the United States did not enter the war until April 1917, Canada, as part of the British Commonwealth, entered in August 1914. Too old to enlist and desiring to do his part for the war effort, Kidner volunteered his time to work with returning injured soldiers. He decided that manual training would be helpful in returning soldiers to some form of work. As part of his efforts, he first interviewed the returning soldiers to understand their needs and employment history. Next, he carefully selected activities that would help them return to productive work, whether it was their previous work or new work.

World War I lasted longer than the Canadians had expected. Initially believing that convalescence would take place in England, Canada was not prepared for the returning soldiers who were disabled. Canada established the Military Hospitals Commission when it became apparent that a significant number of returning soldiers would need continued care. In December 1915, because of his work in technical education and his volunteer work, Kidner was appointed Vocational Secretary of the Military Hospitals Commission. He moved to Ottawa to assume his new position, taking on the responsibility of training and placing ward aides and developing and placing soldiers in work settings. The occupation work consisted of craft activities similar to those used in manual training. These activities were provided bedside, on the wards, and in curative workshops. The returning soldiers progressed to vocational training when they were ready (Friedland, 2007; Friedland & Davids-Brumer, 2007; Friedland & Silva, 2008) (Figure 2-15). Kidner was invited by George Barton to the founding meeting of NSPOT as an international representative. Soon after, the Canadian government

WEDDINGS

Barton-Newton

A quiet wedding took place today at high noon at the North Presbyterian church when Miss Isabel Gladwin Newton, eldest daughter of Mr. and Mrs. Frank E. Newton, of 167 Lewis street, and George Edward Barton of Clifton Springs, were united in marriage. The ceremony was performed by the pastor, Rev. David H. Craver. The bride was attended by her aunt, Mrs. E. B. Hedges, of Westfield, Mass., as matron of honor. The best man was Fitzhugh McGrew, of this city. The wedding march was played by the bride's uncle, E. B. Hedges. Mrs. M. J. Freeman, the organist, played during the recital and the recessional.

The bride was becomingly gowned in a travelling suit of blue with pearl gray hat. She wore a corsage bouquet of white roses and white sweet peas. The matron of honor wore blue georgette crepe over black silk with black lace hat. Her corsage bouquet was pink roses and pink sweet peas.

Mr. and Mrs. Barton left immediately following the ceremony on a short wedding trip and upon their return will be at home at the Consolation House, Clifton Springs, of which Mr. Barton is proprietor.

Figure 2-16. Article reporting the wedding of George Edward Barton and Isabel G. Newton on Monday, May 6, 1918, as a quiet wedding at high noon.

loaned Kidner to the United States as a consultant on developing reconstruction programs. Kidner moved to the United States, where he lived for the rest of his life. After serving as a consultant to the United States government, Kidner worked for the National Tuberculosis Association. He also served a number of years as President of the AOTA.

Isabel Gladwin Newton Barton

Although not noted for her work in the advancement of science and practice in occupational therapy, Isabel G. Newton Barton has a sacred place in the history of the occupational therapy profession in the United States as a founder. She was born on July 21, 1891, in New York. In August 1916, 7 months before the inaugural meeting, Isabel was hired

---

Sidebar 2-3

Founders and Near Founders

In a letter to Mrs. John A. Greene (Marjorie), Director, Boston School of Occupational Therapy, dated May 10, 1938, Eleanor Clarke Slagle named the five founders of AOTA: George Edward Barton, William Rush Dunton, Susan Cox Johnson, Thomas Kidner, and Eleanor Clarke Slagle. Slagle clarified that although Herbert Hall was an early member, he was not a founder, and that Susan Tracy was not a founder but was "elected an active member" and given "all the rights and privileges of an incorporator" at the first meeting (Slagle, 1938a). In retrospect, in light of their contributions to the profession, Peloquin (1991a, 1991b) considers Tracy and Hall to be near founders.

by George Barton as his secretary. She commuted every day from her home in Geneva, New York, to Consolation House in Clifton Springs, New York, on the Auburn Branch of the New York Central Railroad. Isabel was immediately attracted to Barton's personality, his boyish nature, and his sense of humor (Barton, 1968). George Barton and Isabel Newton married on May 6, 1918 (Figure 2-16). They had one son, George Gladwin Barton, who was born on October 16, 1920.

Initially, Barton did not count Isabel as one of the notables who would attend the founding meeting. Later, Barton ensured Isabel's place in history when he wrote to Dunton designating Isabel eligible for active membership in the new society (Barton, 1917b). In March 1917, along with the other notables, Isabel G. Newton became one of the signers of the Articles of Incorporation for the National Society for the Promotion of Occupational Therapy.

As secretary of the new society, Isabel handled Barton's correspondence and maintained the society's records. Isabel also assisted Barton with his writing. The 1920 U.S. Census lists her as an author and a collaborator for technical works. George Barton acknowledged Isabel as his collaborator in his book, *Teaching the Sick* (1919). Isabel, the last survivor of the founding meeting, died on November 4, 1975 (Sidebar 2-3).

Susan E. Tracy

As a nursing student, Susan E. Tracy observed that patients on surgical wards who were occupied in some type of work were happier than those who were not. This impressed her and set her on her life's work. Tracy was characterized as having a warm personality, a big heart, a spontaneous nature, and an unbridled enthusiasm for her work. She graduated from the Massachusetts Homeopathic Hospital in Boston in 1898 (Cameron, 1917). In 1905, after completion of coursework in home economics at Teachers College, she was hired as Director of the Training School for Nurses at Adams Nervine Asylum, located in the Boston area. At the asylum, she used occupations in her work with people with mild mental health issues. She also taught nurses how to select, adapt, and teach crafts based on each patient's needs and conditions and based on the patient's setting or environment, including patients confined to hospital rooms or in restricted positions. She believed that it was important that a person teaching crafts to an invalid have not only knowledge of the

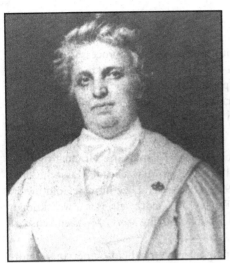

Figure 2-17. Susan E. Tracy. (Printed with permission from the Archive of the American Occupational Therapy Association, Inc.)

craftwork, but also medical knowledge (Tracy, 1910, p. 18).

Tracy stressed the importance of therapeutic use of self in interactions with patients when she wrote:

The value of wise human sympathy, of cheerfulness in work and mien, of tactful dealing with unreasonableness and irritability, of skillful diversion of thought from pessimistic channels, and many other desirable qualifications are emphasized as essential parts of the trained nurse's equipment for her work. (Tracy, 1910, pp. 9-10)

This sentiment was supported by Dr. Daniel H. Fuller, Superintendent of Adams Nervine Asylum, when he wrote, "The personality of the teacher and nurse therefore becomes an important factor. Her real enthusiasm and love for the work react most powerfully on the patient" (Fuller, 1910, p. 5).

William Rush Dunton credited Susan E. Tracy with providing the first course on occupational therapy (Dunton, 1921, p. 15). From 1910 to 1913, Tracy occasionally provided special lectures for nursing students at Teachers College at Columbia University (Slagle, 1938b). She also taught a course in occupation at Massachusetts General Hospital in the spring of 1911 (Dunton, 1921, p. 16). In a letter to Dunton, Tracy indicated that the "occupation study became a recognized part of the curriculum in Adam Nervine Training School for Nurses in the year 1906" (Tracy, 1914). Interest in this course grew through 1912, at which time Tracy left to establish the Experiment Station for the Study of Invalid Occupations. The purpose of the Experiment Station was two-fold. First, it served as a resource center, collecting records and case studies for use by others who were investigating the therapeutic benefit of occupation. Second, Tracy offered coursework, including "demonstrations, exhibitions, [and] private instruction" at Experiment Station for anyone who was interested in learning about this occupation work for invalids (Tracy, 1914).

Whereas some saw economic or commercial value in the sale of objects created by patients, Tracy believed in the therapeutic value of the patient making a purposeful product, not the commercial value (Peloquin, 1991a). In 1910, Tracy published her lectures in the first occupational therapy textbook, *Studies in Invalid Occupations*. Focusing in part on teaching courses for the teacher of occupations, it became a widely used textbook in the early 20th century. Dunton (1917) credits Tracy's book with helping to reignite interest in the therapeutic use of occupation (Figure 2-17).

Tracy was unable to attend the founding meeting because she was in Chicago developing a program at the Presbyterian Hospital of the City of Chicago (Cameron, 1917; Tracy, 1917). Nevertheless, the other founders elected her as an "active member with all the rights and privileges of an incorporator" (Newton, 1917b, p. 19).

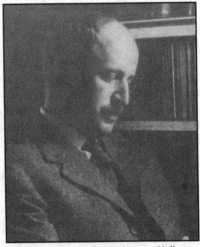

Figure 2-18. Herbert James Hall was born March 12, 1870 in Manchester, New Hampshire where he grew up. Graduating from the Harvard Medical School in 1895, he opened a medical practice in Marblehead, Massachusetts two years after completing his residencies (Printed with permission from the Archive of the American Occupational Therapy Association, Inc.)

Herbert James Hall

The handicrafts combine mild mental effort with simple physical processes, they require the hand and eye to follow the impulse of the mind, and so begin to reestablish the fundamentals of successful living. Occupational therapy may be used with the simple idea of improving morale or for special purposes, such as the development of strength and suppleness in parts which have been injured by accident or disease. (Hall, 1923, p. 3)

Herbert James Hall was born March 12, 1870, in Manchester, New Hampshire. Graduating from Harvard Medical School in 1895, he opened a medical practice in Marblehead, Massachusetts, 2 years after completing his residencies. In December 1897, Hall married Eliza Pitman Goldthwait, who came from a wealthy Boston family. Her brother, Dr. Joel E. Goldthwait, was a well-known orthopedic surgeon (Figure 2-18). Hall was recognized for his untiring work, his keen sense of humor, and his broad-mindedness (AOTA, 1967, p. 292).

Hall was well known for his work with patients suffering from neurasthenia, a nervous condition believed to be brought on by the stresses of daily life, including a faster life pace and increased demands—products of the shift from an agrarian to an industrial society. Many physicians of the times believed that the rest cure, developed by Dr. S. Weir Mitchell, was the best remedy for these stressed conditions. In contrast, Hall theorized that the rest cure, which consisted of a prolonged period of seclusion and restriction from participation in activities, contributed to illnesses. Lack of physical activity allowed one to grow weaker, and lack of participation in activities allowed a person more time to dwell on problems. The work cure, developed by Hall, engaged the mind and hands of patients to help them focus on productive, creative work to forget their problems (Anthony, 2005a; Quiroga, 1995, p. 96; "The Work Cure," 1914). Hall acknowledged the success of asylums that had patients participate in simple work, housekeeping, laundry, kitchen, and farming. Participation in these activities provided a therapeutic benefit to the patient, and also an economic benefit to the institution because it saved the cost of hiring workers to perform these tasks. Hall believed that patients in a higher socioeconomic class would not be interested in these types of work activities. He believed that these patients would find craft activities more appealing. He also believed that these patients should benefit directly from the sale of their craft products (Hall & Buck, 1915, pp. ix-x).

Hall's work cure integrated the arts and crafts philosophy with medicine. By chance in 1904, Hall met Jessie Luther, an artisan who previously worked as director of the Hull House Labor Museum teaching a variety of crafts, including basket weaving, woodcarving, metal work, and pottery. They had a conversation about the treatment of neurasthenia in which they conceptualized a workshop to provide medical treatment to those suffering from neurasthenia. Together they started the Handcraft Shop in Marblehead, Massachusetts. The workshop was first located in an old cobbler shop; then, as more space was required, it was relocated to the Bay View Yacht Club. Luther taught weaving, and other skilled artisans taught basketry, metal work, and pottery to patients.

In an apprentice model, patients worked side by side with skilled artisans making craft products. In the economic-driven society of the times, Hall strongly believed in the importance of creating products to sell. According to Hall, "the more useful the work, the better its therapeutic effect; and conversely, the more trivial and valueless the product of the work, the less effective will it be in the therapeutic sense" (1917, p. 383). Focusing on the process and product, the patient received the benefit of creating an aesthetic piece through use of his or her hands as well as the self-respect of knowing the product had monetary value. Selling products also provided partial income to the patient and took some burden off the family and society for the patient's care (Anthony, 2005a, 2005b; Cabot, 1914; Hall & Buck, 1915; "The Work Cure," 1914).

In 1905, Hall hired Arthur E. Baggs, a skilled potter, to oversee the pottery program at the Handcraft Shop. Although the pottery program was profitable, by 1908 it became apparent that this craft was too difficult for patients. Marblehead Pottery, a commercial venture, was established from the original program to help provide financial support for the Handcraft Shop. Hall eventually sold the Marblehead Pottery business to Arthur Baggs. Recognized by the Marblehead Pottery insignia imprinted on the bottoms of pieces—a rigged sailing ship flanked by the letters M and P for Marblehead Pottery—these pieces have since become valuable art products (Anthony, 2005a; Marblehead Pottery, 2015). Cement work took the place of the pottery program. Molds were used to create cement flower pots, birdbaths, and stepping stones. This venture also proved to be profitable. The Burke Foundation Convalescent Home in White Plains, New York, successfully implemented a similar cement work program for patients with cardiac problems. In the Burke program, cement work activities were graded to provide needed exercise to strengthen, but not overwork, the heart. The program helped return patients to gainful employment (Hall & Buck, 1915, pp. xii-xiii).

Table 2-1
PERSONAL CONTEXTS OF FOUNDERS AND NEAR FOUNDERS

FOUNDER	BIRTHPLACE	RESIDENCE IN 1917	PROFESSION	INTERESTS BROUGHT TO THE TABLE
George Edward Barton *(March 7, 1871– April 27, 1923)*	MA (East)	NY (East)	Architect, author	Environment (architecture, physical context) work simplification, activity analysis (via friendship with Frank Gilbreth)
William Rush Dunton Jr. *(July 24, 1868– December 23, 1966)*	PA (East)	MD (East)	Physician/psychiatrist, author, journal editor, quilter	Moral treatment
Eleanor Clarke Slagle *(October 13, 1870– September 18, 1942)*	NY (East)	IL (Midwest)	Social worker, arts and crafts teacher	Habit training
Thomas Bessell Kidner *(1866–June 14, 1932)*	England	Canada	Architect, educator, vocational secretary	Vocational rehabilitation, manual training
Susan Cox Johnson *(December 29, 1875– January 18, 1932)*	TX (Southwest)	NY (East)	Arts and crafts teacher	Arts and crafts knowledge
Isabel Gladwin Newton Barton *(July 21, 1891– November 4, 1975)*	NY (East)	NY (East)	Secretary, author	Assisted George Barton with starting NSPOT
Susan E. Tracy *(January 22, 1864– September 12, 1928)*	MA (East)	MA (East)	Nurse	Moral treatment, arts and crafts knowledge
Herbert James Hall *(March 12, 1870– February 19, 1923)*	NH (East)	MA (East)	Physician	Work cure

Dr. Hall was awarded a $1,000 grant by Harvard's Proctor Fund in 1905 to study the effectiveness of his work cure and a second grant in 1909 (Anthony, 2005a; Quiroga, 1995, p. 96; Reed, 2005). In 1912, he opened Devereux Mansion in the Devereux section of town. Devereux Mansion, which belonged to the Goldthwait family, was once used as a seaside resort. The family offered the resort to Hall to use as a sanatorium. The mansion had ample rooms and a barn to accommodate the variety of craft activities offered in the Handcraft Shop. One of occupational therapy's early theorists, Hall described a number of concepts used in occupational therapy practice. These included the concepts of grading activities, energy conservation, transferable skills, substitution of new interests in place of old interests associated with illness, and provision of engaging occupations to facilitate participation (Reed, 2005). Dr. Hall's practice primarily treated an upper-class clientele. At times, this caused strained relationships with his peers, who perceived Devereux Mansion to be a resort for the privileged class (Quiroga, 1995, p. 99).

Hall had personal contact with some of the other founders prior to the inaugural meeting. In November 1914, Hall wrote to William Rush Dunton about the possibility of having one of his teachers travel to Sheppard and Enoch Pratt Hospital to instruct workers there about cement work. In this letter, Hall mentioned that Eleanor Clarke Slagle had visited Marblehead to learn about the work and might also provide this instruction at Sheppard and Enoch Pratt (Hall, 1914). Not favored by George Edward Barton, Hall was not invited to the inaugural meeting of NSPOT in Clifton Springs. Hall was elected as an active member by the founders at that meeting (Newton, 1917b). Nevertheless, as a strong, early advocate of occupational therapy, Hall is considered a near founder (Peloquin, 1991a; Schwartz, 2009) (Table 2-1).

Inaugural Meeting of the National Society for the Promotion of Occupational Therapy

The interest in occupational therapy work was spreading throughout the country. Many of those involved with occupation work shared their knowledge, programs, ideas, and successes through various publications, networking, and at professional meetings. One day in 1913, while sharing an evening meal at Dunton's home, William Rush Dunton and Eleanor Clarke Slagle "discovered that each was maintaining an active correspondence with other people throughout the country who were also working in occupational therapy" (Bing, 1961, p. 176). Dunton and Slagle discussed the idea of developing a national organization of the many people engaged in occupational therapy work as a way to exchange ideas and experiences (Bing, 1961, pp. 176-177; Dunton, 1926). Dunton was excited about the possibility of starting an organization promoting occupation work. He already had experience starting organizations such as the Maryland Psychiatric Society and the Haverford Society of Maryland, a group for alumni from his alma mater Haverford College (Bing, 1961, p. 177).

Although Slagle, Dunton, and a few others had entertained the idea of forming an organization, it was the efforts of George Edward Barton and William Rush Dunton that brought the idea to fulfillment. Barton first wrote to Dunton on November 15, 1914, about organizing a conference of those working in invalid occupations (Dunton, 1926). They corresponded for 3 years before the founding meeting of NSPOT. Their letters were delivered across the great distance separating them by trains. A letter from Dunton, a resident of Baltimore, could be delivered to Barton, a resident of Clifton Springs, New York, in 2 days. Frequently, they would respond to a letter they received with an immediate response. The first line of their letter would usually mention the most recent letter received from the addressee. At first, they used formal salutations, addressing each other as Mr.

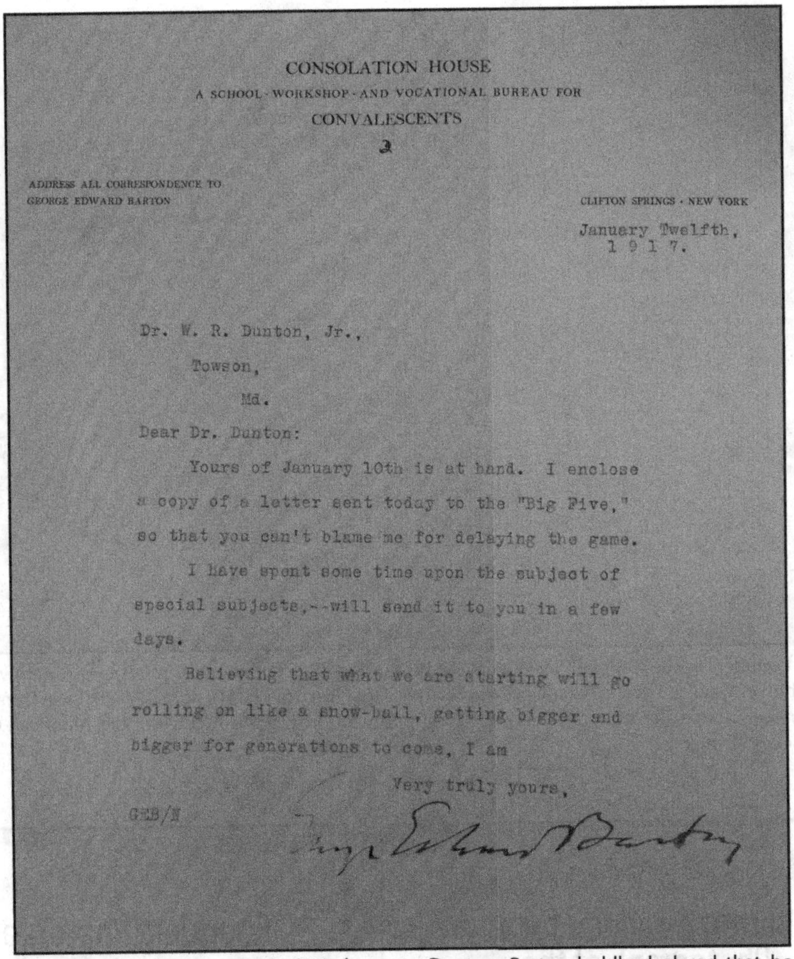

CONSOLATION HOUSE

A SCHOOL - WORKSHOP - AND VOCATIONAL BUREAU FOR

CONVALESCENTS

ADDRESS ALL CORRESPONDENCE TO
GEORGE EDWARD BARTON

CLIFTON SPRINGS · NEW YORK

January Twelfth,
1 9 1 7.

Dr. W. R. Dunton, Jr.,
Towson,
Md.

Dear Dr. Dunton:

Yours of January 10th is at hand. I enclose a copy of a letter sent today to the "Big Five," so that you can't blame me for delaying the game.

I have spent some time upon the subject of special subjects,--will send it to you in a few days.

Believing that what we are starting will go rolling on like a snow-ball, getting bigger and bigger for generations to come, I am

Very truly yours,

GEB/N

George Edward Barton

Figure 2-19. In a January 12, 1917, letter to Dunton, Barton boldly declared that he believed that "what we are starting will go rolling on like a snow-ball, getting bigger and bigger for generations to come…" (Printed with permission from the Archive of the American Occupational Therapy Association, Inc.)

Barton and Dr. Dunton. In time, they became less formal, addressing each other simply as Barton and Dunton.

Barton had very definite ideas about the forming of an organization of occupation workers, including where the first meeting should be held, who should attend, and how the development of the organization should proceed. At one point when correspondence had slowed, Dunton made suggestions about the time and place for a conference to move plans along but was rebuffed by Barton, who, believing his authority had been undermined, threatened to withdraw from the efforts. Dunton's main focus was to get a conference underway, so he assured Barton that he meant no offense and would accept Barton's recommendations. Finally, in January 1917, plans were in place for the meeting to be held that March (Figure 2-19).

Although Barton felt it was best to organize on a local level first, he finally agreed with Dunton's viewpoint that an established national organization could serve as a model to aid the development of state and local associations (Dunton, 1926). Barton believed that to ensure an organization focused on the therapeutic aspects of occupation rather than promoting just an arts and crafts society, it would be advantageous to invite a small number of hand-selected people with similar viewpoints (Barton, 1916a; Dunton, 1926). Both Barton and Dunton agreed to invite Eleanor Clarke Slagle and Susan E. Tracy to the inaugural meeting. Dr. Herbert Hall was considered, but

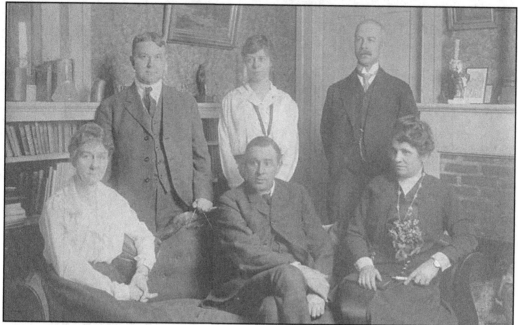

Figure 2-20. Founders of the National Society for the Promotion of Occupational Therapy. Bottom row, left to right: Susan Cox Johnson, George Edward Barton, Eleanor Clarke Slagle. Top row, left to right: William Rush Dunton, Jr., Isabel Gladwin Newton, Thomas Bessell Kidner. (Printed with permission from the Archive of the American Occupational Therapy Association, Inc.)

SIDEBAR 2-4

Barton Arranged for a Photograph of the Founders of the National Society for the Promotion of Occupational Therapy

Understanding the need to publicize the fledgling association, Barton wrote in a letter on February 28, 1917, "I am arranging to have a photograph taken of us all, on one day in order to satisfy the thirst of the newspapers for graphic representation of people who are doing the world's work" (Barton, 1917d). This is now the iconic photograph of the founders of the National Society for the Promotion of Occupational Therapy.

SIDEBAR 2-5

Founders Photograph

In her article about Consolation House and the founding meeting, Isabel Barton reveals that George Edward Barton presented Eleanor Clarke Slagle and Susan Cox Johnson with corsages at the meeting. Mrs. Slagle wore her corsage for the photograph of the founders, whereas Miss Johnson kept her corsage in water in her room. Isabel Barton believed this was a commentary on their personalities. Although Isabel believed both to be strong women, she felt that Mrs. Slagle had more of a flair for style while Miss Johnson was more conservative (Barton, 1968).

Barton and Dunton were not keen on him, questioning the therapeutic value of his work with privileged clientele. Barton suggested Susan Cox Johnson as a better alternative in view of her position as the Director of Occupations for the Department of Public Charities in New York City. Barton asserted that Johnson's position was "by all odds the most important job in the world" (Barton, 1916b). In correspondence leading to the inaugural meeting, Barton refers to the hand-selected group as the Big Five and the Great Five—Barton, Dunton, Slagle, Johnson, and Tracy.

One of the Big Five, Susan E. Tracy, sent her regrets. Although enthusiastically in support of forming the society, she was already obligated to work in Chicago at the Presbyterian Hospital during that time. Thomas Kidner, the Vocational Secretary of the Canadian Military Hospitals Commission, had contacted Barton with a request to meet to discuss Barton's work, so Barton took this opportunity to invite Kidner to the meeting. Barton believed that Kidner's presence would garner international recognition and would be "a feather in our cap" (Barton, 1917c).

Barton insisted the meeting take place in Clifton Springs, writing that "Consolation House, though situated in a small upstate village, is after all one of the most centrally located places in the United States...." (Barton, 1917a). The meeting was originally scheduled to start on March 1, 1917, but Eleanor Clarke Slagle requested a delay until mid-March due to a prior com-

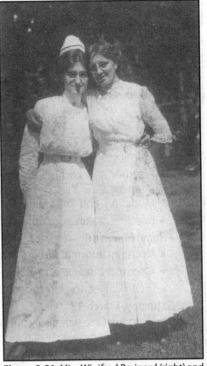

Figure 2-21. Miss Winifred Brainerd (right) and a nurse from the Clifton Springs Sanitarium. (Printed with permission from the Archive of the American Occupational Therapy Association, Inc.)

mitment; therefore, the meeting was rescheduled to start on March 15, 1917. Dunton, Johnson, Kidner, and Slagle arrived in Clifton Springs by train, the main mode of transportation at the time. They were housed in Warfield's Boarding House directly across the street from Consolation House. As usual, Isabel Newton, as Barton's employee, commuted from her home in Geneva (Figure 2-20; Sidebars 2-4 and 2-5).

The agenda for the inaugural meeting was ambitious. On the first day, Barton opened the meeting with a lengthy talk on the "Therapeutic Value of Modeling and Drawing." That evening, application forms for incorporation of NSPOT were completed and submitted to an attorney. On the second day, the founders focused on the organizational structure of NSPOT. Prior to the meeting, Barton planned the general structure of the association and decided who should head up each of the necessary committees based on his perception of their strengths and capabilities. A draft of the constitution was presented. Barton and Dunton had developed the draft prior to the meeting. After discussion, the constitution was adopted. Officers were elected, committees were established, and committee chairs were appointed per Barton's plan. The founders elected 39 people to active membership, 23 as associate members, 15 as sustaining members, and four as honorary members (Newton, 1917b).

On the third day, March 17, the other papers were read and the Articles of Incorporation were signed. A dinner was held at Clifton Springs Sanitarium on Saturday for the founders. The dinner was hosted by Dr. Woodbury, superintendent of the sanitarium; his wife; and Miss Winifred Brainerd, an occupational worker at the sanitarium. Table decorations, including toy wooden animals used as place card holders, had been constructed by patients in the Industrial Room, the craft

SIDEBAR 2-6

Agenda for the Founding Meeting

The *Geneva Daily Times* (March 12, 1917) and the minutes from the founding meeting (Newton, 1917b) recorded the agenda of the founding meeting:

Thursday, March 15
- Morning: Arrivals and acquaintances
- Afternoon: A commemorative photograph was taken of the members of the conference. [G. E. Barton, informal exposition of the Therapeutic Value of Drawing and Modeling, and Preparation of Patients for the Inoculation of the Bacillus of Work]
- Evening: Making out application for Incorporation

Friday, March 16
- Morning: Informal discussion of Constitution
- Afternoon: Business meeting—adoption of the Constitution
- Evening: Election of officers

Saturday, March 17
- Morning: One half hour for each member, informal talk on own work
- Afternoon: Guests of Clifton Springs Sanitarium for midday dinner and inspection of Industrial Department
- Evening: Departures (Newton, 1917b)

SIDEBAR 2-7

Election of Officers and Committee Chairs

The following were elected to office at the founding meeting:
- George E. Barton—President
- Eleanor Clarke Slagle—Vice President
- Isabel G. Newton—Secretary
- William Rush Dunton, Jr.—Treasurer

Committees formed at the founding meeting were as follows:
- Committee on Research and Efficiency—George Edward Barton
- Committee on Installations and Advice—Mrs. Eleanor Clarke Slagle
- Committee on Finance, Publicity, and Publications—Dr. William Rush Dunton, Jr.
- Committee on Admissions and Positions—Miss Susan Cox Johnson
- Committee on Teaching Methods—Miss Susan E. Tracy
- International Committee—Mr. Thomas B. Kidner

Interestingly, these assignments, with the exception of Kidner's assignment, were predetermined by George Edward Barton in a letter to Dunton on February 13, 1917 (Barton, 1917d).

SIDEBAR 2-8

Papers Presented at the Inaugural Meeting

- *The Therapeutic Value of Drawing and Modeling, and Preparation of Patients for Inoculation of the Bacillus of Work*—George Edward Barton
- *History of Occupational Therapy*—William Rush Dunton, Jr.
- *The Work of the Occupational Experiment Station in Chicago*—Eleanor Clarke Slagle
- *The Occupational Work on Blackwell's Island*—Susan Cox Johnson
- *The Difficulties and Results of Re-education of the Crippled Soldier in Canada*—Thomas Bessell Kidner
- *A New Occupation for the Crippled Soldier: The Conservation of the World's Teeth*—Frank B. and Lillian M. Gilbreth (The Gilbreths were not in attendance; the paper was read on their behalf.)

shop at the sanitarium (Dunton, 1917/1967). Kidner, impressed by Miss Brainerd's work, inquired about her availability for work in Canada (Brainerd, 1967) (Figure 2-21; Sidebars 2-6 to 2-8).

The inaugural meeting and activities of the new society were announced in several well-read publications. An advance notice of the meeting was published in the March 8, 1917, edition of the bi-weekly Clifton Springs, New York, newspaper (Figure 2-22), and a summary of the meeting followed in the March 22, 1917, edition. Articles announcing the new society and summaries of the meeting were also published in a number of journals, including *Modern Hospital* ("Leaders in," 1917), *Trained Nurse and Hospital Review* ("A Committee," 1917; "Consolation House Conference," 1917), and *Maryland Psychiatric Quarterly* (Dunton, 1917/1967).

ORGANIZING THE SOCIETY

CLIFTON SPRINGS PRESS.

CLIFTON SPRINGS, N. Y., THURSDAY, MARCH 8, 1917.

First Consolation House Conference Here Thursday.

Burke-Carney Wedding Held On Saturday

Neway Notes Pertaining to Local People

City "Dads" Issue Annual Report And Budget

$14,490.00 Needed For Coming Year

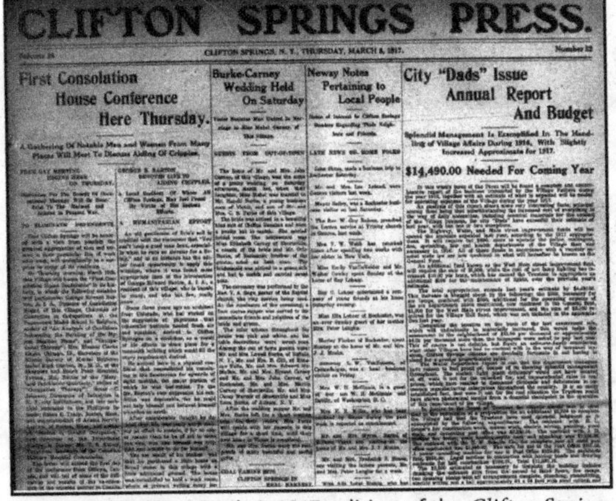

Figure 2-22. The March 8, 1917, edition of the *Clifton Springs Press*, a bi-weekly newspaper in Clifton Springs, New York, published advanced notice of the "First Consolation House Conference," the inaugural meeting of the National Society for the Promotion of Occupational Therapy.

Once the society was formally organized and incorporated, the mundane administrative tasks necessary to get it up and running were started. Consolation House, the official headquarters of the fledgling society, was designated to serve as a reference library and a clearinghouse for those seeking information about occupational therapy. People were asked to send relevant publications to Consolation House to assist in the development of a reference library (Dunton, 1917/1967). Employers interested in finding qualified workers and workers interested in finding open positions were directed to contact Consolation House to share this information.

George Edward Barton and William Rush Dunton worked to choose the colors and letterhead for the official stationery (Barton, 1917f). They settled on a green color

BOARD OF MANAGEMENT	National Society for the Promotion of Occupational Therapy.	COMMITTEES
President, Mr. Geo. Edward Barton. Vice-President, Mrs. Eleanor Clarke Slagle. Treasurer, Dr. W. R. Dunton, Jr. Miss Susan C. Johnson. Miss Susan E. Tracy. ——— Secretary, Miss Isabel G. Newton. Consolation House, Clifton Springs, N. Y.		Committee on Research and Efficiency Chairman, Mr. Geo. Edward Barton, Consolation House, Clifton Springs, N. Y. Committee on Installations and Advice Chairman, Mrs. Eleanor Clarke Slagle, Hotel Alexandria, Chicago, Ill. Committee on Finance, Publicity and Publications Chairman, Dr. Wm. Rush Dunton, Jr., Towson, Md. Committee on Admissions and Positions Chairman, Miss Susan C. Johnson, 9 Livingston Place, New York City Committee on Teaching Methods Chairman, Miss Susan E. Tracy, 870 Centre Street, Jamaica Plain, Boston, Mass. International Committee Chairman, Mr. Thos. B. Kidner, Military Hospitals Commission, Ottawa, Canada.

Figure 2-23. The first letterhead used by the National Society for the Promotion of Occupational Therapy. (Printed with permission from the Archive of the American Occupational Therapy Association, Inc.)

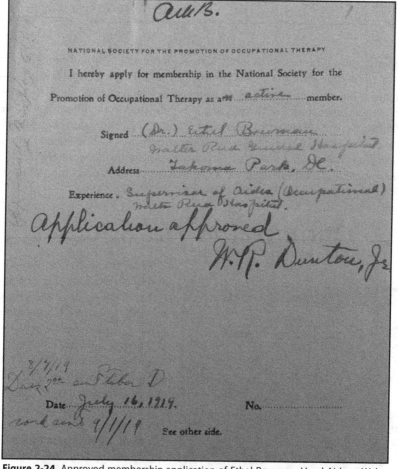

Figure 2-24. Approved membership application of Ethel Bowman, Head Aide at Walter Reed General Hospital. (Printed with permission from the Archive of the American Occupational Therapy Association, Inc.)

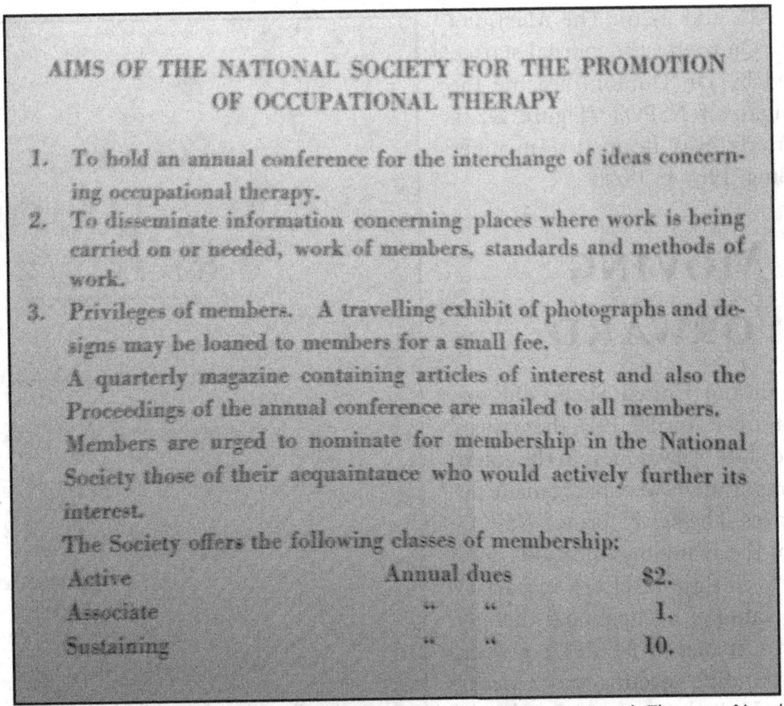

AIMS OF THE NATIONAL SOCIETY FOR THE PROMOTION OF OCCUPATIONAL THERAPY

1. To hold an annual conference for the interchange of ideas concerning occupational therapy.
2. To disseminate information concerning places where work is being carried on or needed, work of members, standards and methods of work.
3. Privileges of members. A travelling exhibit of photographs and designs may be loaned to members for a small fee.

A quarterly magazine containing articles of interest and also the Proceedings of the annual conference are mailed to all members.

Members are urged to nominate for membership in the National Society those of their acquaintance who would actively further its interest.

The Society offers the following classes of membership:

Active	Annual dues	$2.
Associate	" "	1.
Sustaining	" "	10.

Figure 2-25. National Society for the Promotion of Occupational Therapy Aims/Membership Dues. (Printed with permission from the Archive of the American Occupational Therapy Association, Inc.)

THIS IS TO CERTIFY THAT

Mrs. W. R. Dunton, Jr.

IS A Sustaining MEMBER IN GOOD STANDING OF THE

American Occupational Therapy Association

FOR THE YEAR 1928 AND IS ENTITLED TO REGISTER AT THE 1928 ANNUAL MEETING, ON PRESENTATION OF THIS CARD.

1928

Eleanor Clarke Slagle

SECRETARY-TREASURER

(OVER)

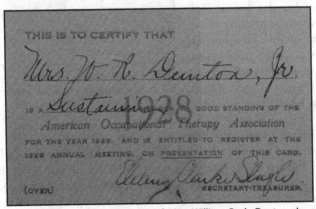

Figure 2-26. Membership card of Mrs. William Rush Dunton, Jr., a sustaining member. (Printed with permission from the Archive of the American Occupational Therapy Association, Inc.)

scheme (Newton, 1917c) (Figure 2-23). Dunton and Isabel Newton collaborated on an application form for membership and a method to maintain a registry of members. Significant effort was put forth by the founders and other supporters to recruit and register new members. The founders wanted to emphasize the therapeutic focus of occupational therapy to distinguish NSPOT from other craft societies and the perception that occupational therapists were merely craft ladies. Therefore, although anyone interested in occupational therapy was eligible to apply for membership, applications were reviewed and approved to ensure the applicants had the experience and background to provide a therapeutic focus in their work (Figure 2-24). The annual membership fees were set at $2 for active members, $1 for associate members, and $10 for sustaining members

(Figures 2-25 and 2-26). The *Maryland Psychiatric Quarterly*, the journal started and edited by Dr. Dunton, became the official organ of NSPOT (Figure 2-27). The quarterly was deemed a member benefit (Bing, 1961, p. 182).

MOVING FORWARD

Although the United States did not declare war until April 6, 1917, there was a heightened state of awareness in the country, and preparations were being made for war readiness. The newly formed NSPOT was one of the many organizations anxious to help in the war effort, in part to prove the value of occupational therapy to society. On March 24, 1917, 1 week after the founding meeting and 2 weeks before the United States declared war against Germany, George Barton sent a letter to Dr. Dunton asking his opinion on offering NSPOT's services to the war effort. Barton had heard a rumor that the Red Cross was contemplating starting a Department of Re-education. He believed that this proposed department had similar aims to occupational therapy (Barton, 1917e). Dunton suggested that Barton should use his discretion to contact the Surgeon General to offer assistance. In a number of letters over the

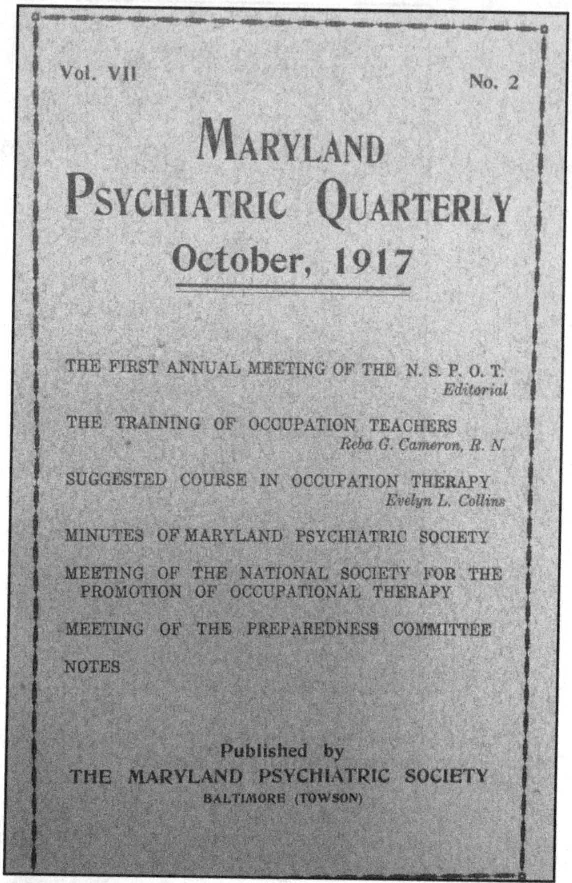

Vol. VII   **No. 2**

MARYLAND
PSYCHIATRIC QUARTERLY
October, 1917

THE FIRST ANNUAL MEETING OF THE N. S. P. O. T.
Editorial

THE TRAINING OF OCCUPATION TEACHERS
Reba G. Cameron, R. N.

SUGGESTED COURSE IN OCCUPATION THERAPY
Evelyn L. Collins

MINUTES OF MARYLAND PSYCHIATRIC SOCIETY

MEETING OF THE NATIONAL SOCIETY FOR THE PROMOTION OF OCCUPATIONAL THERAPY

MEETING OF THE PREPAREDNESS COMMITTEE

NOTES

Published by
THE MARYLAND PSYCHIATRIC SOCIETY
BALTIMORE (TOWSON)

Figure 2-27. Cover of the Maryland Psychiatric Quarterly. This publication, edited by William Rush Dunton, was the official journal of the National Society for the Promotion of Occupational Therapy from 1917 through 1921. (Printed with permission from the Archive of the American Occupational Therapy Association, Inc.)

next few months, Barton requested assistance and advice from Frank Gilbreth, Thomas Kidner, and William Rush Dunton on the potential role of NSPOT in the war effort (Barton 1917h, 1917i, 1917j). He had little luck making contact with any official involved in the war effort, with the exception of a communication with Elliot Wadsworth, Acting Chairman of the American Red Cross. Wadsworth stated that he would bring NSPOT's offer to the attention of Colonel Kean, Director of the Bureau of Medical Services in the United States Army (Barton, 1917g).

The date and place of the first annual NSPOT conference was set at the founding meeting as the first Monday in September 1917 at Consolation House; however, in the summer of 1917, Susan Cox Johnson suggested that New York City would provide a better venue and was more accessible. Dunton was in agreement with the location change; Barton was not. Whether prompted by a perceived slight or by ill health as he claimed, Barton wrote to Dunton indicating he was stepping down as president and suggested that Dunton run for this office (Barton, 1917k). From that time forward, Barton maintained an interest in NSPOT but not an active role. The first annual meeting was held on Labor Day weekend in September 1917 at the Russell Sage Building at 130 East 22nd Street in New York City. Holding the meeting on Labor Day was Dunton's idea. He believed that attendees would be more likely to attend if they missed fewer work days. This did not hold true because only 26 people attended. Realizing that people did not want to give up their holiday, the plan for subsequent annual conferences to be held on Labor Day weekend was abandoned.

Determined to define and promote the role of occupational therapy in the war effort, the theme for the first annual meeting was care of the war wounded. Susan E. Tracy, Susan Cox Johnson, Herbert J. Hall, and William Rush Dunton Jr. all read papers at this conference. Dunton's paper outlined a plan for vocational education for disabled soldiers (Bing, 1961, p. 185). A natural organizer with a strong desire to see this new society grow and flourish, William Rush Dunton Jr. accepted the nomination and election as the second president of NSPOT. Eleanor Clarke Slagle was re-elected as vice president; Louis Haas from Bloomingdale Hospital, White Plains, New York, was elected secretary; and Marion R. Taber from the State Charities Aid Association (New York) was elected treasurer (Bing, 1961, pp. 183, 186).

Dunton, Slagle, Kidner, and a few other attendees met with Dr. Thomas W. Salmon, a neuropsychiatrist and Medical Director of the National Committee on Mental Hygiene, for lunch during the conference (Dunton, 1955). Dr. Salmon was actively involved in planning and organizing medical services for the war effort and was a strong advocate of occupational therapy. This meeting and the leaders' relationship with Dr. Salmon helped to secure occupational therapy's role in World War I working with soldiers suffering from war neuroses.

The work to promote occupational therapy's role in the war effort continued after the first annual meeting. Barton, Slagle, and Johnson all had communications with the Medical Department of the Army. Slagle consulted with the Surgeon General's office and worked with the Red Cross. Dunton consulted with the Nursing Division of the Counsel for Defense. A role for occupation workers was established, and the need was great: 1,000 per General John Pershing's request. Having helped establish a role, the new society worked to meet the need (Report of the President, 1918).

REFLECTION

The Progressive Era in the early 20th century brought a new group of intellectual thinkers, including William James, John Dewey, and Adolf Meyers. These intellectuals developed the philosophical schools of thought of pragmatic psychology; functional psychology, the educational doctrine that emphasized learning by doing; and psychobiology, which provided the basis for the central tenets of occupational therapy. One of the hallmarks of the Progressive Era, the advancement of knowledge, was promoted through experiments, such as the development of programs designed to improve the quality of life of individuals.

Improved economic conditions and changes in the sociocultural and political environments facilitated the development of occupational therapy. Increased emphasis on social responsibility promoted the altruistic activities of upper-class women who worked to help improve quality of life for the disadvantaged. Many of these women became occupation workers or teachers who espoused the ideals of the Arts and Crafts Movement and the Mental Hygiene Movement.

The founders—including two architects (Barton and Kidner), a physician (Dunton), a social worker (Slagle), an arts and crafts teacher (Johnson), and a secretary (Newton)—and the near founders—a nurse (Tracy) and a psychiatrist (Hall)—brought different experiences to the table. Many of the founders were influenced by the thinking of James, Dewey, and Meyers, and in some cases had personal relationships with them. In an era that encouraged sharing of knowledge, the founders gathered to form a new society to share experiences and promote the therapeutic use of occupation. The Founding Vision of NSPOT, as stated in the Certificate of Incorporation (NSPOT, 1917), is reflective of the Progressive Era's emphasis on science and research and the founders' desire to promote the benefits of occupational therapy through networking, conferences, correspondence, and publications in various medical and social service journals (Sidebar 2-9).

Occupational therapy developed from a confluence of ideas with varied rationales behind the therapeutic use of occupations. Occupations were prescribed to exercise certain muscles and promote certain movements, to occupy the mind to help improve focus and substitute healthy thoughts, to develop habits and routines for better living, and to improve self-esteem and self-sufficiency through the sale of handmade products valued by others. The importance of client centeredness and therapeutic use of self was also emphasized as important in achieving successful outcomes. The practice of patient participation in occupations or work as an economic necessity for the operation of some insane asylums soon shifted to the practice of individualized treatment planning in which patients received an economic benefit from sale of their handmade products.

SIDEBAR 2-9

Founding Vision: National Society for the Promotion of Occupational Therapy

---

The particular objects for which this corporation is formed are as follows: The advancement of occupation as a therapeutic measure; for the study of the effect of occupation upon the human being; and for the scientific dispensation of this knowledge. (NSPOT, 1917)

The founders sought to align the new profession with the male-dominated medical profession in an attempt to seek legitimacy. Additionally, it was believed that the sponsorship of the medical profession would help with efforts to provide a scientific basis for the benefits of occupation work and distinguish the female-dominated occupation workers from craft ladies. The therapeutic use of occupation was valued in the Progressive Era. Occupation workers and teachers provided services in a variety of settings, including sheltered workshops, state hospitals, general hospitals, and home services under the direction of physicians. Patient conditions in these settings included neurological and musculoskeletal injuries, crippling diseases, mild to severe mental disorders, cardiac problems, genetic disorders, and systemic diseases such as tuberculosis. Within this context, a firm foundation for occupational therapy was established.

REFERENCES

1875 New York State Census. Town of Stamford, Delaware County, William. J. Clark household, Line 14, June 9, 1875, p. 10.

1880 U.S. Census. Delhi, 1st District, County of Delaware, State of New York, enumeration district (ED) 64, William J. Clark household, Line 8, June 19, 1880, p. 22.

1910 U.S. Census. Washington County, Idaho, Weiser City, enumeration district (ED) 283, Image 1188, Sheet 2B, Line 74, April 1910.

1920 U.S. Census. Washington County, Idaho, City of Weiser, enumeration district (ED) 189, Image 1188, Sheet 1B, Line 95, Slagle household, January 3, 1920.

A committee on therapeutics of occupation. (1917, April). *Trained Nurse and Hospital Review, 58*(4), 226.

Anthony, S. H. (2005a). Dr. Herbert J. Hall: Originator of honest work for occupational therapy 1904-1923 [Part I]. *Occupational Therapy in Health Care, 19*(3), 3-19.

Anthony, S. H. (2005b). Dr. Herbert J. Hall: Originator of honest work for occupational therapy 1904-1923 [Part II]. *Occupational Therapy in Health Care, 19*(3), 21-32.

American Occupational Therapy Association. (1967). Presidents of the American Occupational Therapy Association. *American Journal of Occupational Therapy, 21*(5), 290-298.

Barton, G. E. (1911). *An analysis of the conditions influencing the building of the Myron Stratton Home and recommendations for its foundation and development.* Colorado Springs, CO: Trustees of the Myron Stratton Home.

Barton, G. E. (1914). A view of invalid occupation. *Trained Nurse and Hospital Review, 52*(6), 327-330.

Barton, G. E. (1916a, December 5). [Letter to William Rush Dunton]. Archives of the American Occupational Therapy Association (Series 1, Box 1, Folder 12), Bethesda, MD.

Barton, G. E. (1916b, December 9). [Letter to William Rush Dunton]. Archives of the American Occupational Therapy Association (Series 1, Box 1, Folder 12), Bethesda, MD.

Barton, G. E. (1917a, January 12). [Letter to William Rush Dunton re: suggested location of meeting]. Archives of the American Occupational Therapy Association (Series 1, Box 1, Folder 12), Bethesda, MD.

Barton, G. E. (1917b, January 24). [Letter to William Rush Dunton]. Archives of the American Occupational Therapy Association (Series 1, Box 1, Folder 12), Bethesda, MD.

Barton, G. E. (1917c, February 13). [Letter to William Rush Dunton]. Archives of the American Occupational Therapy Association (Series 1, Box 1, Folder 12), Bethesda, MD.

Barton, G. E. (1917d, February 28). [Letter to William Rush Dunton]. Archives of the American Occupational Therapy Association (Series 1, Box 1, Folder 12), Bethesda, MD.

Barton, G. E. (1917e, March 24). [Letter to William Rush Dunton]. Archives of the American Occupational Therapy Association (Series 1, Box 1, Folder 12), Bethesda, MD.

Barton, G. E. (1917f, April 11). [Letter to William Rush Dunton]. Archives of the American Occupational Therapy Association (Series 1, Box 1, Folder 12), Bethesda, MD.

Barton, G. E. (1917g, June 15). [Letter to William Rush Dunton]. Archives of the American Occupational Therapy Association (Series 1, Box 1, Folder 12), Bethesda, MD.

Barton, G. E. (1917h, June 26). [Letter to Frank B. Gilbreth]. Archives of the American Occupational Therapy Association (Series 1, Box 1, Folder 12), Bethesda, MD.

Barton, G. E. (1917i, June 27). [Letter to William Rush Dunton]. Archives of the American Occupational Therapy Association (Series 1, Box 1, Folder 12), Bethesda, MD.

Barton, G. E. (1917j, July 6). [Letter to Thomas B. Kidner]. Archives of the American Occupational Therapy Association (Series 1, Box 1, Folder 12), Bethesda, MD.

Barton, G. E. (1917k, July 23). [Letter to William Rush Dunton]. Archives of the American Occupational Therapy Association (Series 1, Box 1, Folder 12), Bethesda, MD.

Barton, G. E. (1919). *Teaching the sick*. Philadelphia, PA: W. B. Saunders Company.

Barton, I. G. (1968). Consolation house, fifty years ago. *American Journal of Occupational Therapy, 22*(4), 340-345.

Baum, C. M. (2002). Adolph Meyer's challenge: Focus on occupation in practice and in science. *Occupational Therapy Journal of Research, 22*(4), 130-131.

Bing, R. K. (1961). *William Rush Dunton, Junior—American psychiatrist, a study in self* (Doctoral dissertation). College, Park, MD: University of Maryland.

Bockoven, J. S. (1971). Occupational therapy—a historical perspective. Legacy of moral treatment—1800s to 1910. *American Journal of Occupational Therapy, 25*(5), 223-225.

Burnham, W. H. (1924). *The normal mind: An introduction to mental hygiene and the hygiene of school instruction*. New York, NY: D. Appleton-Century Company Incorporated.

Cabot, R. C. (1914, October 3). Sub-standard workers: Dr. Hall's attack on their problem. *The Survey, 33*, 15-18.

Cameron, R. G. (1917, January). An interview with Miss Susan Tracy. *Maryland Psychiatric Quarterly, 6*(3), 65-66.

Chicago School of Civics and Philanthropy. (1909, July). Announcements 1909-1910 (Bulletin, Vol. 1, No. 1). Chicago, IL: Author. Retrieved from http://babel.hathitrust.org/cgi/pt?id=mdp.39015010775784;view=1up;seq=1

Chicago School of Civics and Philanthropy. (1912, March). Year Book 1912-1913 (Bulletin, Vol. 15). Chicago, IL: Author. Retrieved from http://babel.hathitrust.org/cgi/pt?id=mdp.39015010775784;view=1up;seq=1

Chicago School of Civics and Philanthropy. (1917, December). Special bulletin. In B. Loomis & B. D. Wade (Eds.), *Chicago, occupational therapy beginnings: Hull House, the Henry B. Favill School of Occupations and Eleanor Clarke Slagle* (p. 8). Chicago, IL: University of Illinois Department of Occupational Therapy.

Colorado State Archives. (1911). Record: Marriage license—Agatha J. Farrington and George Edward Barton. Retrieved from https://www.colorado.gov/pacific/archives/archives-search

Colorado State Archives. (1915). Record: Court case—George Edward Barton divorce from Agatha J. Barton. Retrieved from https://www.colorado.gov/pacific/archives/archives-search

Consolation House conference. (1917, May). *Trained Nurse and Hospital Review, 58*(5), 288.

Dewey, J. (1915). *The school and society*. Chicago, IL: University of Chicago Press.

Dobschuetz, B. (2001). Slagle, Eleanor Clarke. In R. L. Schultz & A. Hast (Eds.), *Women building Chicago 1790-1990: A biographical dictionary* (pp. 803-805). Bloomington, IN: Indiana University Press.

Dunton, W. R. (1914, December 2). [Letter to George Edward Barton]. Archives of the American Occupational Therapy Association (Series 1, Box 1, Folder 12), Bethesda, MD.

Dunton, W. R. (1917). History of occupational therapy. *Modern Hospital, 8*(6), 380-382.

Dunton, W. R. (1917/1967). Occupations and amusements. *American Journal of Occupational Therapy, 21*(5), 287-289. (Reprinted from Maryland Psychiatric Quarterly, 1917, 6[4], 91-94.)

Dunton, W. R. (1921). *Occupation therapy: A manual for nurses*. Philadelphia, PA: W. B. Saunders.

Dunton, W. R. (1926). A historical note. *Occupational Therapy and Rehabilitation, 5*(6), 427-439.

Dunton, W. R. (1955, June 2). [Letter to Mrs. Frances Shuff]. Archives of the American Occupational Therapy Association (Series 6, Box 47, Folder 320), Bethesda, MD.

Engagement. (1911, November 22). Colorado Springs, CO: Colorado Springs Gazette.

Favill, J. (1917). *Henry Baird Favill*. Chicago, IL: Privately printed.

Forbush, B., & Forbush, B. (1986). *Gatehouse: The evolution of the Sheppard and Enoch Pratt Hospital, 1853-1986.* Baltimore, MD: J. B. Lippincott.

Friedland, J. (2007). Thomas Bessell Kidner and the development of occupational therapy in the United Kingdom: Establishing the links. *British Journal of Occupational Therapy, 70*(7), 292-300.

Friedland, J., & Davids-Brumer, N. (2007). From education to occupation: The story of Thomas Bessell Kidner. *Canadian Journal of Occupational Therapy, 74*(1), 27-37.

Friedland, J., & Silva, J. (2008). Evolving identities: Thomas Bessell Kidner and occupational therapy in the United States. *American Journal of Occupational Therapy, 62*(3), 349-360.

Fuller, D. H. (1910). The need of instruction for nurses in occupations for the sick. In S. E. Tracy (Ed.), *Studies in invalid occupations* (pp. 1-15). Boston, MA: Whitcomb & Barrow.

Green, J. G. (1934, September). The Emmanuel Movement: 1906-1929. *The New England Quarterly, 7*(3), 494-532.

Hall, H. J. (1914, November 10). [Letter to William Rush Dunton]. Archives of the American Occupational Therapy Association (Series 1, Box 2, Folder 15), Bethesda, MD.

Hall, H. J. (1917). Remunerative occupations for the handicapped. *Modern Hospital, 8*(6), 383-386.

Hall, H. J. (1923). *O.T.—A new profession.* Concord, MA: Rumford Press.

Hall, H. J., & Buck, M. M. C. (1915). *The work of our hands: A study of occupations for invalids.* New York, NY: Moffat, Yard & Company.

Homes for unfortunates. (1914, April). *Journal of American Bankers, 6*(10), 698-700.

Hooper, B., & Wood, W. (2002). Pragmatism and structuralism in occupational therapy: The long conversation. *American Journal of Occupational Therapy, 56*(1), 40-50.

James, W. (1892/1985). Habit. In *Occupational Therapy in Mental Health, 5*(3), 55-67. (Reprinted from *Psychology,* pp. 134-151, by James, W., 1892, New York, NY: Henry Holt and Company)

Johnson, S. C. (1917). Occupational therapy in New York City institutions. *Modern Hospital, 8*(6), 414-415.

Kidner, T. B. (1910). *Educational handwork.* Toronto, CA: The Educational Book Company of Toronto, Limited.

Leaders in work therapy form society. (1917). *Modern Hospital, 8*(5), 356-357.

Levine, R. E. (1987). Looking back: The influence of the arts-and-crafts movement on the professional status of occupational therapy. *American Journal of Occupational Therapy, 41*(4), 248-254.

Lidz, T. (1966/1985). Adolf Meyer and the development of American psychiatry. *Occupational Therapy in Mental Health, 5*(3), 33-53. (Reprinted from *American Journal of Psychiatry,* 1966, 12[3], pp. 320-332)

Lief, A. (1948). *The commonsense psychiatry of Dr. Adolf Meyer.* New York, NY: McGraw-Hill Book Company, Inc.

Loomis, B. (1992). The Henry B. Favill School of Occupations and Eleanor Clarke Slagle. *American Journal of Occupational Therapy, 46*(1), 34-37.

Marblehead Pottery. (2015). Marblehead pottery history. Retrieved from http://marbleheadpottery.net/marblehead_pottery_site/HISTORY.html

Meyer, A. (1922/1977). The philosophy of occupation therapy. *American Journal of Occupational Therapy, 31*(10), 639-642. (Reprinted from *Archives of Occupational Therapy,* 1922, 1, pp. 1-10)

Meyer, A. (1935/1948). The birth and development of the hygiene movement. In A. Lief (Ed.), *The commonsense psychiatry of Dr. Adolf Meyer* (pp. 313-319). New York, NY: McGraw-Hill Book Company, Inc. (Reprinted from *Mental Hygiene,* January 1935, 19, pp. 29-36)

National Committee for Mental Hygiene. (1912). *Origins, objects and plans of the National Committee for Mental Hygiene: Part II. The mental hygiene movement: State societies for mental hygiene.* New York, NY: National Committee for Mental Hygiene.

National Society for the Promotion of Occupational Therapy. (1917). *Certificate of Incorporation.* Clifton Springs, New York: Author.

Newton, I. G. (1917a). Consolation House. *Trained Nurse and Hospital Review, 59*(6), 321-326.

Newton, I. G. (1917b). Report of the secretary: Minutes of the first Consolation House conference. Proceedings of the First Annual Meeting of the National Society for the Promotion of Occupational Therapy (pp. 19-23). Towson, MD: Spring Grove Hospital Press.

Newton, I. G. (1917c, April 11). [Letter to William Rush Dunton]. Archives of the American Occupational Therapy Association (Series 1, Box 2, Folder 13), Bethesda, MD.

Obituary: Gertrude C. Slagle. (1986, April 22). Idaho Press-Tribune.

Occupational Therapy Notes. (1932, April). Obituary: Susan C. Johnson. *Occupational Therapy and Rehabilitation, 11*(2) 152-153.

Peloquin, S. M. (1991a). Looking back: Occupational therapy service: Individual and collective understandings of the founders, part 1. *American Journal of Occupational Therapy, 45*(4), 352-360.

Peloquin, S. M. (1991b). Looking back: Occupational therapy service: Individual and collective understandings of the founders, part 2. *American Journal of Occupational Therapy, 45*(8), 733-744.

Public Welfare Committee. (1917). *Humanizing the greater city's charity: The work of the Department of Public Charities of the City of New York.* New York, NY: Public Welfare Committee.

Quiroga, V. A. M. (1995). *Occupational therapy: The first 30 years: 1900 to 1930.* Bethesda, MD: American Occupational Therapy Association.

Reed, K. L. (1993). The beginnings of occupational therapy. In H. L. Hopkins & H. D. Smith (Eds.), *Willard and Spackman's occupational therapy* (8th ed., pp. 26-43). Philadelphia, PA: J. B. Lippincott Company.

Reed, K. L. (2005). Dr. Hall and the work cure. *Occupational Therapy in Health Care, 19*(3), 33-50.

Reed, K. L., & Sanderson, S. N. (1999). *Concepts of occupational therapy* (4th ed.). Philadelphia, PA: Lippincott Williams & Wilkins.

Report of the President. (1918). In Proceedings of the Second Annual Meeting of the National Society for the Promotion of Occupational Therapy (pp. 15-16). Towson, MD: Sheppard and Enoch Pratt Hospital.

Schwartz, K. B. (2009). Reclaiming our heritage: Connecting the founding vision to the centennial vision. *American Journal of Occupational Therapy, 63*(6), 681-690.

Scull, A., & Schulkin, J. (2009). Psychobiology, psychiatry, and psychoanalysis: The intersecting careers of Adolf Meyer, Phyllis Greenacre, and Curt Richter. *Medical History, 53*(1), 5-36.

Serrett, K. D. (1985). Another look at occupational therapy's history: Paradigm or pair-of-hands? *Occupational Therapy in Mental Health, 5*(3), 1-31.

Slagle, E. C. (n.d). *Experience of Eleanor Clarke Slagle.* Bethesda, MD: Archives of the American Occupational Therapy Association.

Slagle, E. C. (1919a). Department of occupational therapy. *Institutional Quarterly, 10*(3), 29-32.

Slagle, E. C. (1919b). Occupational therapy. In Proceedings of Twentieth New York State Conference of Charities and Corrections, November 11-13, 1919 (pp. 121-135). Syracuse, NY: Organization of the Twentieth New York State Conference of Charities and Corrections.

Slagle, E. C. (1938a, May 10). [Letter to Mrs. John A. Greene]. Archives of the American Occupational Therapy Association (Series 5, Box 24, Folder 162), Bethesda, MD.

Slagle, E. C. (1938b). Occupational therapy. *Trained Nurse and Hospital Review, 100*, 375-382.

The Work Cure. (1914). *Trained Nurse and Hospital Review, 52*(1), 42-43.

Thomson, E. E. (1914, October 17). Illinois opportunity for preventive work in mental hygiene. *The Survey, 33*, 68-69.

Thomson, E. E. (1917). Occupation and its relation to mental hygiene. *Modern Hospital, 8*(6), 397-398.

Tracy, S. E. (1910). *Studies in invalid occupation: A manual for nurses and attendants.* Boston, MA: Whitcomb & Barrows.

Tracy, S. E. (1914, September 18). [Letter to William Rush Dunton]. Archives of the American Occupational Therapy Association (Series 1, Box 2, Folder 21b), Bethesda, MD.

Tracy, S. E. (1917, April 22). [Letter to William Rush Dunton]. Archives of the American Occupational Therapy Association (Series 1, Box 2, Folder 21b), Bethesda, MD.

Training school for occupational therapists. (1918). *Mental Hygiene, 2*(4), 635-636.

United States Corporation Bureau. (1914). Table of cases. *National Corporation Reporter, 47*, p. 819.

3

World War I
1917 to 1920s

Key Points

- Occupational therapy sought legitimacy as a medical profession, aligning with and often working under the supervision of the medical profession.
- In World War I, for the first time in history, the United States government provided reconstruction services for disabled soldiers and sailors to return them to productive, satisfying lives.
- The War Department and Surgeon General's Office established a civilian personnel category of reconstruction aide in occupational therapy to provide services to soldiers and sailors with the American Expeditionary Forces in Europe and for those in the United States.
- Emergency war courses were established to meet the need for reconstruction aides.
- These reconstruction aides, pioneers in occupational therapy, helped to establish the new profession of occupational therapy in the United States.

Highlighted Personalities

- Reconstruction aides in occupational therapy
- Dr. Elliott G. Brackett, orthopedic surgeon
- Dr. Joel E. Goldthwait, orthopedic surgeon
- Dr. Thomas W. Salmon, neuropsychiatrist
- Elizabeth Greene Upham Davis
- Lena Hitchcock, reconstruction aide
- Mrs. Clyde McDowell Myres, reconstruction aide (frequently misspelled as Myers)
- Bird T. Baldwin, psychologist

Key Places

- Pioneer schools in Boston, Philadelphia, St. Louis, and Milwaukee
- Walter Reed General Hospital
- Base hospitals in France
- Base and general hospitals in the United States

Andersen, L. T., & Reed, K. L.
The History of Occupational Therapy: The First Century (pp. 51-88).
© 2017 Taylor & Francis Group.

Key Times/Events

- World War I
- Rehabilitation legislation

Political Events/Issues/Legislation

- War Risk Insurance Act Amendment (Public Law 65-90)
- National Defense Act of 1916 (Public Law 64-85)
- Vocational Education Act of 1917, also known as the Smith-Hughes Act (Public Law 64-347)
- Vocational Rehabilitation Act of 1918, also known as the Soldiers Rehabilitation Act and the Smith-Sears Act (Public Law 65-178)
- Vocational (Industrial) Rehabilitation Act of 1920 (Public Law 66-236), also known as the Civilian Rehabilitation Act, the Smith-Fess Act, and the Smith-Bankhead Act
- United States Veterans Bureau Act of 1921 (Public Law 67-47)

Educational Issues

- Establishing educational qualifications for reconstruction aides and occupational therapists

Association Issues

- Association governed by a Board of five members (1917-1920)

Sociocultural Events/Issues

- Government acceptance of Responsibility to Soldiers
- American Red Cross involvement in World War I
- Junior League funding/support of occupational therapy

Economic Events/Issues

- Economic prosperity in early 1920s

Technological Events/Issues

- Development/advancement of medical equipment such as the x-ray
- Invention of motorized ambulances
- Improved medical treatment for infection control, use of antibiotics
- Development of increasingly destructive weapons of war: highly explosive shells, chemical weapons, poison gases

Practice Issues

- Start of profession's sponsorship by medicine
- Start of physical medicine and rehabilitation
- Differentiation from physical therapy and vocational rehabilitation

INTRODUCTION

"Occupational therapy will someday rank with anesthetics in taking the suffering out of sickness and with antitoxin in shortening its duration."

–Dr. Thomas W. Salmon, 1922

War clouds were on the horizon for the United States in March 1917 when the inaugural meeting was held. Most of Europe was engaged in fighting the Great War, whereas the United States was trying to maintain neutrality. However, less than a month after the founding meeting, the United States declared war on Germany. The founders of the National Society for the Promotion of Occupational Therapy (NSPOT) saw an opportunity for the new society and profession and a responsibility to contribute to the war effort. With the support of physicians advocating for the inclusion of occupational therapy in reconstruction services for disabled soldiers and sailors, they convinced the Medical Department of the Army to establish a new category of personnel: reconstruction aides in occupational therapy. The activities of these reconstruction aides with the American Expeditionary Forces in Europe and at home in the United States impressed many, giving recognition to the new profession.

AMERICA PREPARES FOR WAR

The assassination of Archduke Franz Ferdinand of Austria and his wife Sophie on July 28, 1914, ignited war in Europe. The Central Powers—Germany and Austria-Hungary—were engaged in a war with the Allies, including Russia, France, and the United Kingdom. During the early years of the war in Europe, the United States government maintained a policy of nonintervention and tried to broker peace between the warring nations with little success. Hostile German aggression against American shipping interests and the sinking of the British ocean liner Lusitania in 1915, killing more than 1,100 innocent civilians (including 120 Americans), helped turn public opinion against the stance of neutrality. Anticipating war, many government and private organizations began war preparations. By 1916, the American Red Cross and the United States military were working together on a plan to organize medical personnel and secure equipment and supplies should war break out.

Colonel Jefferson R. Kean, in the new Department of Military Relief, worked with the American Red Cross to organize teams of personnel in various cities and towns in the United States. Many teams were organized in preparation for deployment overseas. When deployed, these teams became mobile units setting up hospital units in various locations for a period of time, then moving to other locations as needed. These teams usually comprised local medical personnel who already worked together. New York Hospital's medical personnel formed one of the first of many base hospital teams organized by Colonel Kean. The desire of the medical personnel to serve was so great that New York Hospital had to decide who could serve in order to maintain adequate staffing at the hospital. The Board of Governors decided that the youngest and oldest workers would be among those chosen to go, leaving a number of middle-aged people to continue to provide services to the home community. Primarily an orthopedic hospital team, this group was deployed to France in August 1917. Base Hospital No. 9, as this group was known, was eventually stationed in Chateauroux, France (Brown, 1920, p. 27).

The American Red Cross played a significant role in raising funds to secure medical equipment and supplies to aid in the care of the sick and wounded soldiers and sailors. In fact, most United States base hospital units deployed to France were organized by the American Red Cross and were often referred to as Red Cross Hospitals (Lynch, Weed, & McAfee, 1923, p. 102). On July 5, 1917, as the Medical Department of the United States Army prepared for war, President Woodrow Wilson officially accepted the American Red Cross offer of assistance (Crane, 1927, p. 229).

On April 6, 1917, the United States was finally provoked to declare war on Germany. Germany's sinking of seven United States merchant ships and the Zimmerman telegram in which the German foreign minister asked Mexico to join Germany in an alliance against the United States were the last straws. The declaration of war resulted in a great expansion of work for all in the military. The combination of the sheer volume of work and overwork of employees resulted in delays, confusion, and errors as America mobilized for war.

In 1917, most travel was by train or ship. Commercial air travel was still in its infancy. The first transatlantic flight by Charles Lindbergh in May 1927 was still a full decade away. However, the Medical Department of the United States Army was more prepared for war than at any other time

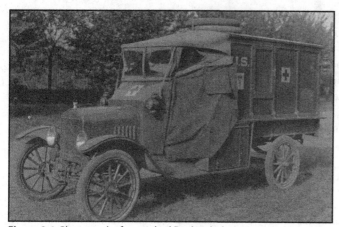

Figure 3-1. Photograph of a standard Ford ambulance.

in history. In spite of this, much more planning and preparation were needed to mobilize for this war overseas. The number and type of medical personnel, the number and sites of hospitals, and the logistics of transporting medical personnel overseas needed to be determined. Planning was needed for supply lines and the housing and feeding of personnel. Preparations and procedures for providing medical care to soldiers, evacuation of soldiers from the front lines, and the assignment and transportation of the wounded to base hospitals were also necessary practical and logistical considerations. The United States had a limited number of ships available to transport military personnel and supplies to Europe. As such, space for military personnel and supplies on these ships was at a premium. Finally, on June 25, 1917, more than 2 months after declaring war, the first American troops of the American Expeditionary Forces reached France.

Technological advances in the early 1900s affected the provision of medical care to injured and ill soldiers and sailors in World War I in both negative and positive ways. World War I weapons were more destructive than ever before. Highly explosive shells and shell fragments, machine guns, and poisonous gases could cause horrific injuries or death (Manring, Hawk, Calhoun, & Andersen, 2009). In contrast, other technological advances helped to save lives. Motorized ambulances were able to more quickly transport injured soldiers to first aid stations and hospitals to receive needed care (Figure 3-1). The use of the Thomas splint, a newly developed traction device used to treat fractured femurs, reduced mortality rates from 80% to 20% (Manring et al., 2009). A new understanding of causes and prevention of infections resulted in new infection control procedures being implemented, saving lives. The new x-ray machine was used for "locating bullets and reading the condition of internal tissues" ("Photography's Aid," 1919), greatly assisting medical care (Figure 3-2).

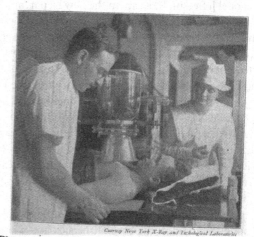

Figure 3-2. Advertisement for an x-ray machine.

RECONSTRUCTION SERVICES
IN THE MILITARY

The Medical Department of the United States Army had the overall responsibility of organizing medical services for wounded soldiers, including acute medical services and reconstructive services designed to return soldiers to maximum functioning. In the spring of 1917, the Surgeon General, Major General William C. Gorgas, and a number of orthopedic surgeons and neuropsychiatrists traveled to England, France, and Canada to survey these allied countries' reconstruction programs. Occupations and activities were provided to convalescents in these programs with great success. Additionally, because the use of occupations and activities were also successful in civilian facilities in the United States, the Medical Department wanted to include these types of services in United States wartime reconstruction programs.

The structures and functions of divisions and departments being established in the Surgeon General's Office were often ill defined and in a constant state of change. Workloads of the office staff had increased significantly, resulting in time delays and errors. A lack of coordinated efforts between divisions and departments compounded the problems. In August 1917, the Surgeon General, having decided that there should be a broad plan of reconstruction comprising all departments of medicine and surgery involved in the problem, created the Division of Special Hospitals and Physical Reconstruction, later renamed the Division of Physical Reconstruction. The division engaged in numerous studies and extensive planning for the reconstruction of soldiers and sailors. Information and literature were gathered about the various medical, vocational, and educational services that might possibly aid in the educational preparation of personnel, the development of facilities, and the securing of equipment that would be required to provide effective reconstruction services. With this information, the Surgeon General's Office developed an extensive plan for physical reconstruction and vocational training.

In January 1918, the Secretary of War, believing the Surgeon General's comprehensive plan would overlap with the programs of other agencies, directed all these agencies to coordinate plans. Representatives from a number of agencies, including the United States Public Health Service, the American National Red Cross, the War Risk Insurance Bureau, and the Federal Board for Vocational Education, met with the Surgeon General's Office for the first time on January 14, 1918. They continued to meet over the next few months (Crane, 1927, p. 36). In August 1918, the final approved plan determined that the military was to restore disabled soldiers and sailors to "full or limited military service." After discharge from the military, the Federal Board of Vocational Education would provide vocational training for disabled soldiers and sailors (Crane, 1927, p. 41).

Initially, the Federal Board of Vocational Education was established to provide for public vocational education to assist the development of semi-skilled workers in agriculture, trades, and industry. When their mission was expanded to include vocational services to disabled soldiers and sailors, the Federal Board of Vocational Education secured the services of Thomas B. Kidner as a Special Adviser on Rehabilitation to assist the establishment of a system of vocational education for disabled soldiers and sailors. Kidner had the experience to advise the United States in setting up a system for the rehabilitation of soldiers and sailors in the United States because he had served as the Vocational Secretary of the Canadian Military Hospitals Commission with the responsibility for rehabilitation of disabled soldiers (Editorial, 1922).

LEGISLATION RELATED TO RECONSTRUCTION AND REHABILITATION SERVICES

Prompted by the progressive thinking of the time, the United States Congress passed a series of laws authorizing a number of educational and rehabilitative programs. With the changes in the early 20th century, these laws took into consideration the need to improve the skill sets of workers to work in new industries, the need to promote economic growth, and the need to improve the quality of life for citizens (Table 3-1).

As war was being fought in Europe, the United States recognized the possibility of being drawn into the conflict. Recognizing the government's social and economic responsibility to ensure a standard of living and quality of life for servicemen and their families, Congress passed a number of laws. The National Defense Act of 1916 (Public Law No. 64-85) provided the opportunity for those in active service to receive instruction "to increase their military efficiency and enable them to return to civil life better equipped for industrial, commercial, and general business occupations." This law also authorized civilian teachers to assist the Army in providing this type of instruction, primarily consisting of vocational education in agriculture or the mechanic arts (National Defense Act, 1921, p. 24).

Table 3-1		
LEGISLATION RELATED TO RECONSTRUCTION AND REHABILITATION SERVICES		
YEAR	**LEGISLATION**	**PURPOSE**
1916	National Defense Act of 1916 (Public Law No. 64-85)	Passed to ensure the country was prepared in case of war; provided opportunity for those in active service to receive instruction to improve military efficiency and develop skills for industrial, commercial, and business occupations in civilian life; provided foundation for vocational re-education
1917	War Risk Insurance Amendments of 1917 (Public Law 65-90)	Provided for rehabilitation, re-education, and vocational training for soldiers and sailors; provided for supplies such as artificial limbs, trusses, and similar appliances
1917	Vocational Education Act of 1917 (Public Law 64-347); also known as the Smith-Hughes Act	Established the Federal Board of Vocational Education, which eventually studied the vocational needs of disabled soldiers and sailors and provided vocational re-education
1918	Vocational Rehabilitation Act of 1918 (Public Law 65-178); also known as the Soldiers Rehabilitation Act and the Smith-Sears Act	Provided for "vocational rehabilitation and return to civil employment of disabled persons discharged from military or naval forces of the United States"
1920	The Vocational (Industrial) Rehabilitation Act of 1920 (Public Law 66-236); also known as the Civilian Rehabilitation Act, the Smith-Fess Act, and the Smith-Bankhead Act	Provided vocational rehabilitation services to civilians physically injured in industrial or occupational accidents
1921	United States Veterans Bureau Act of 1921 (Public Law 67-47)	Consolidated veterans' benefits from the War Risk Insurance Bureau, the United States Public Health Service, and the Federal Board of Vocational Education under the Veteran's Bureau.

The War Risk Insurance Act, first passed in 1914 and amended in 1917 (Public Law 65-90), provided a number of benefits for World War I veterans disabled in the line of duty. Benefits authorized by this law included compensation in cases of service connected disability or death and "courses of rehabilitation, re-education, and vocational training." Additional benefits included "reasonable governmental medical, surgical, and hospital service and with such supplies, including artificial limbs, trusses, and similar appliances as the director may determine to be useful and reasonably necessary." Another amendment in December 1919 authorized the bureau to furnish "wheeled chairs" if reasonably necessary (Public Law 66-104). This law was the first authorize services to assist disabled servicemen return to as productive a life as possible through rehabilitation, re-education, and vocational training (Douglas, 1918).

The Vocational Education Act of 1917 (Public Law 64-347), also known as the Smith-Hughes Act, was passed to provide for public vocational education to assist the development of semi-skilled workers in agriculture, trades, and industry, including the preparation of teachers for vocational education. The Federal Board of Vocational Education (FBVE) was established by this act as federal oversight for state programs. Although when this legislation was passed it did not authorize provision of vocational services to disabled soldiers and sailors, in January 1918 Congress directed the FBVE to study the vocational needs of disabled soldiers and sailors and recommend a plan for their reconstruction.

The Vocational Rehabilitation Act of 1918 (Public Law 65-178), also known as the Soldiers Rehabilitation Act and the Smith-Sears Act, provided for "vocational rehabilitation and return to civil employment of disabled persons discharged from military or naval forces of the United States." Originally, all medical treatment and rehabilitation services were to be provided by the specific military hospitals and centers located in different areas of the country. Once maximum functional potential was achieved, the serviceman would be discharged from the military and could enter a vocational rehabilitation program. Most servicemen were anxious to return home as soon as possible and requested discharge when the war ended, going home instead of to the military hospitals. The Vocational (Industrial) Rehabilitation Act of 1920 (Public Law 66-236), also known as the Civilian Rehabilitation Act, the Smith-Fess Act, and the Smith-Bankhead Act, provided the same vocational rehabilitation services to civilians physically injured in industrial or occupational accidents. Funds were appropriated to assist states to provide these services.

FEDERAL BOARD FOR VOCATIONAL EDUCATION

The FBVE was directed to provide information on the rehabilitation and vocational re-education of injured soldiers and sailors by the United States Senate in January 1918. In response, the FBVE developed a report titled "Training of Teachers for Occupational Therapy for the Rehabilitation of Disabled Soldiers and Sailors." The report was written by Elizabeth Greene Upham, from Milwaukee, Wisconsin. Having overcome a disability of her own, she developed an interest in helping those with disabilities. She was the force behind the start of a training course in invalid occupations at Milwaukee-Downer College in 1913 (Jones, 1988). Upham wrote the report when she was working as a research assistant for the FBVE. She understood that the benefits of occupational therapy were more abstract, of greater variety, and more complex than those of physiotherapy (massage, exercise, hydrotherapy, and electrotherapy), so in addition to providing curricular information, the report effectively described the benefits of occupational therapy and clarified the difference between occupational therapy and vocational education.

The report described three phases of recovery: (1) the acute stage, (2) the convalescence stage, and (3) the vocational training or education stage. The acute stage primarily involved medical and/or surgical care, and therapy in this phase consisted of invalid, bedside, or ward occupations, which were mainly diversional in nature to improve mental outlook. Occupational therapy was of utmost importance in the second phase, the convalescence stage, to enable the disabled soldier to regain functional control of the body, both physical and mental, and to help prepare the soldier for vocational training and/or for civilian life. Once the disabled soldier had sufficiently recovered, he entered the third stage, the vocational training stage, to participate in a prescribed course of study to learn a vocation. Occupational therapy provides the vital link between medical treatment and vocational training, enabling the soldier to participate in vocational training (Upham, 1918, pp. 11-13). Canadian statistics from the war indicated that 80% of disabled soldiers were able to return to a former occupation after treatment in a curative workshop. Twenty percent needed full or partial vocational training (Upham, 1918, p. 18). The report by Elizabeth Greene Upham advocated the need for occupational therapists, not only as a war measure but as essential for industrial accidents and civilian disabilities such as mental illness (Upham, 1918, p. 68).

RECONSTRUCTION AIDES IN OCCUPATIONAL THERAPY

The reconstruction aides in occupational therapy were known by a variety of names: occupational aides, occupational therapists, occupational therapeutists, occupational teachers, reconstruction aides in occupational therapy, and re-aides (Sidebar 3-1).

A memo from the Surgeon General dated January 5, 1918, makes the first mention of occupational aides. The memo describes occupational aides' services as purely medical and necessary to provide "early ward occupation" to prepare convalescents for subsequent vocational treatment (Crane, 1927, p. 57). Although the work was described as a purely medical function, these occupational aides were placed under the supervision of an educational director, in contrast to physiotherapy, which was under medical direction. Instructions provided by the Surgeon General

---

SIDEBAR 3-1

Alternate Names for Occupational Therapy

The following are names sometimes used to describe occupation as a therapeutic agent before the term *occupational therapy* became widely accepted.

- Work cure
- Curative work
- Curative occupation
- Invalid occupations
- Diversional occupation
- Diversional therapy
- Cheer-up work
- Therapeutic diversion
- Reconstructive activities
- Re-education
- Finger therapy

- Activity therapy
- Ergotherapy
- Reconstruction therapy (part of WWI Army program)
- Curative therapy
- Work therapy
- Industrial therapy
- Functional therapy
- Therapeutic occupation
- Occupational remediation
- Remedial occupation

in March 1918 stated that "all therapeutic work, excluding physiotherapy, was to be classed as occupational therapy..." (Crane, 1927, p. 79). Reconstruction work took place in hospitals, general hospitals, and base hospitals set up in the United States and Europe. The types of occupation work included the following: "(a) bedside occupations to take the patient's attention from his disability and occupy his mind. At first diversional ... these became ... vocational, economic or social in value, (b) Ward, shop, or farm occupations and study to occupy the patient's time in worth-while work, and thus develop in him a good mental attitude toward his disability, his treatment, and the hospital, (c) Ward, classroom, or farm operations and study in preparation for reeducation..." (Crane, 1927, p. 86).

There were three classifications of occupational therapy aides: (1) Class A were experts in one or more lines of work, including social work and library service, and were teachers in "industrial and fine arts, general science, English, commercial branches, free-hand drawing and design, mechanical drawing, telegraphy and signalling, French, manual training, agriculture (gardening and floriculture), music, plays, and games, mathematics"; (2) Class B were teachers or craftsmen in "one or more lines of knitting (hand, machine, rake), weaving, clay and papier-maché modeling, wood carving and toy making, metal working, jewelry, and engraving"; and (3) Class C were informed on "military procedures in hospitals, the War Department's program for physical reconstruction of disabled soldiers, regulations as to insurance, pensions, and other benefits, under the War Risk Insurance Bureau, and opportunities offered by the Federal Board for Vocational Training" (Crane, 1927, p. 58; Haggerty, 1918).

Curative shops were established in connection with each hospital to provide light work for disabled soldiers in preparation for retraining in new occupations or vocations (Crane, 1927, p. 29). Occupational therapy was to be medically prescribed.

No patient was to be assigned ward occupational work until the ward surgeon had entered on his clinical record the fact that he was physically fit for such work, and no patient was to be assigned to work in the shop, on farms, etc., except on written prescription of the proper medical officer, such prescription to state the functional result to be obtained, the length of time the patient should work, whether the work should be light or heavy, and whether indoors or outdoors (Crane, 1927, p. 79).

The original plan specified that men should teach "manual activities required by occupations," preferably men who had overcome a similar disability, or at least men with experience in the occupation to be taught (Crane, 1927, p. 21). Although the Army allowed for female nurses, the belief was that nurses had the appropriate education and qualifications, whereas other women, including those providing reconstructive and therapeutic services, would be detrimental to the discipline and morale of troops (Crane, 1927, p. 32; Russell, 1918). With a shortage of men to fill these positions, by December 1917, after careful study, the Medical Department decided to employ Women's Auxiliary Medical Aides as civilian personnel to carry out this reconstructive work in hospitals (Crane, 1927, p. 57). To fill the need for these occupational aides, the Division proposed to establish educational programs to train 1,000 women for occupational work by October 1, 1918 (Crane, 1927, pp. 57-58; Lynch et al., 1923, p. 474). These civilian employees were commonly known as reconstruction aides. Male civilians were also approved for hire as reconstruction aides (Table 3-2, Sidebar 3-2, Figure 3-3).

Neuropsychiatric Services

With war officially declared, Dr. Thomas W. Salmon, a psychiatrist and the Medical Director of the National Committee on Mental Hygiene, recognized the need to plan for medical care of soldiers and sailors suffering from psychiatric disorders (Figure 3-4). He wrote to the Rockefeller Foundation on May 1, 1917, asking for funds and support to visit England and France to learn how the Allies dealt with the nervous and mental disorders suffered by soldiers and sailors sent to war (Salmon, 1917b). The Rockefeller Foundation granted Dr. Salmon's request.

Table 3-2 MILITARY TIMELINE FOR RECONSTRUCTION SERVICES	
April 6, 1917	The United States declares war on Germany
Spring 1917	General Gorgas, the Surgeon General of the United States; neuropsychiatrists; and orthopedic surgeons visit England, Canada, and France to learn about those countries' reconstruction programs for soldiers. The focus is to learn specifically about the organization of programs and problems encountered (McDaniel, 1968, p. 69).
June 25, 1917	The first American troops, the American Expeditionary Forces, reach France.
July 1917	The American Orthopedic Association officially offers their services to the Surgeon General (Lynch et al., 1923, p. 424).
July 12, 1917	In a letter from a military official to the military director of the Red Cross regarding planning for reconstruction services, the concept of reconstruction aides is introduced (Lynch et al., 1923, p. 431).
August 22, 1917	The Division of Special Hospitals and Physical Reconstruction organizes, with Major Edgar King named as Chief. Later, Colonel Frank Billings becomes Chief. This Division includes the Special Section of Education, which includes curative workshop functions and occupational therapy, and the Special Section of Physiotherapy (Lynch et al., 1923, p. 474).
November 7, 1917	Original plan for the reconstruction of soldiers is submitted, specifying that enlisted men with disabilities teach those with like disabilities.
December 1917	The War Department approves of hiring women and men as reconstruction aides. These reconstruction aides will be "employees at large" of the Medical Department cooperating with the Division of Orthopedic Surgery (Lynch et al., 1923, p. 474).
December 1917	The neuropsychiatric service of the American Expeditionary Forces begins under the supervision of Dr. Thomas Salmon.
January 5, 1918	A memo from the Surgeon General makes the first mention of occupational aides. A proposal is submitted to establish educational programs to train 1,000 women for occupational work by October 1, 1918 (Crane, 1927, pp. 57-58).
January 1918	Physical therapist Marguerite Sanderson, a former employee of Dr. Joel Goldthwait, is appointed first supervisor of reconstruction aides in occupational therapy and physical therapy. Her primary duties include recruiting and training personnel.
January 30, 1918	In response to a Senate resolution, a report written by Elizabeth Greene Upham titled "Training of Teachers for Occupational Therapy for the Rehabilitation of Disabled Soldiers and Sailors" is submitted to the United States Senate.
February 15, 1918	Dr. Elliott Gray Brackett (Chief, Division of Orthopedic Surgery) initiates occupational therapy services in Walter Reed Army Hospital with three occupational therapy aides (Crane, 1927, p. 96; McDaniel, 1968, p. 77).
April 1918	First described as a "purely medical function" in a January 5, 1918, memo, the Surgeon General places occupational aides under the direction of the educational service, compared with physiotherapy, which is under medical direction (Crane, 1927, p. 58).
April 29, 1918	The designation occupational therapy for therapeutic work, mental or manual, is discarded, being thereafter included in the term curative workshop schedule.
May 1918	Reconstruction programs start at Fort McHenry, Maryland; Fort McPherson, Georgia; and Lakewood, New Jersey. By July, an additional 21 sites are selected to participate in the program.
May 18, 1918	Base Hospital No. 117, a specialized neuropsychiatric hospital unit comprising five reconstruction aides in occupational therapy, sails for Europe. They arrive in La Fauche, France, on June 16, 1918.
July 1918	Dr. Joel Goldthwait writes a letter stressing the need for large numbers of aides trained in bedside occupations.

(continued)

Table 3-2 (continued)	
MILITARY TIMELINE FOR RECONSTRUCTION SERVICES	
July 31, 1918	The Surgeon General's Office designates 26 general hospitals for the rehabilitation of soldiers in the United States, including Walter Reed General Hospital, Fort McHenry #2 (MD), Fort McPherson #6 (GA), Otisville #8 (NY); Lakewood #9 (NJ), Oteen #19 (NC), Whipple Barracks #20 (AZ), Fort Des Moines #26 (IA), Fort Sheridan #28 (IL), Fort Snelling #29 (MN), and Carlisle #31 (PA). In August 1918, additional sites are added, including Fort Sam Houston (TX), Fort Riley (KS), Camp Custer (MI), Camp Gordon (GA), Camp Grant (IL), Camp Jackson (SC), Camp Kearney (CA), and Camp Dix (NJ).
August 13, 1918	Requested by Chief Surgeon of the American Expeditionary Forces, Dr. Joel Goldthwait, 27 reconstruction aides (13 occupational therapy and 14 physical therapy) arrive at Base Hospital #9 in Chateauroux, France. On September 15, 1918, seven reconstruction aides in occupational therapy transferred to Base Hospital #14 in Beau Desert (Crane, 1927, p. 65).
August 1918	Dr. Thomas Salmon requests more reconstruction, writing, "The Reconstruction Aides, especially those working in handicrafts, are worth their weight in gold" (McDaniel, 1968, p. 85; Myers, 1948). General Pershing, at the behest of Surgeon General Gorgas, cables, "Send over a thousand of these aides as soon as you can get them ready" (Myers, 1948; Quiroga, 1995, p. 164).
November 11, 1918	Armistice Day; World War I ends. (For the purposes of the history of the Medical Department of the United States Army in the World War, the period of war activities extends from April 6, 1917, to December 31, 1919 [Bailey, Williams, & Komora, 1929, p. v].)
June 20, 1919	The Division of Physical Reconstruction ceases to exist, becoming the Section on Physical Reconstruction in the Division of Hospitals in the U.S. Public Health Service (Crane, 1927, p. 50).
January 1922	Reconstruction aides transfer to the United States Veterans Bureau within the U.S. Public Health Service.
December 1926	The Surgeon General recommends the term *reconstruction aide* be abolished, in part to eliminate confusion about the respective roles of occupational therapy and physical therapy (McDaniel, 1968, p. 91).

SIDEBAR 3-2

Carry On Magazine

Carry On: A Magazine on the Reconstruction of Disabled Soldiers and Sailors, was a collaborative effort of the American Red Cross and the Surgeon General's Office. The main purpose was to educate disabled soldiers and sailors and the public about the benefits of restoring the soldiers and sailors to meaningful, productive lives through rehabilitation. The first issue was published in June 1918 and the last in July 1919 (see Figure 3-3).

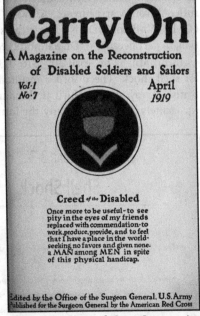

Figure 3-3. Cover of *Carry On* magazine, Volume 1, Issue 7, with Creed of the Disabled.

Soldiers suffering from shell shock were of foremost concern to Dr. Salmon. Technologically advanced highly explosive shells were now being used in battle. The use of highly explosive shells has implications not only for physical injury and death, but for psychological damage from the shell shock. Initially it was believed that the concussion from these highly explosive shells physically affected soldiers' nervous systems, causing a nervous disorder. Closely examining hundreds of cases, Dr. Salmon found that soldiers who had not been involved in battle and were not exposed to bursting shells also suffered from nervous disorders. In his view, the term *shell shock* was a

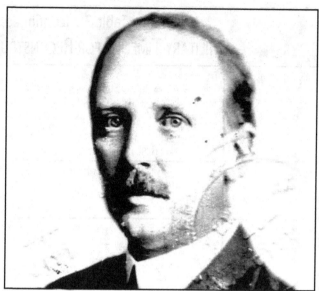

Figure 3-4. Dr. Thomas W. Salmon.

misnomer because a definitive physiological or psychological etiology had not been determined (Salmon, 1917a). The more acceptable medical term for soldiers' nervous disorders was *war neuroses* or *functional war neuroses* (Crane, 1927, p. 162; Salmon, 1917a). The term *shell shock* continued to be used, often with a broad brush to label soldiers suffering from mental and nervous disorders as a result of the stresses of war. A century later, *posttraumatic stress disorder* is the preferred medical term.

In World War I, some suffering from war neuroses were thought to be malingerers. Worse, some who, under the stress of war, froze in place or fled their posts were charged with cowardice or desertion and were executed. The British military executed 306 British soldiers for cowardice or desertion in World War I. Ninety years later, many of these soldiers executed were believed to have suffered from war neuroses. All were pardoned posthumously in 2006 by the British government (Taylor-Whiffen, 2011). No American soldiers were executed in World War I for cowardice or desertion, in part because of Dr. Salmon's recognition of the need for medical care, not punishment.

In Britain, as of April 30, 1916, 1,300 officers and 10,000 soldiers were admitted to hospitals for shell shock. The disorder resulted in "one-seventh of the discharges for disability from the British Army, or one-third if discharges for wounded are excluded" (Salmon, 1917a). Salmon was acutely aware of not only the human aspect of this disability, but also the economic impact from loss of fighting military personnel and the cost to provide medical care. Salmon believed it was vitally important for troop morale and staffing to provide effective medical treatment for these soldiers as soon as possible to return them to the front or discharge them to a productive civilian life (Salmon, 1917a) (Sidebar 3-3).

The symptoms of war neuroses included hysterical paralysis, hysterical blindness, hysterical deafness, tics, tremors, gait disturbances, disorders of speech, confusion, amnesia,

---

SIDEBAR 3-3

Shell Shock

Dr. Salmon, illustrating how the effects of battle can affect a man's behavior and the fine line between heroism and cowardice, was quoted as saying:

When a man breaks he starts to run; when he runs toward the enemy he is shot by them and dies a hero; when he runs toward his own lines he is shot by his comrades and dies a coward. The impulse is the same in both cases. (Johnson, 1945)

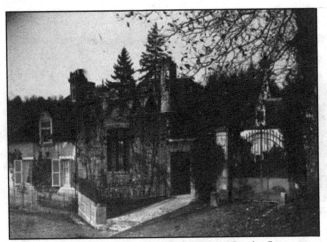

Figure 3-5. Grounds of Base Hospital No. 117 in La Fauche, France.

hallucinations, and anxiety. Salmon advocated for the use of occupations to treat soldiers suffering from war neuroses. He believed that using meaningful occupations, using the principle of learning by doing, would help in re-education and in restoring thought, will, feeling, and lost or impaired functions (Salmon, 1917a).

Dr. Thomas Salmon was a strong advocate of the occupational therapists' role with soldiers suffering from war neuroses. He insisted that occupational therapy be included as part of the neuropsychiatric services. Dr. Salmon was personally and professionally acquainted with Eleanor Clarke Slagle. He, as many others, recognized her as an authority in occupational therapy work. Desiring to offer the best occupational therapy services, he offered Slagle "...a position in charge of all re-educational work with over-seas psychiatric cases" to work under his direction (Slagle, n. d.). Slagle decided she would better serve the war effort by staying in the United States to help establish training schools (Slagle, n.d.). She stayed in the United States and established the Red Cross School in Chicago.

Base Hospital No. 117 was organized in March 1918, at Camp Crane, Pennsylvania, to serve as a neuropsychiatric base hospital. Under the supervision of Dr. Salmon, the hospital team consisted of officers, enlisted men, and nurses who had had previous experience with mental and nervous diseases. The unit trained at Camp Crane until May 17, 1918, when it proceeded by rail to the port of embarkation in Hoboken, New Jersey. The unit set sail from Ellis Island on May 18, 1918. Traveling via England, they finally arrived at their destination of La Fauche, France, on June 16, 1918. La Fauche, a village southeast of Paris in the foothills of the Vosges Mountains, was a mere 30 miles from the front lines. The base hospital group included five civilian reconstruction aides, among the first to arrive in France. The group of reconstruction aides in occupational therapy consisted of Mrs. Clyde McDowell Myres, who had volunteered at Blackwell's Island and worked at Bloomingdale Hospital for mental patients; Amy Drevenstedt, who taught the History of Art at Hunter College; Corrine Dezeller, who taught woodworking to exceptional children in a New York City public school; Laura LaForce, a graduate nurse who taught basket making and weaving in New York City Hospital for Children; and Eleanor Hope Johnson, a psychologist (Johnson, 1945; Myers, 1948).

Mrs. Myres, a 43-year-old widow, was placed in charge of the aides. In time, additional reconstruction aides in occupational therapy were sent to work at Base Hospital No. 117 (Figures 3-5 and 3-6).

Predicting that there would be a lack of tools and supplies available in France, these women had gathered what they could in the United States, including hammers, saws, soldering irons, pliers, files, looms, yarns, paints, and brushes. On arriving in La Fauche, and with

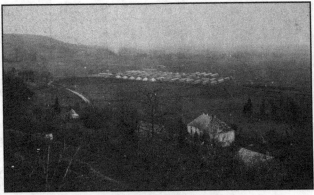

Figure 3-6. Bird's eye view of Base Hospital No. 117.

building supplies in short supply, they set up shop, making use of discarded materials such as trashed beds and wooden boxes to make work and seating areas. Luckily, a short time after the initial workshop was set up, a representative of the Red Cross arranged for a new Red Cross hut and occupational therapy workshop outfitted with new tools (Myers, 1948; Schwab, 1919) (Figure 3-7).

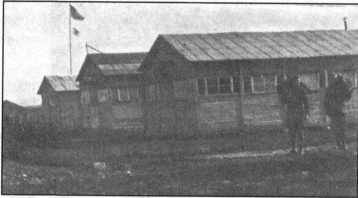

Figure 3-7. Red Cross hut and occupational therapy workshop at Base Hospital No. 117.

The soldiers suffering psychological and physical effects (e.g., hysterical paralysis, tics, tremors) of war neuroses participated in a range of activities such as wood carving, metal work, weaving, painting, sketching, building the base hospital roads, and farming (Schwab, 1919). Recovering soldiers engaged in tinsmithing, where they made tin candlesticks, flower holders, cookie cutters, toys, ashtrays, and other creative products. With limited supplies, the reconstruction aides made use of trash such as empty tin cans for construction of craft projects (Myers, 1948). Mrs. Clyde Myres, called Mother Myres by the soldiers, recalled the endless supply of empty tin cans used for craft projects in the occupational therapy workshop (Dallas Woman's Work, 1958; Thatcher, 1919, pp. 9-11). Although the work of the soldiers in the occupational therapy workshop produced numerous types of craft projects, Mrs. Myres firmly believed that "the great thing fashioned in that shop was not toy or souvenir, but steadiness of hand, power of concentration, ability to make manual and moral adjustments, and renewal of self-confidence and courage" (Myres, 1919, p. 138) (Figures 3-8 and 3-9).

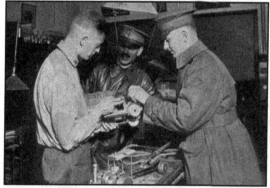

Figure 3-8. Soldiers making toys and other creative objects out of tin cans.

Initially, Dr. Salmon had difficulty convincing the military authorities that this type of therapeutic service was needed; however, once the reconstruction aides arrived, the workshop at Base Hospital No. 117 was an immediate success. In addition to observation of improved troop morale and increased participation in occupations, reports indicated that 93% of soldiers admitted to Base Hospital No. 117 were returned to duty, with 20% returning to field duty. Only 7% were sent home to the United States (Thayer, 1919). Meta Anderson, one of the

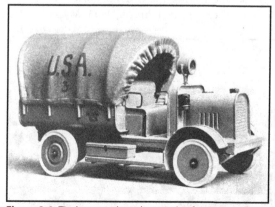

Figure 3-9. Tin Army truck made entirely of tin cans.

reconstruction aides assigned to Base Hospital No. 117, described the activities at the workshop as follows:

The workshop was considered a sort of specialized therapy directed to a more definite end, planned to treat some definite symptom or to meet some special indication, while the other work was regarded as a kind of therapeutic background underlying the whole scheme of curative effort. The physiological and psychological needs were met by the use of muscular effort in the production of tangible articles. The handling of the tools and the various movements of sawing, nailing, screwing, and hammering, and the finer and more coordinated movements of wood carving, metal work of various kinds, weaving, and tinning as well as much more delicate and more emotionally inspired technique of painting, sketching, and printing, supplied the essential training that the paralysis, tremors, and other symptoms needed (McDaniel, 1968, p. 90).

Dr. Salmon sang the praises of occupational therapy. In August 1918, he sent a request for more occupational therapists, writing, "The Reconstruction Aides, especially those working in handicrafts, are worth their weight in gold" (McDaniel, 1968, p. 85; Myers, 1948). Dr. Salmon maintained his supportive relationship with the profession of occupational therapy after the war ended, frequently speaking at state and national association meetings. Sadly, occupational therapy lost a strong advocate when Dr. Thomas Salmon was lost in a sailing accident in 1927.

Orthopedic Services

In the summer of 1916, the orthopedic section of the American Medical Association (AMA) and the American Orthopedic Association (AOA) formed committees to study the preparedness of the United States to provide orthopedic services in the event of war. The committees were charged with determining the needs of orthopedic hospitals with regard to equipment and supplies as well as a plan to reconstruct or rehabilitate disabled soldiers (Lynch et al., 1923, p. 424). Both committees were chaired by Dr. Joel E. Goldthwait of Boston (Crane, 1927, p. 3; Goldthwait, 1917a; Orr, 1921, p. 12). Goldthwait was commissioned as a major in the Medical Reserve Corps of the United States Army in May 1917 and sent to Europe to study the provision of orthopedic services by the British Army (Crane, 1927, p. 4). His brother-in-law, Dr. Herbert J. Hall, provided occupational therapy services at Devereaux Mansion, a home that had belonged to the Goldthwait family for generations.

During World War I, the Canadian government was one of the first to accept responsibility for the reconstruction, rehabilitation, and re-education of disabled soldiers and sailors. Dr. Goldthwait was among the first in the United States to advocate for a similar commitment. In view of humanitarian and economic considerations, Goldthwait argued that it was important to provide not only acute medical care to save lives but also reconstruction services to help disabled soldiers and sailors lead productive lives again. Through reconstruction, injured soldiers and sailors might return to active military duty, or, if not able to return to active duty, reconstruction would enable disabled soldiers or sailors to learn new occupations and vocations. Rather than remaining dependent on others and deteriorating mentally, these injured soldiers and sailors could become productive citizens leading full lives.

Goldthwait asserted that providing occupation to disabled soldiers in curative workshops would help "lessen the monotomy" experienced during long periods in recovery and, if the occupation were carefully selected and graded, it would provide a "distinct benefit to the affected part" (Goldthwait, 1917b, p. 682). Goldthwait maintained that using an injured extremity in an occupation helps to "stimulate circulation and general tone"; for example, for a patient who has a stiff wrist, "the use of a carpenter's plane will necessitate the use of the fingers as well as the use of the wrist" (Goldthwait, 1917b, p. 683). Repeated strokes of the plane can encourage increased movement (Goldthwait, 1917b, p. 683). Dr. Goldthwait hand-selected the orthopedic surgeons for Base Hospital No. 9 in Chateauroux, France. Base Hospital No. 9 became the orthopedic center of the American Expeditionary Forces (Brown, 1920, p. 73). In August 1918, 13 reconstruction

aides in occupational therapy arrived to work at Base
Hospital No. 9 (Hoppin, 1933,
p. 51) (Figure 3-10).

Dr. Elliott Brackett agreed
that engagement in an occupation to prevent "mental
inertia" kept soldiers in a
better mental state for recovery and return to function
and that the physical benefit of mobilization of joints
and using muscles facilitated
return to function (Brackett,
1919, p. 163). Brackett recognized that special knowledge
was needed to provide carefully selected occupations
and specially adapted tools

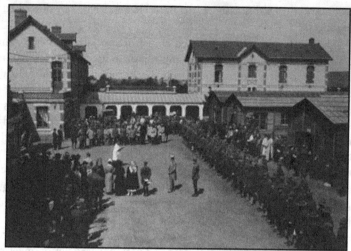

Figure 3-10. Fourth of July celebration on the grounds of Base Hospital No. 9 in Chateauroux, France.

for exercise that focused on making a tangible end product (Brackett, 1919). Brackett maintained that "the effect of a distinct occupation on these men, who are necessarily detained in medical institutions for protracted periods, sometimes for many months, is seen in the eagerness and in the quickness with which they take up their occupation after their discharge" (Brackett, 1919, p. 166).

Colonel Brackett started an occupational therapy program at Walter Reed General Hospital in February 1918 as an experiment. This experiment was designed as a model program to determine the standards for an occupational therapy shop and school. Major Bird T. Baldwin, a psychologist, was named the director. The goal of occupational therapy was to assist each patient with improving physical function, making him self-reliant and self-respecting and enabling him to work to contribute to society economically.

The Department of Occupational Therapy consisted of five sections: (1) an administrative sec-
tion, (2) a psychological and statistical section, (3) a general or academic section, (4) a technical section, and (5) a recreational section. The psychological section was responsible for completing evaluations on the patients. These evaluations consisted of interviews, surveys, psychologi-
cal tests, vocational surveys and tests, and measurements of movement. The technical section provided vocational training and craft activities, including "chair caning, cardboard construc-
tion work, woodwork, block printing, rush seating, brush making, bookbinding, modeling, rug making, stenciling, mop making, designing post cards, plasticine modeling, drawing, leather work, hand knitting, rake knitting, frame knitting, machine knitting, weaving, basketry, bead work, making colonial mats, netting, cord work, crocheting, and embroidery" (Baldwin, 1919b; Crane, 1927, pp. 91-97).

Baldwin was one of the first to advance the use of the biomechanical model in occupational therapy. When using the biomechanical model, treatment activities were selected based on spe-
cific, repetitive movements required by the activity—movements that would increase range of motion and strength. The activities were also selected based on one of the tenets of occupational therapy: engaging occupations, including play, activities of daily living, and work activities, are most effective to improve function. An advantage of using carefully selected activities was that "the patient's attention is repeatedly called to the particular remedial movements involved; at the same time the movements have the advantage of being initiated by the patient and of forming an

integral and necessary part of a larger and more complex series of motions," in contrast to passive mechano-therapy, which usually focused on individual movements (Baldwin, 1919a, p. 5). Baldwin developed an apparatus to measure joint range of motion (now known as a goniometer). This apparatus was modified to measure motion of various joints. Measurements were taken at regular intervals to record progress and to document the effectiveness of occupational therapy. By monitoring these regular assessments, patients were provided with hope and motivation for recovery (Baldwin, 1919a, pp. 11-15).

A school was started at Walter Reed in 1918 to train the reconstruction aides in occupational therapy. The curriculum included lectures and practical experience under the supervision of more experienced aides. The school's existence was short lived. First, the planned start of the school was delayed by the influenza epidemic. Then, the school was discontinued in late 1918 when the armistice was signed (Baldwin, 1919b). Still, many of the aides who gained experience at Walter Reed went on to serve in general and base hospitals in Europe and United States.

Tuberculosis Care

Tuberculosis was a significant public health problem during World War I. Concerned about the spread of this infectious disease through the troops, the Medical Department of the Army set out to examine 1.2 million soldiers for the disease. By March 1918, they recommended the discharge of 9,600 diagnosed with tuberculosis. Of the 2 million men who were drafted for the service after the end of March 1918, 12,500 were found to have tuberculosis and were not accepted for service (Lynch et al., 1923, p. 373). From September 1917 through June 1919, there were 1,600 military deaths attributed to tuberculosis (Lynch et al., 1923, p. 377). By 1922, compensation was given to more than 36,000 World War I veterans who contracted tuberculosis while in the service (Drolet, 1945).

The Medical Department established nine special hospitals for soldiers with tuberculosis, selecting sites in areas where the climate was thought to be favorable for recovery (Crane, 1927, p. 192). Between December 1918 and April 1919, a total of 10,036 soldiers suffering from pulmonary tuberculosis were registered for educational work (including occupational therapy), second only to soldiers with orthopedic injuries, who numbered 17,062 (Crane, 1927, p. 261). Prior to World War I, occupational therapy was incorporated into treatment programs of a number of tuberculosis sanatoriums, such as Arequipa Sanatorium in California, which embraced Herbert J. Hall's work cure. The work of reconstruction aides in occupational therapy with soldiers with tuberculosis solidified the role of occupational therapy in treatment for patients with tuberculosis.

Patients with tuberculosis were classified by physical condition. Reconstruction aides in occupational therapy provided graded activities, under medical supervision, based on this classification. Class D patients had extensive inactive lesions and persistent temperatures above 99° and were confined to bed. These patients were provided with bedside handicrafts such as knitting, embroidery, crocheting, and raffia weaving. Class C patients had dyspnea, excessive coughing, and extensive inactive lesions and also participated in bedside handicrafts, although for longer periods of time. Class B patients with little evidence of active disease and participated in workshop activities and outdoor activities such as carpentry, wood carving, plumbing, gardening, and automobile repair. Class A patients had no evidence of active disease and participated in graded work activities to facilitate return to full work (Crane, 1927, pp. 189, 192-194).

RECRUITMENT OF RECONSTRUCTION AIDES IN OCCUPATIONAL THERAPY

Qualifications

Initially, the military sought candidates for reconstruction aides in occupational therapy with the following qualifications:

> Good teachers, knowledge and skill in the (specific) occupation to be taught, attractive, and forceful personality, teaching ability, sympathy, tact, judgment, [and] industry." By June 1918, hospital training was required. Additionally, candidates needed to be United States citizens, 25-40 years of age, 60-70 inches in height, between 100 and 195 pounds, and have the ability to pass the Army Nurse Corps physical exam. (Haggerty, 1918; McDaniel, 1968, p. 72) (Exceptions to the age range were made on occasion.)

Both single and married women were eligible to apply; however, if appointed, married women were primarily assigned in the United States. By August 1918, to ensure higher standards and competence, graduation from a secondary school was required. Applicants who graduated from normal school or college with comparable technical training were given preference (Haggerty, 1918; McDaniel, 1968, p. 72).

Classification and Salaries

Reconstruction aides in occupational therapy were selected by the Surgeon General's Office and issued a letter of appointment. Generally, appointments were made for the duration of the war. The reconstruction aides were considered civilian employees and had no military status. There were two classes of occupational therapy aides: those working with patients with orthopedic injuries and those working with patients with war neuroses. The starting salary was $50 per month for regular aides and $65 per month for head aides. Overseas duty warranted an additional $10 per month. Reconstruction aides were provided with meals, lodging, and laundry. An allowance of $62.50 per month was allowed if meal, lodging, or laundry was not available. Travel allowances were also provided (Haggerty, 1918; McDaniel, 1968, p. 72).

Uniforms

Reconstruction aides were required to have a street uniform and a hospital uniform. The Red Cross supplied uniforms to those reconstruction aides who were going overseas (Figure 3-11). The street uniform was a dark gray Norfolk suit with a dark brimmed hat. The hospital uniform was a belted blue chambray dress with detachable white collars and cuffs covered by a white butcher's apron (Figures 3-12 to 3-14). The uniform was often described by reconstruction aides as less than attractive. Reconstruction aide Lena Hitchcock opined that "some misguided male in the Surgeon General's office designed our hideous street uniforms" (Hitchcock, n.d., p. VIII).

```
                        WAR DEPARTMENT
                   Office of The Surgeon General
                          Washington

              INSTRUCTIONS FOR RECONSTRUCTION AIDES

                       OVERSEAS SERVICE.

      Immediately on reporting in New York City, Reconstruction Aides
   should go to the Representative of Nursing of the Red Cross at 44 East
   23rd Street and present their travel orders as a means of identification.

      The following equipment will be supplied by the Red Cross, without
   coat, to each aide.  Any article in List A which the aide may have purchased
   elsewhere, in advance, will be deducted and no allowance will be made for
   such deductions.

                           LIST A.

            TO BE PROVIDED BY RED CROSS TO RECONSTRUCTION AIDES
            WITH MILITARY ESTABLISHMENTS FOR "OVERSEAS SERVICE".

         1   Pr. Gloves                              $1.25
         1   Souwester                                1.20
         1   Rain Coat                                7.65
         1   Pr. Rubber Boots                         2.65
         1   Gray Sweater                             4.25
         2   Prs. Woolen Tights                       5.00
         3   Prs. Outing Flannel Pajamas              7.50
         4   Suits Woolen Underwear                  10.00
         ½   Doz. Merino Stockings                    3.00
         ⅝   Doz. Cotton Stockings                    1.80
         3   Prs. Shoes (1 Black; 2 tan)             27.00
         3   Blue Chambray Uniforms                  15.00
        12   Sets Collars and Cuffs                   3.84
         2   Prs. Cuff Links                           .75
         4   Caps                                      .44
         1   Blanket (steamer)                        7.00
         1   Sleeping Bag                             9.00
         1   Hold-All                                 3.85
                                                   $111.18

      All street uniforms must be purchased by the aides from the Red Cross,
   who will supply articles mentioned in List B at cost.

                           LIST B.

              TO BE PROVIDED BY RECONSTRUCTION AIDE.

         1   Norfolk Suit                           $32.50
         1   Black Velour Hat                         2.50
         1   Black Straw Hat                          2.50
         2   Shirt Waists, White-Wash                 4.20
         1   Flannel or Silk Waist                    5.00
         1   Ulster                                  30.00
             Metal "R.A." one half inch in height     .50
                                                    $77.20

         1   Cape (optional).
```

Figure 3-11. Instructions for reconstruction aides—overseas service re: obtaining required clothing. (Printed with permission from the Archive of the American Occupational Therapy Association, Inc.)

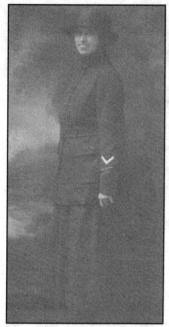

Figure 3-12. Reconstruction aide in occupational therapy Mildred Pierce in a street uniform. (Printed with permission from the Archive of the American Occupational Therapy Association, Inc.)

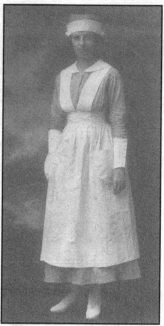

Figure 3-13. Reconstruction aide in occupational therapy Mildred Pierce in a hospital uniform. (Printed with permission from the Archive of the American Occupational Therapy Association, Inc.)

EXPERIENCES OF RECONSTRUCTION AIDES IN OCCUPATIONAL THERAPY

Reconstruction aides came from many different areas of the country and had a variety of experiences and backgrounds. Whereas some reconstruction aides had experience in health care and/or craftwork, some were just out for the adventure of traveling and working in a new profession. Reconstruction aides were assigned to general hospitals (Figure 3-15, Sidebar 3-4) in the United States and to base hospitals in Europe (Figure 3-16, Sidebar 3-5). Initially, reconstruction aides were not well received at military hospitals because the nature of the work was not understood or appreciated. Further, it was believed that the presence of these women would be disruptive. This was quickly debunked as the reconstruction aides proved their worth (Crane, 1927, p. 81). The worldwide influenza pandemic of 1918 resulted in a significant number of civilian and military deaths. The influenza outbreaks and other illnesses often required reconstruction aides to work as nursing assistants, caring for the sick rather than providing therapeutic activities (Crane, 1927, p. 64). Reconstruction aides at Base Hospital No. 8 in Savenay, France, were often assigned to make plaster bandages and gauze dressings for the injured soldiers (Crane, 1927, p. 72).

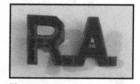

Figure 3-14. A reconstruction aide pin that belonged to Winifred Brainerd, OTR. (Copyright © Dr. Lori T. Andersen.)

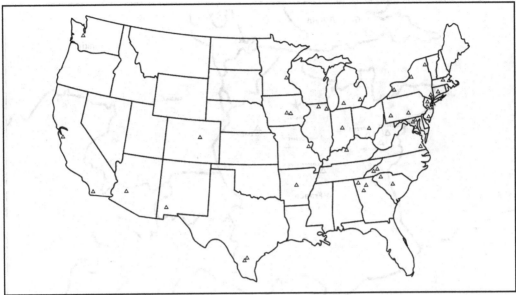

Figure 3-15. Selected general, base, camp, and other hospitals in the US where reconstruction aides worked.

SIDEBAR 3-4

Selected General, Base, Camp, and Other Hospitals in the US

Atlanta, GA - Camp Gordon

Atlanta, GA - Fort McPherson, General Hospital No. 6

Ayers, MA - Camp Devens

Baltimore, MD - Evergreen – Roland Park, General Hospital No. 7

Baltimore, MD - Fort McHenry, General Hospital No. 2

Bayard Station, NM - Fort Bayard

Bergen County, NJ - Camp Merritt

Biltmore, NC - General Hospital No. 12

Boston, MA - Parker Hill, General Hospital No. 10

Buffalo, NY - Fort Porter

Cape May NJ - General Hospital No. 11

Carlisle, PA - Carlisle Barracks

Chicago IL - Fort Sheridan, General Hospital No. 28

Chillicothe, OH - Camp Sherman

Columbia, SC - Camp Jackson

Denver, CO - Fitzsimmons General Hospital, General Hospital No. 21

Des Moines, IA - Camp Dodge

Des Moines, IA - Fort Des Moines, General Hospital No. 26

Detroit, MI - Ford Hospital, General Hospital No. 36

Fort Oglethorpe, GA - General Hospital No. 14

Hampton, VA - General Hospital No. 43, Debarkation Hospital No. 51

Indianapolis, IN - Fort Benjamin Harrison, General Hospital No. 25

Kalamazoo, MI - Camp Custer

Lakewood, NJ - General Hospital No. 9

Little Rock, AR - Camp Pike

Louisville, KY - Camp Zachary Taylor

New Haven, CT - General Hospital No. 16

Oswego, NY - Fort Ontario, General Hospital No. 5

Oteen, NC - General Hospital No. 19

Pierce County, WA - Camp Lewis

Pittsburgh, PA - Parkview Station, General Hospital No. 24

Plattsburg, NY - Plattsburgh Barracks, General Hospital No. 30

Pocantico Hills, NY – Eastview, General Hospital No. 38

Prescott, AZ - Whipple Barracks, General Hospital No. 20

Rahway, NJ – Colonia, General Hospital No. 3

Rockford, IL - Camp Grant

San Diego County, CA - Camp Kearney

San Antonio, TX - Camp Travis

San Antonio, TX - Fort Sam Houston, General Hospital No. 1

San Francisco, CA - Letterman General Hospital, at the Presidio

Spartanburg, SC - Camp Wadsworth, General Hospital No. 42

St. Louis MO - Jefferson Barracks, General Hospital No. 40

St. Paul, MN - Fort Snelling, General Hospital No. 29

Staten Island, NY - Fox Hills, General Hospital No. 41

Suffolk County, NY - Camp Upton

Washington, DC - Walter Reed General Hospital

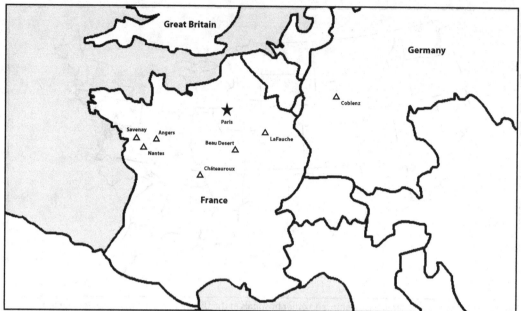

Figure 3-16. Selected base, camp and evacuation hospitals in Europe where reconstruction aides worked.

SIDEBAR 3-5

Selected Base, Camp, and Evacuation Hospitals in Europe

Angers, France - Base Hospital No. 85	Chateauroux, France - Base Hospital No. 9
LaFauche France (Neuropsychiatric Service) - Base Hospital No. 117	Savenay, France - Base Hospitals No. 8, No. 69, No. 88
Beau Desert, France - Base Hospitals No. 14, No. 114, No. 121	Coblenz, Germany - Evacuation Hospitals No. 16, No. 27
Nantes, France - Evacuation Hospital No. 31	Savenay, France (Neuropsychiatric Service) - Base Hospital No. 214

The reconstruction aides who went overseas with the American Expeditionary Forces were often put in harm's way. Two reconstruction aides in occupational therapy told of harrowing times traveling to France via Liverpool, England. Mrs. Clyde Myres' ship performed evasive zig-zag maneuvers toward the end of its transatlantic voyage to avoid being torpedoed by a submarine (Myers, 1948). Twenty-nine-year-old Lena Hitchcock sailed to Europe on the British ship *Walmer Castle*, fortunately surviving a submarine attack (Hoppin, 1933, p. 51) (Figure 3-17, Figure 3-18).

Eva McLagan (Mrs. Burrell B. Mink) of Drain, Oregon, a reconstruction aide in physiotherapy who was assigned to a base hospital in France, described the devastation of war:

> The work of salvaging was not yet complete, and to unaccustomed eyes, the desolation was almost unbelievable. Where graveyards had been blown up by explosives, human bones, partly clothed in some instances, were lying about, and the earth pock-marked by a mass of deep shell holes. Heaps of barbed-wire entanglements, wrecked tanks, piles of scrapped war machinery were in evidence, and as we followed along the line of advance, piles of bricks marked the places where houses had been. (Hoppin, 1933, p. 70)

Space was limited in hospital facilities, so the occupational therapy rooms and curative workshops were often confined to corners of small rooms. These areas were often converted to hospital rooms when convoys of injured soldiers arrived. Limited equipment and supplies required

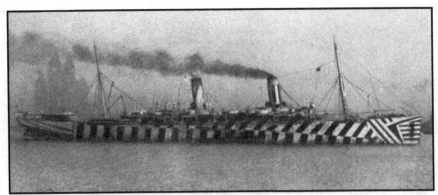

Figure 3-17. The *Walmer Castle*, the British ship that reconstruction aide Lena Hitchcock sailed on, was one of the dazzle ships painted with a geometric pattern as a camouflage. This camouflage made it difficult for German warships to determine the speed and direction of these dazzle ships.

reconstruction aides to be resourceful in finding materials, at times using personal funds to purchase supplies. Stationed at Base Hospital No. 9 in Chateauroux, France, Lena Hitchcock described the state of affairs there:

> We were sent to Base 9, Chateauroux, where we were not at first wanted …. At first we did nothing but Nurses' Aide duty, gradually working in as O.T.s, salvaging tin, wood (cigar boxes), old linen (which we dyed), and other materials from the dump heap. Our community box containing tools and materials had disappeared in transit. I had taken wood tools, leather tools, nut picks, and a small bead and bed loom in my trunk. These tools we copied in the blacksmith shop, begged others from the Engineers and Aviation Camp nearby, and out of our own pockets bought the necessary things and materials. (Hoppin, 1933, p. 51) (Figure 3-19)

Hitchcock reported that although initially scorned, the reconstruction aides soon gained the respect of the military (Figures 3-20 to 3-23):

> We never received any money for materials from the Government the entire time my group worked overseas yet the work turned out in spite of obstacles, was of a very high order, and on the strength of the good achieved by this small group of O.T.s, curatively and by way of morale—after an inspection by the Chief Surgeon of the A.E.F., General Ireland, Dr. Goldthwait was permitted to cable home for additional aides. (Hoppin, 1933, p. 51)

Ward work included knitting, simple weaving, block printing, bead work, wood carving, leatherwork, embroidery, plaques, tiles, worsted and raffia work on canvas, and beading. Shop work included tin work, brass work, and wood carving. Proceeds from the sale of products were often used to buy more supplies. Initially confined to ward work, reconstruction aides were gradually allowed to run classes in the curative workshops. Given one free afternoon each week, the reconstruction aides often spent this time shopping for the patients in the nearby village of Chateauroux. Sunday was a day of rest for all (Crane, 1927, p. 68-69).

The spirit, sense of adventure, and humor of these pioneers in occupational therapy are evident in a number of accounts given by reconstruction aides (Carlova & Ruggles, 1961; Hoppin, 1933). Ora Ruggles, a reconstruction aide in occupational therapy, credits her pioneering spirit to her parents, who settled in western Nebraska in the late 1800s (p. 14). Ora was recruited to serve as a reconstruction aide and was assigned to Fort McPherson in Georgia, where she worked with soldiers with tuberculosis and those who had undergone amputations. Her arrival at Fort McPherson was met with resistance by doctors and officers, who believed that she would not be able to do any good for the soldiers (p. 51). Undeterred, Ora set about developing an occupational therapy program but soon ran into

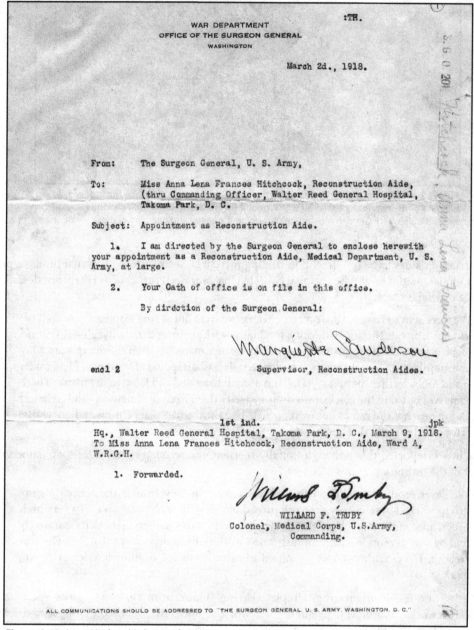

Figure 3-18. Lena Hitchcock's letter of appointment as a reconstruction aide. The letter is signed by Marguerite Sanderson, Supervisor of Reconstruction Aides. Miss Sanderson, a physical therapist, was a former employee of Dr. Joel Goldthwait. (OHA 97: Angier and Hitchcock Collection. Otis Historical Archives, National Museum of Health and Medicine.)

another roadblock: a lack of crafts supplies. Determined, resourceful, and rebellious, she worked around Army red tape to find a source for the supplies (p. 54).

Frances Lafaye Locke of Fort Lyon, Colorado, described the camaraderie among the aides and the hardships they endured:

> Sent to Camp Travis, January 15, 1919 …. We lived in a long dormitory and none of us got much sleep. There was always someone coming in and we all got up to listen to their experiences …. It was an adventure. We never thought that getting up before

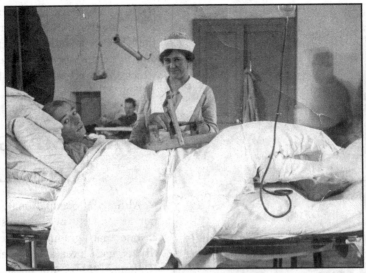

Figure 3-19. Reconstruction aide Lena Hitchcock providing bedside occupation therapy to a soldier at Base Hospital No. 9 in Chateauroux, France. The soldier, having lost his right arm in battle, is using a one-handed loom. (OHA 97: Angier and Hitchcock Collection. Otis Historical Archives, National Museum of Health and Medicine.)

daylight in a cold room, your shoes so damp that they were hard to get on, and poor food were hardships. (Hoppin, 1933, p. 63)

Eunice M. Cates of Aspinwall, Pennsylvania, spoke humorously of her dedication to her work:

On my tombstone (if one should be erected in my memory) I expect the inscription to read something like this: 'Eunice M. Cates, Faithful Unto Death—A Re-Aide O.T.,' while, instead of the symbolic cross and crown, the angel will hold in one hand a leather pocketbook, a reed tray or a pair of book ends, perhaps, in the other—'Form 1216.' (Hoppin, 1933, p. 24)

The reference to Form 1216, a change of address form, is apparently a reference to her many moves while in service. This humorous request was not fulfilled; Eunice M. Cates' tombstone only includes her name, year of birth, and year of death.

Marie E. Ryan (Mrs. Meredith B. Murray) of River Forest, Illinois, also spoke of numerous relocations while serving, some due to the closing of hospitals as patients were discharged:

Entered the Army March 15, 1919 …. Ordered to Ft. Oglethorpe; helped to organize school there. Hospital closed in June. Ordered to Parker Hill, as Head Aide; found it closed and after a skirmish trying to get straightened out ordered to Plattsburg Barracks to stay until it closed in September. Then to Colonia for a brief six week; off again when it closed to Fort Bayard where I had charge of Ward and School academic work. Stayed until it was taken over by P. H. in June 1920…. (Hoppin, 1933, p. 88)

Helen Bradley, a reconstruction aide in physical therapy from Kansas City, Missouri, shed some light on how reconstruction aides in occupational therapy were regarded. She traveled with a group of reconstruction aides in physical therapy to Fort Sam Houston in San Antonio, Texas:

It was only after they got to the old Army post that the high pitch of their enthusiasm was dropped and then not for long. No one from the C.O. to the Chief Nurse had expected them. One good looking young lieutenant said he'd heard of them—that they taught the boys to make little baskets. And that idea was so fixed in the doctors' minds that they were most disappointed, and felt that these PT girls should at least

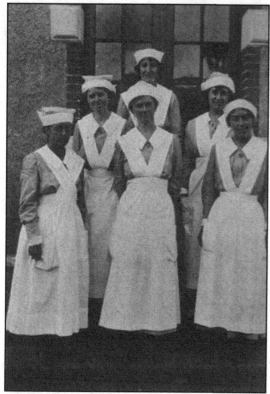

Figure 3-20. Reconstruction aides in occupational therapy at Base Hospital No. 9, Chateauroux, France. Pictured from left to right are Louise L. Green, Hope Gray, Susan Hills (center), Elizabeth Melcer, Lena Hitchcock, and Daphne Dunbar.

try to do OT work. It was some time before the first of the OTs arrived and the PTs were awfully glad to see them and to help share the problems with which they were confronted (Hoppin, 1933, p. 17).

WAR EMERGENCY SCHOOLS

Although occupational therapy was not an entirely new profession, but rather one that "gradually developed by justifying itself over a long period of years" (Upham, 1918, p. 48), no standard qualifications for people providing occupational therapy nor standards for length or content of courses had been set. The Chicago School of Civics and Philanthropy, the Henry B. Favill School, the program at Teachers College of Columbia University, and the school at Sheppard and Enoch Pratt were a few of the programs and schools offering training for occupational workers. At the inaugural meeting of NSPOT, the founders decided that membership would be restricted to those with certain qualifications and knowledge to ensure a therapeutic focus. To this end, a teaching committee was appointed to establish standards for education and training; however, the war broke out prior to completion of their charge.

After the Surgeon General's Office called for reconstruction aides in occupational therapy, several war emergency courses were established. The call for these aides offered an opportunity for a number of schools and programs to develop programs and enroll students. However, with the lack of set standards, there was no quality control on the training. To seek legitimacy in enrolling students, many of these schools and programs sought the approval of the Surgeon General's Office (Russell, 1918). The Surgeon General's Office initially approved the program at Teachers College, Columbia University, directed by Susan Cox Johnson; the Boston School of Occupational Therapy, directed by Mrs. Joel Goldthwait; the War Services Classes in New York City, directed by Mrs. Howard Mansfield (Figure 3-24); and the program at Walter Reed Hospital

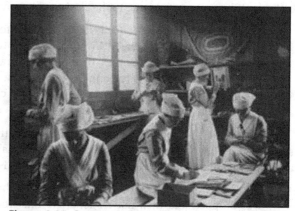

Figure 3-21. Reconstruction aides making preparations in the occupational therapy workshop at Base Hospital No. 9, Chateauroux, France.

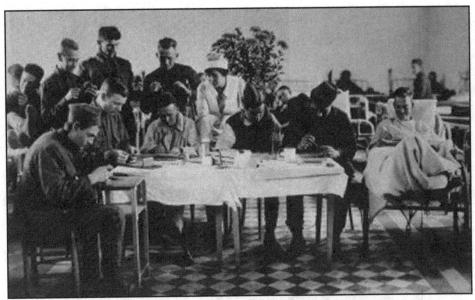

Figure 3-22. Class in occupational therapy at Base Hospital No. 9 in Chateauroux, France.

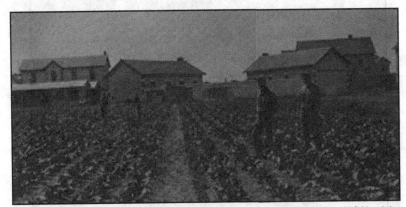

Figure 3-23. Occupational therapy in the hospital garden at Base Hospital No. 9 in Chateauroux, France.

(Crane, 1927, p. 59; McDaniel, 1968, p. 76). In January 1918, the Surgeon General's Office offered guidance for the development of a curriculum to train reconstruction aides in occupational therapy. The suggested curriculum described a basic 10-week course that included 310 hours in craft work, including weaving, wood carving, woodworking, basketry, bookbinding, and leatherwork. By September 1918, the Surgeon General's Office recognized that the suggested curriculum needed to be expanded to include more time and course work in medical disorders, hospital practice, and theory to ensure that reconstruction aides in occupational therapy had the knowledge and skills to work with injured and ill soldiers (McDaniel, 1968, pp. 75-76).

In April 1918, James E. Russell, the Dean of Teachers College, Columbia University, was named as head of the Education Section in the Division of Physical Reconstruction (Crane, 1927, p. 45). One of the first tasks he encountered was handling the large number of requests for approval of war emergency curricula for reconstruction aides in occupational therapy. With a lack of staff to review such requests and no solid information about training/educational standards and standard qualifications, he suspended the Surgeon General's Office involvement in any recognition or

Bulletin No. 1: EXCERPTS, PRINTED IN NEW YORK CITY, APRIL 27, 1918

TRAINING CLASSES FOR RECONSTRUCTION AIDES IN
OCCUPATIONAL THERAPY FOR MILITARY
HOSPITALS

A circular of information dated March 27, 1918, and issued by the Medical Department, United States Army, says: "There is immediate need in our Military Hospitals for trained women to furnish forms of occupation to convalescents and to give patients the therapeutic value of activity. This will be particularly essential in the case of the disabled soldier."

It is with these needs in mind and with the approval of the Surgeon General, United States Army, that arrangements are being completed to establish here on or about June 1st, special classes for the training of Reconstruction Aides in Occupational Therapy.

There is a distinct field for this work, and it is the purpose in these special classes to study the problem and develop it under the ablest of instructors, so that those who graduate will not only have a practical understanding of what may be made in hospital wards that is worth making and has material as well as therapeutic value, but will be prepared to cooperate intelligently with the hospital authorities in restoring the patients to health and activity.

The handicrafts approved by the Surgeon General's office include

    Hand Weaving
    Basketry
    Block Printing
    Simple Wood Carving
    Book Binding
    Toymaking
    Modeling - suitable to bedside work
    Handwork
    Design

Practice teaching in hospitals will be an essential part of the course.

The importance of the work is obvious, and the qualifications demanded for the service are of a high order. It offers very special opportunities to women skilled in Crafts who possess these qualifications and who desire to serve their country. It also offers a fine opportunity to women as yet untrained to make themselves efficient either as volunteers or as professionals in a work for which the medical profession predicts a growing demand long after the war is over.

Two courses for intensive training will be immediately organized. The short course, from eight to ten weeks, will be for those skilled in one or more of the Crafts, and

presupposes a knowledge of design and color. The longer course will be for those who are untrained and will last from twelve to fifteen weeks according to individual requirements.

The Classes will be limited in number: the chief object in establishing them is to graduate well-equipped Aides.

It is very necessary, therefore, that all who register for training should realize the importance of taking sufficient time to prepare themselves adequately for their work.

COMMITTEE ON ORGANIZATION

Mrs Howard Mansfield, Director
Mrs Cornelius J Sullivan, Assistant Director

Mrs Ripley Hitchcock
Miss Anna Maxwell
Mrs John D Rockefeller Jr
Mrs Charles Sprague Smith
Mrs Ripley Weisse

Miss Maude M Mason
Mrs Grayson M P Murphy
Mrs James C Rogerson
Mrs Willard Straight

Affiliated Committee on Arts and Handicrafts

Mrs Hitchcock   Chairman
Miss Mason   Secretary

Figure 3-24. Draft of a bulletin recruiting students for Mrs. Howard Mansfield's war emergency course. (Printed with permission from the Archive of the American Occupational Therapy Association, Inc.)

certifications. He appealed to the National Society for the Promotion of Occupational Therapy to develop standards for training schools to assist the Surgeon General's Office in finding qualified candidates (Russell, 1918).

WAR EMERGENCY COURSES AND PIONEER SCHOOLS

Many of the war emergency courses and early pioneer schools had short lives. The schools that survived the early years and later became accredited schools include the Boston School of Occupational Therapy, the school at Milwaukee-Downer College, the St. Louis School of Occupational Therapy, and the Philadelphia School of Occupational Therapy.

Boston School of Occupational Therapy

In 1918, General Gorgas, in consultation with Colonel Elliott G. Brackett, formed a committee to set up a training school for reconstruction aides in occupational therapy. Notable members of the committee included Herbert J. Hall; Mrs. Joel Goldthwait, wife of Dr. Joel E. Goldthwait and sister-in-law of Herbert Hall; and Miss Minnie Brackett, Dr. Elliott Brackett's sister. The committee established the Boston School of Occupational Therapy and became the first board of trustees. Mrs. Joel Goldthwait served as chairperson of the school (McDaniel, 1968, p. 76). The committee developed a 12-week curriculum that included "training in simple crafts and lectures on hospital procedure," in spite of the Army's desire for a shorter 8-week curriculum to quickly meet the urgent need (Robinson, 1943, p. 2). All 123 women who completed the program served in a military hospital. Open for about 12 months, the school closed its doors when the war ended and the emergency was over (Robinson, 1943, pp. 1-2) (Figure 3-25).

Recognizing the benefit of occupational therapy and the civilian population's need for occupational therapy services, the school was reopened in the fall of 1919 with Miss Ruth Wigglesworth and Mrs. John (Marjorie) Greene as directors. When Miss Wigglesworth left in 1924 to get married, Mrs. Greene, secretary of the original Boston School of Occupational Therapy, became the sole director. The curriculum was expanded to 12 months, including 3 months of practical work experience

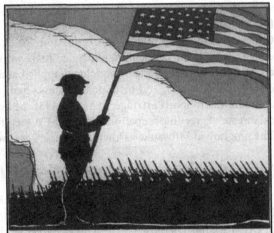

"*In the Service of the Flag*"

BOSTON SCHOOL OF OCCUPATIONAL THERAPY

CERTIFIED BY
SURGEON GENERAL, U. S. A.

FOR THE PURPOSE OF TRAINING WOMEN TO BECOME APPLICANTS AS RECONSTRUCTION AIDES IN OCCUPATIONAL THERAPY FOR MILITARY HOSPITALS

A FULL-TIME INTENSIVE DAY COURSE FOR WOMEN; TWELVE WEEKS LONG; COMMENCING ABOUT APRIL 22, 1918
HOURS, 8.30 A.M. TO 4.30 P.M. FIVE DAYS A WEEK; 8.30 A.M. TO 12 M. ON SATURDAYS

CONDUCTED AT
FRANKLIN UNION
BERKELEY AND APPLETON STREETS

Figure 3-25. Boston School of Occupational Therapy recruitment poster. (Printed with permission from the Archive of the American Occupational Therapy Association, Inc.)

under supervision to more fully prepare graduates. The first 9 months were dedicated to medical, social science, and craft work. Anatomy, kinesiology, physiology, psychology, social service lectures, and instruction in a number of crafts were included in the curriculum. Students learned about principles and theories of occupational therapy, ethics, and record keeping. Practical work consisted of experiences in settlement houses, psychopathic hospitals, tuberculosis hospitals, general hospitals and district work. In particular, the work in settlement houses was deemed important for students "to learn of the actual home and community life, habits, and traditions of the various nationalities that make up America" (Greene & Wigglesworth, 1921, p. 568; Robinson, 1943). The Boston School of Occupational Therapy is now part of Tufts University.

Milwaukee-Downer College

In September 1918, at the urging of Elizabeth Greene Upham Davis, Milwaukee-Downer College opened an 18-week war emergency course in occupational therapy with Charlotte Partridge as director. Hilda Goodman from Canada was hired to run the fieldwork program. The students learned about design and crafts, in addition to having a number of prominent physicians and specialists provide medical lectures. One-half day per week was spent observing practical application of occupational therapy concepts in a general hospital setting. Recognizing the need for occupational therapy beyond reconstruction of soldiers and sailors, Milwaukee-Downer College continued to offer a course of study in occupational therapy after the war emergency ended. In 1921, the curriculum expanded to 32 weeks at the graduate level, plus a 12-week affiliation. Coursework included physiology (applied anatomy, kinesiology, medical lectures on heart disease, tuberculosis, and orthopedics), abnormal psychology, and occupational therapy theory and administration (Partridge, 1921). In 1931, Milwaukee-Downer College offered the first baccalaureate degree in occupational therapy ("A step forward in the education," 1931; Jones, 1988). The program at Milwaukee-Downer College was discontinued in 1972.

St. Louis School of Occupational Therapy

First known as the St. Louis Training School for Reconstruction Aides, the St. Louis School of Occupational Therapy started in December 1918 under the direction of the Missouri Association of Occupational Therapy. The St. Louis chapter of the Junior League, an organization of socially connected young women, donated $5,000 to help start the school (Medicine in St. Louis Hospital, 1919, p. 3). Initially, Dr. G. Canby Robinson, who was Dean of Washington University School of Medicine, and Mrs. Elias Michael (nee Rachel Stix), chairperson of the instruction committee of the St. Louis Women's Committee of the Council of National Defense, assisted in organizing a board of trustees for the occupational therapy school. The committee requested Eleanor Clarke Slagle to review the school plans and curriculum they had developed. Slagle visited the school on November 7, 1918, approved the plans and curriculum, and recommended a director for the school: Alice H. Dean, a graduate of the Henry B. Favill School.

In spite of the fact that the armistice ending World War I was signed 4 days later on November 11, 1918, the group continued with plans to open the school, believing that the need for occupational therapy would continue. The school was renamed St. Louis School of Occupational Therapy in early December 1918, shortly after the first class started. The curriculum "consisted of 40 hours of lectures in medical and socio-vocational topics, nine weeks of hospital practice, and nine weeks of craft classes" ("Occupational therapy in St. Louis," 2009). Starting in June 1919, the school was directed by the Missouri Association of Occupational Therapy. In September 1920, program length increased to 6 months, followed by 3 months of hospital work (Kidder, 1921; Missouri Association for Occupational Therapy, 1923; Occupational therapy in St. Louis, 2009). The St. Louis School of Occupational Therapy is now part of Washington University School of Medicine in St. Louis (Figure 3-26).

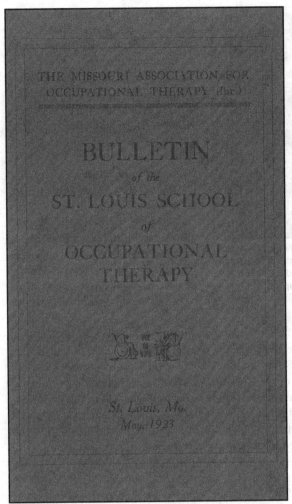

Figure 3-26. St. Louis School brochure, 1923. (Copyright © Dr. Lori T. Andersen. Reprinted with permission.)

Philadelphia School of Occupational Therapy

The Philadelphia School of Occupational Therapy opened in the spring of 1918 to educate women for service as reconstruction aides through intensive coursework (Quiroga, 1995, p. 82). In 1921, the school expanded the length of the curriculum, offering a 9-month course in occupational therapy, with Florence Wellsman Fulton serving as the chairperson. Seven months were spent on campus attending lectures in anatomy, kinesiology, and personal and social hygiene. Students also spent a considerable number of hours learning crafts such as weaving, reed basketry, wood construction, chair caning, pottery, block printing, and book binding. Two months of field experience in general and tuberculosis hospital settings and work with the Visiting Nurse Society followed (Fulton, 1921). For many years, the authors/editors of the well-known textbook *Principles of Occupational Therapy* (later editions were known as Willard and Spackman's *Occupational Therapy*) were mainstays of the school. Helen Willard was chairperson and Clare Spackman served on the faculty. Eventually the Philadelphia School became part of the University of Pennsylvania. The school was discontinued in 1981.

ARMISTICE: NOVEMBER 11, 1918

The process to mobilize for war was far from complete but well under way when the Armistice, signaling the end of World War I, was signed on November 11, 1918. Prior to the Armistice, few reconstruction aides were needed in the United States because disabled soldiers and sailors were not yet returning home in large numbers. With the Armistice, anticipating that wounded and ill servicemen would now be returning home, the Medical Department of the Army shifted focus to ensure general hospitals and camp hospitals in the United States were prepared to receive and care for these men. Reconstruction aides began to return from Europe (Crane, 1927, p. 54). At the beginning of 1919, there were 1,700 soldiers receiving services under the Bureau of War Risk Insurance. By the end of the year, 50,000 soldiers had been discharged from military service due to neuropsychological disorders and another 24,500 due to tuberculosis. With the Armistice and the change in priorities, the Army set in motion the plan for continued medical care and reconstruction services to accommodate the influx of returning soldiers. This included setting up general and base hospitals in the United States (Crane, 1927, p. 249).

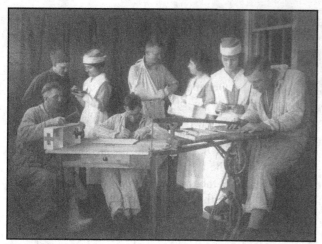

Figure 3-27. Reconstruction aides in occupational therapy in uniform at Camp Grant, Rockford, Illinois, in April 1919. From left to right are Carolyn Bean, Otilla Koehler, and Jeannette Moody. (Printed with permission from the Archive of the American Occupational Therapy Association, Inc.)

Ideally, soldiers and sailors were to be sent to general hospitals or camps closest to their homes. Some of the hospitals were general in nature, providing services for varied diagnoses. Other hospitals and camps provided specialized services for those with speech defects, hearing disorders, blindness, and tuberculosis. Mrs. T. Harrison Garrett offered her estate Evergreen in Roland Park, Maryland, to the government. United States General Hospital No. 7 in Roland Park provided rehabilitation for soldiers who were blinded (Zimmerman, 1918). Other general hospitals such as Fort Bayard (Bayard Station) in New Mexico provided care for those with tuberculosis (Crane, 1927, p. 7) (Figures 3-27 and 3-28).

Initially, the Medical Department's projected need for reconstruction aides was significant; they anticipated the need for 1,000 in 1918 and another 4,000 within the next year (Russell, 1918, p. 115). This changed with the signing of the Armistice. Just as the war effort had gradually ramped up in 1917, in 1919 it began to ramp down. Instead of being sent overseas to work with the American Expeditionary Forces, reconstruction aides were assigned to work in general hospitals in the United States. Reconstruction aides returning from Europe went to general hospitals in the United States or, if requested, were discharged from military service.

Although the exact number of reconstruction aides in occupational therapy who served is not known, various reports from World War I give an indication of the numbers. Mrs. Eleanor R. Wembridge, working in the Surgeon General's Office as the supervisor of reconstruction aides in occupational therapy, reported that on January 1, 1919, there were 455 reconstruction aides. Of this number, 358 were serving in the United States and 97 were serving with the American Expeditionary Forces (McDaniel, 1968, p. 91). At the end of February 1919, 22 occupational therapy aides were serving in various base hospitals in France, including Angers, Nantes, and Savenay (Crane, 1927, p. 66). On April 30, 1919, there were a total of 1,070 reconstruction aides serving (Billings, 1920, p. 9), and by July 1919, there were more than 1,300 in service (Crane, 1927, p. 60).

Soldiers and sailors were discharged to general Army hospitals and from the military when they recovered or reached maximum functional gains. As the census in a hospital decreased, the hospital was closed. Many times when a hospital closed, reconstruction aides were relocated to a hospital that was still open. In March 1919, congressional action authorized transfer of

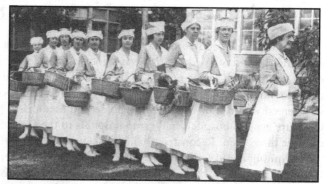

Figure 3-28. Reconstruction aides often used baskets to transport supplies to hospital wards and patient bedsides. It was a quiet way to transport supplies to the wards and helped maintain a quiet, comfortable environment for recovery. (Printed with permission from the Archive of the American Occupational Therapy Association, Inc.)

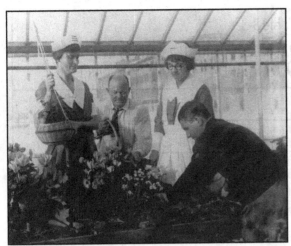

Figure 3-29. Helen Willard (holding basket) at Edward Hines Hospital in Maywood, Illinois, circa 1924. Edward Hines Hospital was first one of the United States Public Health Service hospitals, then part of the Veterans Bureau, and finally part of the Veterans Administration Hospital system. (Printed with permission from the Archive of the American Occupational Therapy Association, Inc.)

the general hospitals and medical activities of the Medical Department of the Army to the United States Public Health Service. On June 20, 1919, the Division of Physical Reconstruction in the Medical Department of the Army ceased to exist, and its functions were transferred to the Section on Physical Reconstruction in the Division of Hospitals in the United States Public Health Service (Crane, 1927, p. 50) (Figure 3-29).

In a time when few women worked outside the home, many reconstruction aides in occupational therapy continued in the workforce after World War I, some in the hospitals that the Medical Department of the Army had transferred to the United States Public Health Service. A number were discharged from military service to continue careers, start new careers, or get married and start families (Table 3-3; Figures 3-30 and 3-31).

United States Veterans Bureau Act of 1921 (Public Law 67-47) consolidated the benefits that veterans received from various federal agencies, including the War Risk Insurance Bureau, the United States Public Health Service, and the Federal Board of Vocational Education. With this change, reconstruction aides in occupational therapy, who first worked for the Medical Department of the United States Army and then for the United States Public Health Service, finally worked for the United States Veterans Bureau.

REFLECTION

The new profession of occupational therapy, beginning to flourish during the Progressive Era, was further propelled when the United States entered World War I. A spirit of patriotism swept the country. Many organizations were anxious to help with the war effort, including the new profession of occupational therapy. The founders reached out to the government to offer services, believing that participation in the war effort would promote the new profession.

The United States government, recognizing its social responsibility and the economic benefit to be gained from caring for soldiers disabled in war, passed legislation that provided for reconstruction services. Although at times it was a political battle, the Medical Department of the Army worked with a number of other government and private agencies to establish programs for the rehabilitation of those disabled in war. Several physicians, including Dr. Thomas Salmon, Dr. Joel Goldthwait, and Dr. Elliott Brackett, advocated for and successfully facilitated the inclusion of occupational therapy services in base hospitals in Europe and the United States. With this, occupational therapy's alignment with and sponsorship by the medical profession became solidified.

The Medical Department of the Army created a new category of civilian personnel called reconstruction aides in occupational therapy to provide rehabilitation services to injured and ill soldiers. Initially, because of gender issues, the Army was reluctant to hire women as reconstruction aides. Later, because of lack of manpower and the need to provide care, the Army accepted women in these positions, at least for the duration of the war. Initially rebuffed, the reconstruction aides working with the American Expeditionary Forces in Europe, as well as those working in general

Table 3-3

ACTIVITIES OF INDIVIDUAL RECONSTRUCTION AIDES IN OCCUPATIONAL THERAPY DURING AND AFTER WORLD WAR I

Mrs. Mary L. Abbey of Chicago, Illinois	"Served in Fort Sheridan…in the spring of 1923, went to Great Lakes' Naval Hospital where 607 ex-service men were hospitalized…"
Eleanor Abrams of New York City	"Walter Reed. Artist, illustrating covers for the Literary Digest. 'The Italian Garden,' 'Easter Lilies,' and 'Bermuda Garden' were some of the subjects."
Julia Standish Alexander of New York City	"Entered service October 11, 1918. Sailed for France on November 11, 1918. Stationed at Savenay, Base No. 8 and Base No. 88, and Mesves, Base No. 24. Sent to Army of Occupation, Coblenz, April 16, 1919. Stationed at Evacuation Hospital No. 26, Bad-Neuenahr, Germany. Sailed for U.S. on July 2, 1919. At Fort McHenry, resigned from service and received discharge October 28, 1919. Other positions since 1919: O.T. Dept., New York Neurological Institute, N.Y.C. Civil Service, Public Health Hospitals–Polyclinic and Marine, Head Aide."
Jennie K. Allen of Chicago, Illinois	"Carlisle and Camp Bouregard…in charge of O.T. Department at Cook County Hospital, the largest hospital in the world, and President of the Illinois Ass'n of Occupational Therapy."
Madeleine Ashley (Mrs. John Owen Carter) of Los Angeles, California	"Graduate of the Boston School of Occupational Therapy. Stints at Colonia, Camp Gordon, Fort McPherson, Fox Hills, Polyclinic Hospital (U.S. Public Health Service), U.S. Veteran's Hospital in Bronx, NY, U.S. Naval Hospital in Chelsea, MA … taught craft work for one year to sub-normal children in one of the Los Angeles Public Schools…[taught] chair caning and weaving in the State of California Industrial Work Shop for the Blind, in Los Angeles."
Carolyn Bean of Milwaukee, Wisconsin	"Camp Grant, 1919, and Fort Sheridan…in charge of special service work at Mendota State Hospital, Mendota, Wis." (see Figure 3-28).
Mildred Orr Beaton (Mrs. Calvin Hemingway Burks) of Charles City, Iowa	"First graduate, St. Louis School of Occupational Therapy. Camp Lee and Oteen."
Ethel Bowman of Baltimore, Maryland	"Walter Reed…Chief Aide in charge of O.T. Department…professor of psychology at Goucher College, Baltimore, Md."
Belva Cuzzort of Washington, DC	"Walter Reed, 1918; Fort Sheridan…first president of the National Association of Ex-Military Aides … 1920 to 1925."
Mabel Corinne Dezeller (Mrs. Henry M. Lucas) of Cleveland Heights, Ohio	"A.E.F., Base Hospitals 117 and 114, March 4, 1918, to June 1919; Fox Hills, June 1919 to June 1920."
Amy Drevenstedt of New York City	"Head Aide, Coblenz, 1919. Artist and illustrator. Her original greeting cards and illustrations are well known." (She also served at Base Hospital No. 117.)
Hope Gray of Boston, Massachusetts	"Appointed June 19, 1918. Base 9, Chateauroux, France, August 5, 1918, to February 1, 1919. Base 69, Savenay, France, February 1 to February 24, 1919. Base 114, Beau Desert, near Bordeaux, February 24 to May 11, 1919. Hampton, Va., May 24 to June 14, 1919. Honorable discharge about June 16, 1919" (see Figure 3-21).
Louise L. Green of Detroit, Michigan	"A.E.F., Base 9, Chateauroux. Head Aide, O.T., Base 8, Savenay, France" (see Figure 3-22).
Susan W. Hills of Newton Highlands, Massachusetts	"In 1921 was doing work in O.T. for Dr. Goldthwait of Boston." (O.T. Head Aide at Base Hospital No. 9 in Chateauroux, France [see Figure 3-21].)
Lena Hitchcock of Washington, DC	"Walter Reed…Base 9, Chateauroux…Base 114, Beau Desert, Bordeaux" (see Figures 3-16, 3-20, and 3-21).
Nellie Holland of Oak Park, Illinois	"Fort Sheridan, 1919 to December 31, 1920…Edward Hines Jr. Hospital, Hines, Ill., 1921. St. Louis School of O.T., 1924."

(continued)

Table 3-3 (continued) **ACTIVITIES OF INDIVIDUAL RECONSTRUCTION AIDES IN** **OCCUPATIONAL THERAPY DURING AND AFTER WORLD WAR I**	
Eugenia Hume of Atlanta, Georgia	"Oteen, 1918 to 1919. Established a department at Decatur, Ga., in the Masonic Home for Crippled Children."
Otilla Koehler of Davenport, Iowa	"Served at Camp Grant" (see Figure 3-28).
Geraldine Lermit of St. Louis, Missouri	In January 1917, enrolled in a 6-month Bedside Occupations course given at the American Red Cross training center. Assigned to Fort Porter, October 1918 to January 1919, then to Camp Pike. Worked for U.S. Public Health Service at General Hospital No. 4 in Chicago, then for the US Veterans Bureau Hospital No. 30 in St. Louis. "Director of the Missouri Association for Occupational Therapy and the St. Louis Training School of Occupational Therapy."
Gracia Loehl (Mrs. Gerald J. Maloney) of St. Peter, Minnesota	"Camp Devens...Fort McPherson...Fort Sam Houston...director of O.T. at Glen Lake Sanatorium, a T.B. institution near Minneapolis."
Jessie Luther of Providence, Rhode Island	"Chief Aide at Butler Hospital, Providence, R. I." (She previously worked with Dr. Herbert J. Hall at the Handcraft Shop in Marblehead, Massachusetts.)
Mary E. Merritt of Westfield, New Jersey	"A.E.F, fall of 1918; Army of Occupation, summer of 1919. Public Health Service and Veteran's Bureau; Director of O.T. Department, Bellevue Hospital, N.Y.C."
Marjory Moffatt (Mrs. Frank F. Spierling) of Chicago, Illinois	"Camp Custer, February 25 to April 29, 1919; Fort Porter, April 30 to October 24, 1919; Hampton, October 29 to December 6, 1919; Chicago P. H. Hospital, January to October 1920."
Marie Mohr of Buffalo, New York	"Camp Custer, January 13, 1919. Eastview, April 18, 1919. Fort Porter, July 18, 1919. Fort McHenry, October 26, 1919 to April 14, 1920."
Jeannette L. Moody of Meriden, Connecticut	"Served at Camp Grant, February 1919; Colonia, October 1919 to 1922; P.H.S. 41, New Haven, Conn., March 1922 to 1924...Special Classes for Mentally Retarded Children, Meriden, Conn." (see Figure 3-28).
Elizabeth Wells Robertson of Highland Park, Illinois	"Hospital for Shell-Shocked Soldiers, Magill University, Montreal, Canada, under direction of Invalided Soldiers Com. of Canada, summer of 1918. Head Aide, Fort Sheridan...Supervisor of Art, Districts 11 and 12, Chicago."
Harriet Robeson of Boston, Massachusetts	"Camp Custer, Eastview and Colonia, November 1919 to October 1920. Director of Aides, P.H.S., Washington, DC..with the State Dept. of Mental Hygiene, N.Y.C."
Ora G. Ruggles of Olive View, California	"Fort McPherson, 1918...Americanization Dept. of the Los Angeles City School System."
Meta N. Rupp (Mrs. Humphrey M. Cobb) of Waverly Place, New York City	"Camp Upton, January 1 to July 1, 1919. Fox Hills, July 1, 1919 to June 1, 1920. After discharge, associated with the Amer. O. T. Ass'n." (Meta Cobb later became Executive Director of the American Occupational Therapy Association in 1938.)
Helen Tanquary Smith (Mrs. Frank Smith) of Washington, DC	"Mrs. Smith was the first O.T. Aide. She began service at Walter Reed in February 1918...Cape May, January to April 1919...Carlisle, April to July 1919. She now has a very attractive studio, at 2 Dupont Circle, in Washington. She specializes in lamp shades, traveling to Europe to procure rare parchments and other unusual materials for her work."
Mary Louise Speed of Louisville, Kentucky	"Served from October 31, 1918, to August 18, 1919." Assigned to Oteen, then in Public Health Service, Greenville, South Carolina, then Lake City, Florida. Resigned in May 1922 to travel in Europe. "Received B.S. in Landscape Architecture...Gave a 10-day course in 'Garden Making for the Occupational Therapist' at the Boston School of O.T....writes for garden magazines."

(continued)

Table 3-3 (continued)
ACTIVITIES OF INDIVIDUAL RECONSTRUCTION AIDES IN OCCUPATIONAL THERAPY DURING AND AFTER WORLD WAR I

Marjorie Taylor of Milwaukee, Wisconsin, Milwaukee-Downer College	"Lakewood."
Helen Willard of Ambler, Pennsylvania	"Entered the service October 1918. Assigned to Boston for special course in P.T. at Harvard Medical School and Children's Hospital." Served at Robert Breck Brigham Hospital, Parker Hill, from December 1918 to February 1919; Camp Meade from February to April 1919; Fort Oglethorpe from April to June 1919; Ford Hospital in Detroit from June to July 1919; and Walter Reed. Discharged from military service September 1919. October 1920, assigned to Edward Hines Jr. Hospital, Hines, IL, as Assistant Superintendent of Aides in charge of both physical therapy and occupational therapy departments. In 1923, qualified with Civil Service as Chief Aide in Occupational Therapy and became Occupational Director as well as Chief Aide in Physical Therapy (see Figure 3-30).
Elizabeth K. Wise of Rochester, New York	"In 1921 promoted O.T. in Rochester, N.Y., under the Rochester Tuberculosis Association." (Elizabeth K. Wise endowed a scholarship for occupational therapy students.)
Excerpts taken from Laura Brackett Hoppin's book *The History of World War Reconstruction Aides*, 1933.	

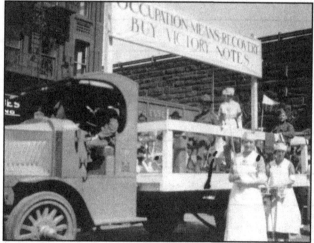

Figure 3-30. Photograph from the collection of Lena Hitchcock. Victory notes were sold to help pay for the war. [OHA 97: Angier and Hitchcock Collection. Otis Historical Archives, National Museum of Health and Medicine.]

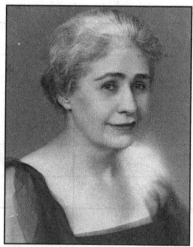

Figure 3-31. After World War I, Lena Hitchcock worked at Walter Reed General Hospital; Children's Hospital in Washington, DC; and as Director of Occupational Therapy for the DC Society for Crippled Children. She also served as President of the Women's Overseas League. She was proud that her experience in occupational therapy had gained her registration with the American Occupational Therapy Association. (Photo from Lloyd Notes and Facts, Volume II, Second Edition, 2010, courtesy of the authors.)

and base hospitals in the United States, established the worth of the profession. These reconstruction aides made great strides toward defining the role of occupational therapy in treatment of patients with neuropsychiatric problems, orthopedic problems, and tuberculosis. They established the worth of the profession and made great strides in defining the role of occupational therapy in the treatment of patients with neuropsychiatric problems, orthopedic problems, and tuberculosis.

The projected need for reconstruction aides in occupational therapy offered opportunities and economic incentives for schools to develop instructional training programs. Many programs and schools were established throughout the country, if only temporarily. However, a lack of set educational standards left many graduates ill prepared to provide occupational therapy services. This in turn spurred the start of efforts to establish educational standards to ensure competence of graduates.

The Army was very influential in defining the role of occupational therapy in the early years of the profession. Part of the Division of Special Hospitals and Physical Reconstruction in the Medical Department of the Army, occupational therapy was considered a medical service. Reconstruction aides in occupational therapy worked in a medical model, supervised by physicians who wrote prescriptions for treatment. Occupational therapy was part of the Division of Special Hospitals and Physical Reconstruction's Educational Department along with academic and vocational training and education. There was some confusion between the role delineation of occupational therapy and vocational trainers in preparing the disabled soldiers and sailors to return to work. The Division clarified these roles, indicating that occupational therapy provided prevocational activities to prepare patients for vocational education programs.

REFERENCES

A step forward in the education of occupational therapists. (1931). Occupational therapy notes. *Occupational Therapy and Rehabilitation, 10*, 204-206.

Bailey, P., Williams, F. E., & Komora, P. O. (1929). *The Medical Department of the United States Army in the World War: Volume X: Neuropsychiatry in the United States.* Washington, D.C.: U. S. Government Printing Office.

Baldwin, B. T. (1919a). Occupational therapy applied to the restoration of the function of disabled joints. Walter Reed Monograph printed by the Department of Occupational Therapy, Walter Reed General Hospital. Printed on the authority of the Surgeon General of the Army.

Baldwin, B. T. (1919b, January 30). Report of the Department of Occupational Therapy: Walter Reed General Hospital. Tacoma Park, DC: Published by Authority of the Commanding Officer.

Brackett, E. G. (1919, March). Productive occupational therapy in the treatment of the disabilities of the extremities. *Pacific Coast Journal of Nursing, 15*(3), 163-167.

Brown, R. S. (1920). *Base Hospital No. 9 A.E.F.: A history of the work of the New York hospital unit during two years of active service.* New York, NY: New York Hospital.

Carlova, J., & Ruggles, O. (1961). *The healing heart: The story of Ora Ruggles, pioneer in occupational therapy.* New York, NY: Julian Messner, Inc.

Crane, A. G. (1927). The medical department of the United States Army in the World War: Volume XIII: Part One: Physical reconstruction and vocational education. Washington, DC: U.S. Government Printing Office.

Dallas woman's work: Craft therapy began at end of first war. (1958, October 15). *Dallas Morning News,* p. 19.

Douglas, P. H. (1918, May). War Risk Insurance Act. *Journal of Political Economy, 26*(5), 461-483.

Drolet, G. J. (1945, July). World War I and tuberculosis: A statistical summary and review. *American Journal of Public Health, 35*(7), 689-697.

Editorial. (1922). A brief account of the sixth annual meeting of the American Occupational Therapy Association held at Atlantic City, N.J., September 25 to 29, 1922. *Archives of Occupational Therapy, 1*(5), 419-427.

Fulton, F. W. (1921). The Philadelphia School of Occupational Therapy. *Modern Hospital, 16*(6), 572-574.

Greene, M. B., & Wigglesworth, R. (1921). Boston School of Occupational Therapy. *Modern Hospital, 16*(6), 568-570.

Goldthwait, J. E. (1917a). Correspondence: The orthopedic preparedness of the nation. *American Journal of Orthopedic Surgery, 15*(3), 219-220.

Goldthwait, J. E. (1917b). The place of orthopedic surgery in war. *American Journal of Orthopedic Surgery, 15*(10), 679-686.

Haggerty, M. E. (1918). Where can a woman serve?: A big field is open for reconstruction aides. *Carry On, 1*(3), 26-29.

Hitchcock, A. L. (n.d.). *The great adventure: Being the tale of Hope Gray and Lena Hitchcock: The elephant's nest, crossing the sea, the A.E.F. and finally the end of the great adventure.* Unpublished manuscript.

Hoppin, L. B. (1933). History of the World War reconstruction aides. Millbrook, NY: William Tyldsley.

Jones, J. L. (1988). Early occupational therapy education in Wisconsin: Elizabeth Upham Davis and Milwaukee-Downer College. *American Journal of Occupational Therapy, 42*(8), 527-533.

Johnson, E. H. (1945). Reminiscences of World War I: Base Hospital 117. *American Journal of Orthopsychiatry, 15*(4), 607-620.

Kidder, I. (1921). St. Louis School Occupational Therapy. *Modern Hospital, 17*(1), 65-67.

Lynch, D., Weed, F. W., & McAfee, L. (1923). The Medical Department of the United States Army in the world war: Volume I: The Surgeon General's Office. Washington, DC: United States Government Printing Office.

Manring, M. M., Hawk, A., Calhoun, J. H., & Andersen, R. C. (2009). Treatment of war wounds: A historical review. *Clinical Orthopaedics and Related Research, 467*(8), 2168-2191.

McDaniel, M. L. (1968). Occupational therapists before World War II (1917-1940). In R. S. Anderson, H. S. Lee, & M. L. McDaniel (Eds.), *Army Medical Specialist Corps* (pp. 69-97). Washington, DC: Office of the Surgeon General, Department of the Army.

Medicine in St. Louis Hospital. (1919, February 16). *St. Louis Post-Dispatch*, pp. 3, 13.

Missouri Association for Occupational Therapy. (1923). Bulletin of the St. Louis School of Occupational Therapy. St. Louis, MO: Author.

Myers, C. (1948). Pioneer occupational therapists in World War I. *American Journal of Occupational Therapy, 2*(4), 208-215.

Myres, C. M. (1919). The occupational therapist in overseas service, Neuropsychiatric Division. In Proceedings of the Third Annual Meeting of the National Society for the Promotion of Occupational Therapy (pp. 133-139). Towson, MD: Sheppard and Enoch Pratt Hospital.

National Defense Act. (1921). The National Defense Act approved June 3, 1916. Washington, DC: Government Printing Office.

National Defense Act of 1916 (Public Law 64-85) (1916).

Occupational Therapy in St. Louis. (2009). Bernard Becker Medical Library Digital Collection. Retrieved from http://beckerexhibits.wustl.edu/mowihsp/health/OTstl.htm

Orr, H. W. (1921). *An orthopedic surgeon's story of the Great War.* Norfolk, NE: The Huse Publishing Co.

Partridge, C. R. (1921). Milwaukee-Downer College gives O.T. course. *Modern Hospital, 17*(1), 64-65.

Photography's aid in the mending of men. (1919, January). *Modern Hospital, 12*(1), 109.

Quiroga, V. A. M. (1995). *Occupational therapy: The first 30 years: 1900 to 1930.* Bethesda, MD: American Occupational Therapy Association.

Robinson, R. A. (1943). The Boston School of Occupational Therapy: Alumnae Luncheon, May 22, 1943. Bethesda, MD: Archives of the American Occupational Therapy Association. (Series 12, Box 101, Folder 732).

Russell, J. E. (1918). Occupational therapy in military hospitals. *American Journal of Care for Cripples, 7*(2), 112-116.

Salmon, T. W. (1917a). Care and treatment of mental diseases and war neuroses ('shell shock') in the British Army. *Mental Hygiene, 1*(4), 509-547.

Salmon, T. W. (1917b). Personal correspondence to The Rockefeller Foundation on May 1, 1917. Retrieved from http://rockefeller100.org/files/original/151dd97bd0530e402e49faf420b82f4d.pdf

Schwab, S. I. (1919). The experiment in occupational therapy at Base Hospital 117, A.E.F. *Mental Hygiene, 3*, 580-593.

Slagle, E. C. (n.d.). Experience of Eleanor Clarke Slagle. Bethesda, MD: Archives of the American Occupational Therapy Association (Series 1, Box 1, Folder 11).

Taylor-Whiffen, P. (2011, March 3). Shot at dawn: Cowards, traitors or victims? BBC. Retrieved from http://www.bbc.co.uk/history/british/britain_wwone/shot_at_dawn_01.shtml

Thatcher, E. (1919). *Making tin can toys.* Philadelphia, PA: J. B. Lippincott Company.

Thayer, W. S. (1919, December). The medical aspects of reconstruction. *American Journal of the Medical Sciences, 158*(6), 765-773.

United States Veterans Bureau Act of 1921 (Public Law 67-47)(1921).

Upham, E. G. (1918). Training of teachers for occupational therapy for the rehabilitation of disabled soldiers and sailors. Washington, DC: Federal Board for Vocational Education.

Vocational Education Act of 1917 (Public Law 64-347) (1917).

Vocational Rehabilitation Act of 1918 (Public Law 65-178) (1918).

Vocational (Industrial) Rehabilitation Act of 1920 (Public Law 66-236) (1920).

War Risk Insurance Act Amendment (Public Law 65-90) (1917).

Zimmerman, W. H. (1918). Our first blinded soldier: He is being re-educated and will make good. *Carry On, 1*(1), 13-14.

4

Standard Setting
1920s to 1940s

Key Points

- The desire to upgrade professional status prompted the move to establish minimum standards for courses of training in occupational therapy.
- The Society worked to distinguish occupational therapy as a medical profession, separating themselves from crafts persons.
- The National Register and a procedure for the accreditation of training schools were put in place as mechanisms to ensure the high standards of the profession.
- Due to the economic conditions of the Great Depression, the military was ill prepared to provide occupational therapy services at the start of World War II.

Highlighted Personalities

- Susan E. Tracy
- Susan Cox Johnson
- William Rush Dunton, Jr., President, September 1917 to 1919
- Eleanor Clarke Slagle, President, 1919 to 1920
- Herbert J. Hall, President, 1920 to 1923
- Thomas Kidner, President, 1923 to 1928

Key Places

- New York City—Association headquarters
- Boston School of Occupational Therapy
- Philadelphia School of Occupational Therapy
- St. Louis School of Occupational Therapy
- Milwaukee-Downer College

Andersen, L. T., & Reed, K. L.
The History of Occupational Therapy: The First Century (pp. 89-123).
© 2017 Taylor & Francis Group.

Key Times/Events

- Name of the Society changed to the American Occupational Therapy Association in 1921
- Occupational Therapy Pledge adopted in 1926
- Eleanor Clarke Slagle resigned as American Occupational Therapy Association Secretary-Treasurer in 1937
- Annual meetings held in conjunction with American Hospital Association from 1922 to 1937

Political Events/Issues

- Health care for reconstruction aides
- 19th Amendment to the Constitution ratified in 1920, giving women the right to vote
- National Economy Act of 1933 (Public Law 73-2)
- Social Security Act of 1935 (Public Law 74-271)

Educational Issues

- Minimum Standards for Courses of Training in Occupational Therapy adopted in 1923, revised in 1927 and 1930
- National Register established in 1931
- First National Directory published in 1932
- American Medical Association's Council on Medical Education and Hospitals published *Essentials of an Acceptable School of Occupational Therapy* and began accrediting schools

Sociocultural Events/Issues

- Improved social and political status for women
- Military status for occupational therapy

Economic Events/Issues

- Increased consumerism in early 1920s, an age of prosperity and excess
- Stock market crash of 1929
- The Great Depression of the 1930s

Technological Events/Issues

- First solo transatlantic flight completed by Charles Lindbergh in 1927
- Start of commercial air travel
- Widespread use of radio and talking pictures (movies) for entertainment

Practice Issues

- *Principles of Occupational Therapy* written in 1918
- Differentiation of occupational therapy from crafts teachers
- Sponsorship by medical profession

Association Issues

- Association managed by a 10-member Board of Management

INTRODUCTION

"If a normal man cannot be idle without becoming mentally and physically unfit, how much more important is it that people who are slowly convalescent or chronically ill should have the opportunity for wholesome work. It seems inconceivable that we should have so long missed this vital point in our care of invalids."

–Editor of *Modern Hospital* (1922)

Post-World War I ushered in the Roaring Twenties with a spirit of optimism; movements in support of women's rights, including women's right to vote; and the advancement of manufacturing, transportation, and communication technologies. Talking movies and radio were major forms of entertainment. By the end of the 1920s, with President Herbert Hoover in office, the economy went into a recession. The stock market crashed in 1929, causing the Great Depression, which would last until the start of World War II. The difficult economic times had significant implications for all, including occupational therapy. Unemployment reached 25% throughout the nation and as high as 80% to 90% in some cities. Hoovervilles, poorly constructed shanty towns, began to emerge in many areas to house the unemployed (Figure 4-1). The election of Franklin Delano Roosevelt in 1932 brought hope to the country with his promise of a New Deal—a series of domestic programs designed to get the country back on its feet. Additionally, President Roosevelt's wife, Eleanor, had an agenda and a national stage for promoting social justice. In this

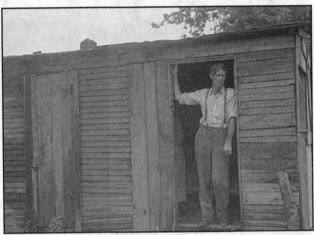

Figure 4-1. With 25% unemployment in the Great Depression, many people out of work ended up living in Hoovervilles, so called because of the anger toward President Herbert Hoover, under whose watch the Great Depression occurred.

environment, the leaders of occupational therapy set a course to obtain improved professional status for the profession by starting a professional journal and establishing standards of training, a National Register, and a method of accrediting training schools.

ESTABLISHING A FIRM FOUNDATION

William Rush Dunton Jr., Eleanor Clarke Slagle, Herbert J. Hall, MD, and Thomas B. Kidner all provided dedicated leadership guiding the fledgling Society through the formative years. When George Edward Barton decided not to run for reelection, Dr. Dunton agreed to step in to keep the Society going. He served for 2 years, from September 1917 to September 1919. He continued serving on various committees and as editor of the official journals of the Society until he was in his 80s. At the third annual meeting, Eleanor Clarke Slagle was the first woman elected President of the National Society for the Promotion of Occupational Therapy (NSPOT, 1919, p. 36) (Figure 4-2). Nominated for a second term at the fourth annual meeting, she was defeated by Dr. Herbert Hall by one vote (NSPOT, 1920c, p. 26). Hall, honoring his opponent in his first speech as President, noted the closeness of the election and mentioned that the late vote cast for Slagle would have resulted in a tie (NSPOT, 1920a, p. 39). In 1921, Mrs. Slagle was elected Secretary-Treasurer just as the offices were combined (Second Day—Afternoon Session, 1922, p. 223). She held this office on a volunteer basis until her resignation in 1937.

Dr. Hall's illness in 1922 required that Thomas Kidner step in to fulfill the presidential duties. When Hall died in February 1923, Kidner was elected outright as President and served through 1928. He was succeeded by Dr. C. Floyd Haviland (Figure 4-3). The untimely death of Haviland on New Year's Day 1930, coupled with the death of Vice President Dr. Burt W. Carr 2 weeks later, required Kidner to fill in once again until the election of new officers (Figure 4-4). Dr. Joseph Doane was President from 1930 to 1938. A past President of the American Hospital Association (AHA), he helped to strengthen the alliance between AHA and the American Occupational

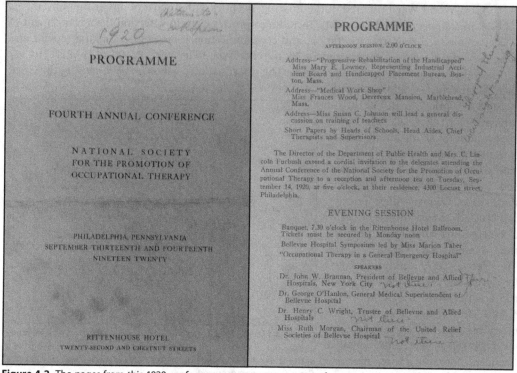

Figure 4-2. The pages from this 1920 conference program represent conference goers through the years who have attended conferences to participate in new experiences. In the upper right-hand corner, this conference goer has penciled in the program: "Skipped this + went sight-seeing." (Printed with permission from the Archive of the American Occupational Therapy Association, Inc.)

Therapy Association (AOTA, 1967b). Early attempts to establish a House of Delegates as part of the Society's management structure met with difficulties in determining representation of various groups. Additionally, because of the limited ability of delegates to travel to attend meetings, it was decided to have a 10-member Board of Management, comprising nine members and the President, run the association (Editorial, 1922b). The House of Delegates was later reinstated in 1938 to act as a recommending body to the Board of Management (AOTA, 1938; Jones, 1992).

Developing Principles of Occupational Therapy

William Rush Dunton Jr. began the discussion of formalizing the profession's underlying principles when he read a paper titled "The Principles of Occupational Therapy" at the second annual meeting in 1918 (Dunton, 1918). After his address, Dunton moved to appoint a committee to formally establish the principles of the profession. Eleanor Clarke Slagle; Dr. William L. Russell of Bloomingdale Hospital in White Plains, New York; and Mr. Norman L. Burnette of the Invalided Soldiers Commission

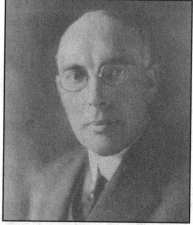

Figure 4-3. Dr. C. Floyd Haviland served as President of the AOTA from 1928 to 1930. Haviland was a close professional colleague of Eleanor Clarke Slagle whom he recruited to the position of Director of Occupational Therapy for the New York State Department of Mental Hygiene. A visionary and enthusiastic leader with common sense and unselfish devotion, Dr. Haviland died unexpectedly of pneumonia in 1930 while traveling in Egypt. (Printed with permission from the Archive of the American Occupational Therapy Association, Inc.)

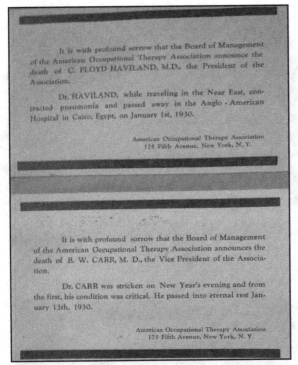

It is with profound sorrow that the Board of Management of the American Occupational Therapy Association announce the death of C. FLOYD HAVILAND, M.D., the President of the Association.

Dr. HAVILAND, while traveling in the Near East, contracted pneumonia and passed away in the Anglo-American Hospital in Cairo, Egypt, on January 1st, 1930.

American Occupational Therapy Association
175 Fifth Avenue, New York, N. Y.

It is with profound sorrow that the Board of Management of the American Occupational Therapy Association announces the death of B. W. CARR, M. D., the Vice President of the Association.

Dr. CARR was stricken on New Year's evening and from the first, his condition was critical. He passed into eternal rest January 13th, 1930.

American Occupational Therapy Association
175 Fifth Avenue, New York, N. Y.

Figure 4-4. In an unusual set of circumstances, both the President, Dr. C. Floyd Haviland, and the Vice President, Dr. Burt W. Carr of AOTA, died in a period of 2 weeks. Thomas B. Kidner once again stepped in to fulfill the role of President. (Printed with permission from the Archive of the American Occupational Therapy Association, Inc.)

in Toronto, Canada, were appointed to the committee. Fifteen principles were developed based on Dr. Dunton's paper (Dunton, 1919a). Many of these principles still apply today (Figure 4-5; Sidebar 4-1).

Society Name Change

In 1920, Herbert Hall suggested changing the name of the Society (Dunton, 1955; Editorial, 1946). As President of NSPOT in 1920, Eleanor Clarke Slagle presented this suggestion to the membership at the fourth annual meeting held at the Hotel Rittenhouse in Philadelphia, Pennsylvania (Figure 4-6). In recounting the activities of NSPOT and the tasks at hand, she questioned the name of the Society: "Do we longer need the descriptive phrase 'for the promotion' of occupational therapy?" (Slagle, 1920b, p. 2). Following up on Slagle's suggestion, Louis Haas, Secretary of NSPOT, requested members to provide suggestions for a new name for the Society. Haas noted that at this time in the life of NSPOT, "we do not need to be promoted nearly as much as we need development" (Haas, 1920, p. 4). Later in the meeting, Thomas B. Kidner moved to empower the Board of Directors to "receive suggestions as to a better name, shorter, more convenient name, with power to act; that is to say, to decide on a name" so that it could be presented and voted on at the next annual meeting (Kidner, 1920b, pp. 24-25).

In preparation for the upcoming annual meeting scheduled to be held in Baltimore, Maryland, the July 1921 issue of the *Maryland Psychiatric Quarterly* published the proposed constitutional changes for members to consider. President Herbert J. Hall highlighted the name change: "You will note that the name of the Society is changed to the American Occupational Therapy Association, certainly an advantage over the old cumbersome designation" (Hall, 1921, p. 18). At the annual meeting, although there was much discussion about the proposed constitutional changes affecting governance of the Society, there is no record of any discussion about the name change. The members voted on the morning of October 20, 1921, to accept the amended constitution, and as such, a new name for the Society: the American Occupational Therapy Association (AOTA, 1921; First Day—Morning Session, 1922, p. 64) (Figures 4-7 to 4-10).

ACTIVITIES OF THE FOUNDERS

George Barton and Isabel Newton Barton curtailed their activities in the new Society within the first year. Susan Cox Johnson and Susan Tracy were very active initially, both major forces in shaping educational standards. Thomas Kidner was instrumental in establishing a National Register and initiating efforts to start an accreditation program for training schools. Eleanor Clarke Slagle and William Rush Dunton continued to be involved in Association activities for many years, shaping the Association and the new profession.

To the members of the National Society for the Promotion of

Occupational Therapy:

Your Committee on Principles has agreed upon the following as
representing the basic principles of occupational therapy:

(1.) Occupational therapy is a method of treating the sick or
injured by means of instruction and employment in productive
occupation.
(2.) The objects sought are to arouse interest, courage, and
confidence; to exercise mind and body in healthy activity; to
overcome functional disability; and to re-establish capacity for
industrial and social usefulness.
(3.) In applying occupational therapy, system and precision are
as important as in other forms of treatment.
(4.) The treatment should be administered under constant medical
advice and supervision, and correlated with the other treatment
of the patient.
(5.) The treatment should, in each case, be specifically directed to the individual needs.
(6.) Though some patients do best alone, employment in groups
is usually advisable because it provides exercise in social adaptation and the stimulating influence of example and comment.
(7.) The occupation selected should be within the range of the
patient's estimated interests and capability.
(8.) As the patient's strength and capability increase, the type
and extent of occupation should be regulated and graded accord-
ingly.
(9.) The only reliable measure of the value of the treatment is
the effect on the patient.
(10.) Inferior workmanship, or employment in an occupation which
would be trivial for the healthy, may be attended with the greatest benefit to the sick or injured. Standards worthy of entirely normal persons must be maintained for proper mental stimulation.
(11.) The production of a well-made, useful, and attractive article
or the accomplishment of a useful task, requires healthy exercise
of mind and body, gives the greatest satisfaction, and thus produces the most beneficial effects.
(12.) Novelty, variety, individuality, and utility of the products
enhance the value of an occupation as a treatment measure.
(13.) Quality, quantity, and saleability of the products may prove
beneficial by satisfying and stimulating the patient but should
never be permitted to obscure the main purpose.
(14) Good craftmanship, and ability to instruct are essential
qualifications in the occupational therapist; cheerful outlook
and manner are equally essential.
(15.) Patients under treatment by means of occupational therapy
should also engage in recreational or play activities. It is advisable that gymnastics and calisthenics, which may be given for
habit training, should be regarded as work. Social dancing and all
recreational and play activities should be under the definite head
of recreations.

Figure 4-5. Photograph of typed list of 15 principles. (Printed with permission from the Archive of the American Occupational Therapy Association, Inc.)

Eleanor Clarke Slagle

Eleanor Clarke Slagle earned the title Mother of Occupational Therapy by virtue of her dedication and work to promote the profession. By the early 1920s, Slagle had already served a number of
years as the Chairperson of the Committee on Installations and Advice. In this role, Slagle advised
organizations about developing occupational therapy programs and training schools, assisted

---

SIDEBAR 4-1

Definition of Occupational Therapy

"Occupational therapy may be defined as any activity, mental or physical, definitely prescribed and guided for the distinct purpose of contributing to and hastening recovery from disease or injury." (Pattison, 1922)

After presenting his paper at the fifth annual conference, Pattison asked for feedback on his definition of occupational therapy: "I want to know if there is not someone who wants to put up a rifle and shoot holes through that definition..." Discussion ensued about the necessity of a medical prescription and whether that was a qualification to make occupation therapeutic (Second Day—Morning Session, 1922, p. 158).

---

with placement of capable occupational therapists in open positions, and gave numerous talks to various clubs, organizations, and schools. Requests for information about occupational therapy came from all over the United States and from a number of foreign countries. Through her volunteer activities in the Society and her work activities, Slagle developed an extensive professional network. She was appointed consultant to the Department of Reconstruction in the Public Health Service in 1920, providing her with the opportunity to meet with numerous government officials and promote occupational therapy (Slagle, 1918, 1919, 1920a). She continued in an ambassador role for occupational therapy with her election as Secretary-Treasurer of AOTA in 1921.

On July 1, 1922, Slagle was appointed Director of Occupational Therapy for the New York State Department of Mental Hygiene. Slagle had been recruited to the position by C. Floyd Haviland, a psychiatrist who later became President of AOTA (AOTA, 1967b) (Sidebar 4-3).

Returning to her home state, Slagle took up residence in New York City. For a time, she managed Association affairs from her apartment, keeping documents and files in her kitchen. Finally, the Board of Managers voted to rent office space to establish an official headquarters. The Association leased a room in an office building from the National Health Council. The building, located at 370 Seventh Avenue in New York City, housed a number of other health organizations, including the National Committee for Mental Hygiene, the National Tuberculosis Association, the National Organization for Public Health Nursing, the National League of Nursing Education, and the American Social Hygiene Association. The close proximity to these organizations offered opportunities for networking and strategic alliances (Report of Secretary-Treasurer, 1922, pp. 49-50). In November 1925, the office was moved to the Flatiron Building at 23rd Street and 5th Avenue because that location was easier to find and offered a larger office and more exposure (Board of Management, 1926a).

Slagle continued to respond to requests about occupational therapy, handle membership applications, and correspond with a number of states seeking to establish state societies of occupational therapy. She also continued with speaking

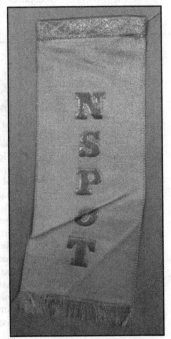

Figure 4-6. An NSPOT conference ribbon from the scrapbook of Dr. William Rush Dunton Jr. (Printed with permission from the Archive of the American Occupational Therapy Association, Inc.)

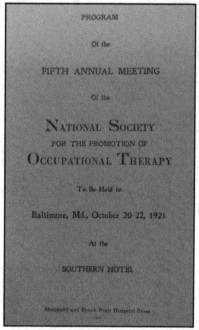

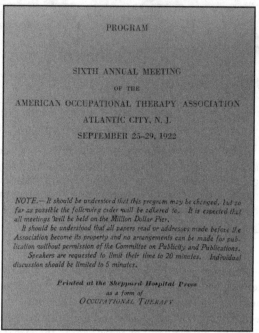

Figure 4-7. Program from the fifth annual meeting showing the name as the Society. (Printed with permission from the Archive of the American Occupational Therapy Association, Inc.)

Figure 4-8. Program from the sixth annual meeting showing the name change of the Society to the American Occupational Therapy Association. (Printed with permission from the Archive of the American Occupational Therapy Association, Inc.)

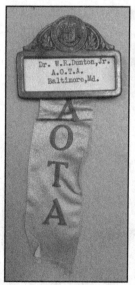

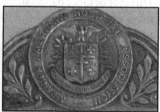

Figure 4-9. (A) This AOTA conference ribbon is from the scrapbook of Dr. William Rush Dunton Jr. of Baltimore, Maryland. (B) A closer view shows "Member American Hospital Association" embossed around the insignia at the top of the ribbon holder. Several AOTA conferences were held in conjunction with the American Hospital Association. (Printed with permission from the Archive of the American Occupational Therapy Association, Inc.)

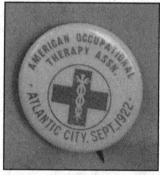

Figure 4-10. AOTA Button – 1922 is from the 5th Annual Meeting held in Atlantic City, NJ after the name was changed from NSPOT to AOTA. (Printed with permission from the Archive of the American Occupational Therapy Association, Inc.)

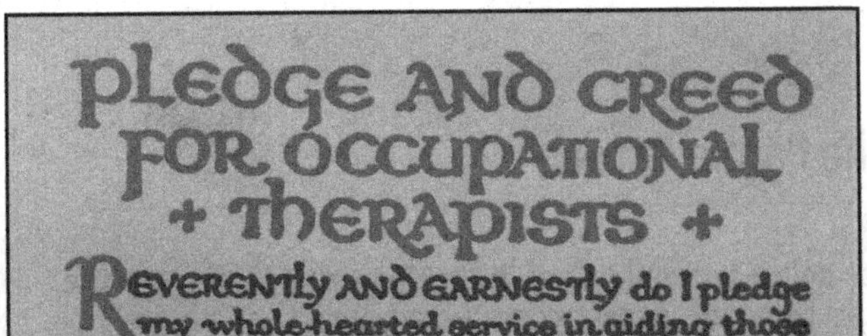

PLEDGE AND CREED FOR OCCUPATIONAL + THERAPISTS +

REVERENTLY AND EARNESTLY do I pledge my whole-hearted service in aiding those crippled in mind and body.

To this end that my work for the sick may be successful. I will ever strive for greater knowledge, skill and understanding in the discharge of my duties, in whatsoever position I may find myself.

I solemnly declare that I will hold and keep inviolate whatever I may learn of the lives of the sick.

I acknowledge the dignity of the cure of disease and the safeguarding of health in which no act is menial or inglorious.

I will walk in upright faithfulness and obedience to those under whose guidance I am to work, and I pray for patience, kindliness and strength in the holy ministry to broken minds and bodies.

Figure 4-11. Pledge and Creed. (Printed with permission from the Archive of the American Occupational Therapy Association, Inc.)

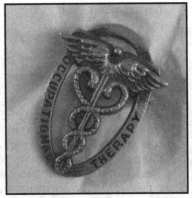

Figure 4-12. An early occupational therapy pin that belonged to Winifred Brainerd. (Copyright © Dr. Lori T. Andersen.)

SIDEBAR 4-2

Pledge and Creed for Occupational Therapists

In December 1924, Mrs. Marjorie B. Greene of the Boston School of Occupational Therapy wrote to President Thomas Kidner expressing the desire to adopt a Pledge and Creed for occupational therapists (Greene, 1924). Modeled after the Pledge and Creed of the American Hospital Association, the Pledge and Creed was formally adopted by the AOTA Board of Management at its 10th annual meeting in Atlantic City, September 26, 1926 (Board of Management, 1926b) (Figure 4-11).

---

engagements and visits to institutions, public gatherings, clubs, and associations. As Secretary-Treasurer of AOTA and Director of Occupational Therapy for the New York State Department of Mental Hygiene, Slagle connected with a number of important people in health care institutions and agencies (Report of Secretary-Treasurer, 1922).

Slagle knew the importance of networking and collaborating with community organizations. Mrs. George Hewitt, a friend and colleague of Slagle, was president of the New York State Federation of Women's Clubs. This organization was one of the state federations of the General Federation of Women's Clubs, a philanthropic and educational organization. In a speech given at the fourth annual meeting of NSPOT, Mrs. Hewitt noted that the Federation and Society shared similar purposes, such as improving child welfare and public health. At a time when women had just won the right to vote, Mrs. Hewitt understood the political power of the state federation with 275,000 members and the national organization with 2 million members. She offered the Federation's support to NSPOT in any legislative initiatives (First Day—Afternoon Session, 1920, pp. 32-33). Slagle took charge of the Occupational Therapy Committee of the General Federation. A highly sought-after speaker, she gave talks throughout the United States on the benefits and successes of occupational therapy (Sidebar 4-4; Figure 4-13).

SIDEBAR 4-3
The Parole Carpet

A 1926 article written by Florence Kelley and published in the *New York Times* tells the story of the "parole carpet," a hooked rug craft project constructed out of used garments by psychiatric patients in a state hospital. Patients worked together on this project as part of their occupational therapy to help them regain health so that they could be "paroled," or allowed to go home. The project gained the interest of the patients who wanted to work on it. The activity facilitated cooperation and resocialization because several could work on it at one time. It also provided motivation and incentive. One day, Eleanor Clarke Slagle, Director of Occupational Therapy for the State Hospital Commission, encountered a patient working feverishly on a simple task. When she inquired about his hurried pace, he replied:

> I must get this done first and then there are two other things I must do before I'll be ready to work on the parole carpet. And after I work on that I can go home! I must hurry and finish this! (Kelley, 1926)

SIDEBAR 4-4
"Former Hobart Girl Is Honored"

A newspaper article in the *Stamford Mirror-Recorder* (New York) on January 8, 1931, reported that Eleanor Clarke Slagle was honored for her work in occupational therapy at a recent national conference held in New Orleans. The presiding official at the meeting "predicted that because of her work, Mrs. Slagle's name would stand out in history" ("Former Hobart girl honored," 1931) (Figure 4-13). It has!

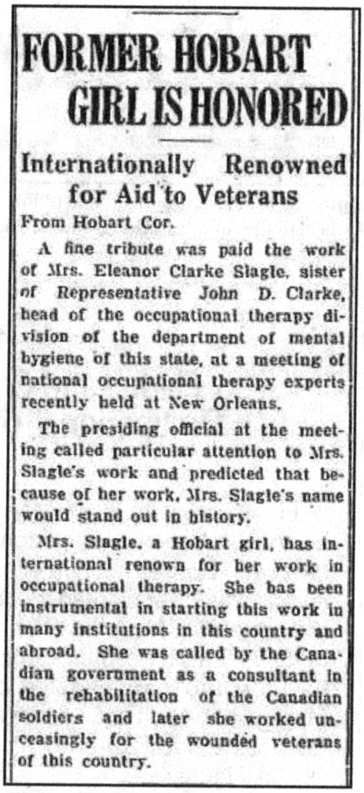

FORMER HOBART GIRL IS HONORED

Internationally Renowned for Aid to Veterans

From Hobart Cor.

A fine tribute was paid the work of Mrs. Eleanor Clarke Slagle, sister of Representative John D. Clarke, head of the occupational therapy division of the department of mental hygiene of this state, at a meeting of national occupational therapy experts recently held at New Orleans.

The presiding official at the meeting called particular attention to Mrs. Slagle's work and predicted that because of her work, Mrs. Slagle's name would stand out in history.

Mrs. Slagle, a Hobart girl, has international renown for her work in occupational therapy. She has been instrumental in starting this work in many institutions in this country and abroad. She was called by the Canadian government as a consultant in the rehabilitation of the Canadian soldiers and later she worked unceasingly for the wounded veterans of this country.

Figure 4-13. The Thursday, January 8, 1931, issue of the *Stamford Mirror-Recorder* in Stamford, New York, published this prophetic article: "Former Hobart Girl Honored." Her name does stand out in history: the Eleanor Clarke Slagle Lectureship.

Dr. William Rush Dunton

Dr. Dunton's work life at Sheppard and Enoch Pratt Hospital began to change in 1918. On December 21, 1918, a disgruntled physician, Dr. Noboru Ishida, shot and killed another physician, Dr. George B. Wolff, in Dr. Dunton's office. The Board of Trustees were critical of the hospital Superintendent, Dr. Edward N. Brush, for not recognizing signs of mental illness in Dr. Ishida. This prompted Dr. Brush's resignation, effective April 1, 1920. The new Superintendent, Dr. Ross Chapman, wanted to make administrative changes throughout the hospital. He replaced Dunton as Director of the Occupational Therapy Department and assigned him to be in charge of research (Bing, 1961, pp. 210-211). Dr. Chapman then hired Dr. Henry Stack Sullivan, a rising psychiatrist, in 1922. This signaled a paradigm shift in the treatment of those with mental

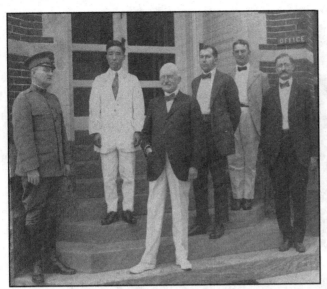

Figure 4-14. Physicians on staff at Sheppard and Enoch Pratt Hospital in 1918. From left to right: Dr. George Franklin Sargent; Dr. Noboru Ishida; Dr. Edward N. Brush, Superintendent; Dr. George Baney Wolff (murdered by Dr. Ishida); Dr. William Rush Dunton Jr.; and Dr. L. Gibbons Smart. (Printed with permission from the Archive of the American Occupational Therapy Association, Inc.)

illness because Sullivan favored the psychodynamic theories proposed by Sigmund Freud, which were gaining popularity. Freud believed that the etiology of mental illness was within the person. This was not consistent with Dr. Dunton's views, which considered the environment or context to contribute to mental illness. Sullivan developed his own theory of psychiatry based in part on Freud's teachings. Sullivan's theory emphasized the importance of interpersonal relationships. Poor interpersonal relationships were believed to be the cause of mental illness. Dr. Sullivan had difficulty with interpersonal relationships with his coworkers. He was perceived to be critical, demanding, and sarcastic (Forbush & Forbush, 1986, p. 61). The differences in ideology and poor working relationships prompted Dr. Dunton to resign his position at Sheppard and Enoch Pratt Hospital in 1924. A new opportunity quickly presented itself when he was offered the opportunity to become the Medical Director of Harlem Lodge, a small, private psychiatric sanitarium in Catonsville, Maryland (Bing, 1961, pp. 211-212) (Figure 4-14).

In spite of the difficulties at work, Dr. Dunton maintained active participation in AOTA. As Chair of the Committee on Publicity and Publications, Dunton began and was editor of *Archives of Occupational Therapy*, published by Williams & Wilkins, from 1922 to 1924. Individuals could subscribe to the journal for $5 per year. Previously, articles about occupational therapy had been published in journals such as *Modern Hospital, Trained Nurse and Hospital Review*, and *Maryland Psychiatric Quarterly*; however, it became increasingly difficult to get these journals to accept occupational therapy papers. The goal of *Archives of Occupational Therapy* was to provide a journal to preserve the important papers and discussions of AOTA and to give occupational therapists access to professional literature specific to occupational therapy (Committee on Publicity and Publications, 1922; Editorial, 1922a). In 1924, the name of the journal was changed to *Occupational Therapy and Rehabilitation*. The name change was meant to communicate the expanded scope of the journal, which was to provide a resource and forum for all people involved in rehabilitation services (Dunton, 1925c). Subscription fees were incorporated into membership dues by a vote of the membership at the annual meeting in 1925 (Committee on Publicity and Publications, 1925) (Figures 4-15 and 4-16).

SETTING EDUCATIONAL STANDARDS

Amid the backdrop of World War I, the newly formed NSPOT was gaining its footing, defining directions and tasks to move the Society and profession forward. As the Society desired to emphasize the therapeutic nature of occupation, active membership was restricted to those "actually using occupation as a therapeutic agent, or who are teaching, supervising, or superintending such work." A person who was "desirous of doing such work—i.e., pupils, social workers, nurses, etc." could apply for associate membership (NSPOT, 1917, pp. 1-2).

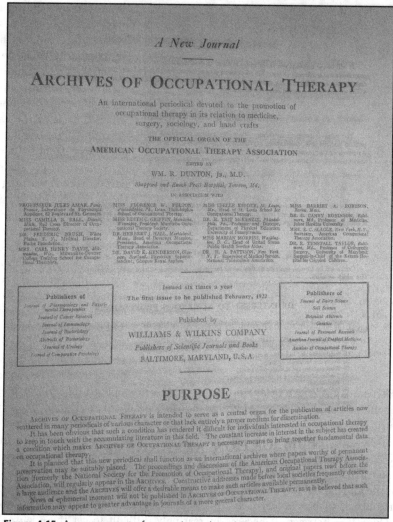

Figure 4-15. Announcement of a new journal: *Archives of Occupational Therapy*. The Archives were published from 1922 through 1924. (Printed with permission from the Archive of the American Occupational Therapy Association, Inc.)

Two standing committees established by NSPOT's constitution played significant roles in setting qualifications for occupational therapists and educational standards for training schools. First, the Committee on Teaching Methods, chaired by Susan E. Tracy, was formed to "investigate the different methods in vogue, to prepare outlines of methods of teaching, both in public classes and in nurses' training schools, etc." (NSPOT, 1917, p. 10). Second, the Committee on Admissions and Positions, chaired by Susan Cox Johnson, was formed to "receive all applications for admission to the Society and after proper consideration to present them, if eligible, to the Board" (p. 9). This committee was also designated to be an employment bureau, placing members in institutions in need of an occupational teacher.

Shortly after the founding meeting, Susan E. Tracy named her committee members and provided an outline of a training curriculum to Dr. Dunton (Tracy, 1917). To accomplish their charge, Tracy's committee began to survey institutions about the therapeutic use of occupation in their facilities and gathered information about the types of facilities and organizations, programs offered, methods (activities) used by occupation workers, types of patients seen, and number of hours spent providing treatment (Committee on Teaching Methods, 1917, 1918, 1919). Tracy believed that understanding the scope of occupational therapy practice was preliminary to developing educational standards.

Susan Cox Johnson asked for clarification of duties of the Chair and Committee on Admissions and Positions at the annual meeting in 1918, indicating that she was gravitating to establishment of standards for training. Johnson stated:

> If the word 'Positions' is to be more widely interpreted to cover all matters concerning the fitness of teachers to fill positions creditably and the conditions under which they serve, or in other words to set standards for qualifications of teachers and terms of service, then the present Chairperson would find herself more closely allied with her interests and general duties and so the more able to serve the society." (Committee on Admissions and Positions, 1918, p. 18)

The Board of Management approved her request to charge the Committee with the duty "To formulate and present to the Board of Management for approval, standards by which teachers shall be judged as qualified to hold certain positions in the field of occupational therapy..." (p. 19).

Discussion ensued on whether occupational therapy should be provided by specially trained nurses who had a strong medical background or by people who had strong knowledge and expertise in crafts. Reba G. Cameron, Superintendent of Nurses and occupational instructor at Taunton State Hospital, Massachusetts (Cameron, 1915), and Adelaide Nutting, Director of the Department of Nursing and Health of Columbia University, considered occupational therapy as a special branch of nursing training that should be taken after general education has given the student nurse a firm foundation (Dunton, 1919b, p. 80). Cameron (1917), a friend and colleague of Susan E. Tracy, wrote that "Miss Tracy is firmly of the opinion that occupational therapy is nurse's work, and she also believes that every training school for nurses should, as part of the curriculum, include a course in occupation" (p. 66).

Susan Cox Johnson had a background in design, worked as an arts and crafts teacher, and taught occupations

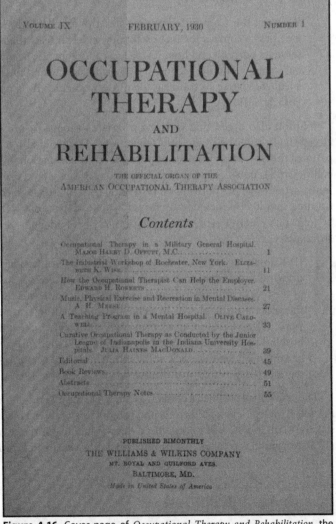

Figure 4-16. Cover page of *Occupational Therapy and Rehabilitation,* the official journal of AOTA from 1925 through 1946. (Printed with permission from the Archive of the American Occupational Therapy Association, Inc.)

courses. She believed the field of occupational therapy was becoming a distinct specialty as the war caused occupation to be swept out of the hands of the nurses and to a group foreign to hospitals (Johnson, 1918). Nurses no longer had the time to devote to extra training in therapeutic use of occupations, nor the time to implement occupation programs in hospitals (Johnson, 1917). There was a need to train a new classification of worker, one with medical knowledge and skill in crafts and teaching (Adams, 1922).

In trying to bring two factions together, Johnson asserted:

> What seems to be a difference of opinion among those who are working with the same ends in view, is often NOT A REAL difference but is due to the failure to keep always before us, the several natural divisions of the work and the different purposes of each, as well as the fact, that each must overlap and mere one into the other instead of being separate and aloof. No standards for training teachers can be set without recognition of these different elements. (Johnson, 1918, p. 44)

Johnson also wanted to avoid alienating reconstruction aides, most of whom trained in time-limited war emergency courses to fill an urgent need. Eager to move the profession forward, Johnson acknowledged:

> Whereas the Committee appreciates the excellent work accomplished through the emergency courses for reconstruction aides, it feels that if occupational therapy is to serve its purpose and hold its place as a therapeutic agent in civilian hospitals of various types, it should become a real profession which must be dignified by a long and adequate course of training for those who enter it. (Committee on Admissions and Positions, 1919, p. 18)

Johnson also urged that training programs should be provided by colleges and schools that already had established value and reputations. This would improve the professional status of occupational therapy. Many courses required to train occupational therapists were already provided by colleges and schools. Sharing of faculty and facilities would provide additional economic benefits. Johnson qualified her position on providing training through colleges and schools, indicating that training should also include supervised hospital experience (NSPOT, 1920b, pp. 54-55).

Johnson's committee described the essentials of adequate training for occupational therapists as follows:

> (1) Knowledge and skill in a fairly wide range of handcrafts, games and recreations, drawing and design, and certain academic and commercial subjects; (2) understanding of the more commoner mental and physical conditions from which patients suffer and the general principles of hygiene and therapeutic treatment required for occupation work; (3) understanding of the social and economic conditions commonly related to hospital problems; (4) understanding and practice of teaching methods which would be employed with the sick and handicapped and general on hospital organization and regime. (Committee on Admissions and Positions, 1919, p. 19)

The committee outlined a standard course of study based on these essentials, recommending that the Society adopt it as a guide only and recognizing that "the methods and principles of teaching the sick were still in a state of unorganized knowledge" (Committee on Admissions and Positions, 1919, p. 24). No action was taken (Committee on Admissions and Positions, 1919; NSPOT, 1920b, p. 52).

Minimum Standards for Courses of Training in Occupational Therapy

The Society became more earnest in developing standards for training, recognizing that the reputation of the profession was based on the work of occupational therapists and that inadequate preparation of occupational therapists would reflect poorly on the profession's image as a whole. In 1921, Dr. Herbert J. Hall, NSPOT President, appointed Susan Cox Johnson as chair of a new Committee on Education charged with the duty to work "toward the establishment of uniform standards in the training and certification of aides and the advancement of professional status of the occupation aide" (Committee on Admissions and Positions, 1922, p. 76). Miss Ruth Wigglesworth, Director of the Boston School of Occupational Therapy, replaced Susan E. Tracy as Chairperson of the Committee on Teaching Methods.

Miss Wigglesworth's committee also took to task the charge of developing uniform standards. The 10 members of the committee, all school representatives, went to work gathering information about existing schools and opinions regarding the requirements for entrance, minimum length for a course of study, and length of practical work (Committee on Teaching Methods, 1922; Round Table on Training Courses, 1923).

At a roundtable discussion on training courses, it became clear that the Association wanted to differentiate between occupation therapists who had required training and crafts teachers who did not (Round Table on Training Courses, 1923). To make this distinction, Miss Wigglesworth advised that:

> Schools must emphasize the fact that they are not training teachers of occupation therapy, but occupation therapists. Nurses are not teachers in the sense indicated, and this phrase used by some, again implies teaching teachers of crafts and not that we are training medical workers. Now is the tie to make the point clear. (Committee on Teaching Methods, 1922, p. 64)

Discussion and debate continued as the Association sought to achieve a middle ground, perhaps best defined by Miss Idelle Kidder, Director of the Missouri Association for Occupational Therapy and affiliated with the St. Louis School of Occupational Therapy. Kidder expressed that "courses should not be lengthened too rapidly to seriously hinder hospitals in being able to open occupational therapy departments, nor the standards be lowered by shortening courses so that existing and future departments cannot continue with well-trained aides" (Third Day, Morning Session, 1922, p. 228).

To move the issue of training forward, Mr. Kidner, who had taken over as President for the ailing Hall, worked with Mrs. Slagle and Miss Wigglesworth to develop a draft of the Minimum Standards of Training. The draft was based on the numerous reports, discussions, and suggestions received over the past several years. The draft was discussed and revised at the June 1923 Board meeting and approved by the membership at the annual meeting in Milwaukee on October 30, 1923 (Board of Management, 1923; AOTA, 1924).

The adoption of the Minimum Standards required that candidates for admission to training courses have a high school education or equivalent and be at least 20 years old at graduation. The length of training programs was set at no less than 12 months, including at least 8 months of theoretical and practical work and at least 3 months of supervised hospital practice training. The Board also proposed that, in the future, it would be advisable to establish short postgraduate training courses (AOTA, 1924).

The Board of Managers had indicated that from time to time, the Minimum Standards would need to be revised. This occurred in 1927, when the Minimum Standards were revised to increase the practice training from 3 months to 6 months (Kidner, 1928). The Minimum Standards were revised again in 1930 to increase the total length of the educational program from a minimum of 12 months to 18 months, which included 9 months of theoretical and technical work and at least 9 months of hospital practice training under competent supervision (New Minimum Standards..., 1930).

Two of the founders who had taken on the monumental task of moving the profession forward by setting Minimum Standards of Training stopped participating in Society activities in the early 1920s. Miss Susan E. Tracy dropped out of Association activities approximately 1 year before passage of the Minimum Standards, and Miss Susan Cox Johnson around the time the Minimum

Standards were approved. Tracy was likely very involved with her teaching activities around the country. Johnson lost her teaching position at Teacher's College in 1924 when the occupational therapy program was closed due to lack of enrollment (Quiroga, 1995, p. 221). Tracy died in 1928 of a stroke (Presbyterian Hospital of Chicago, 1929), and Johnson died in 1932 of pneumonia (Occupational Therapy Notes, 1932).

ESTABLISHING A NATIONAL REGISTER

The Society recognized that the first step in establishing a National Register was to develop Minimum Standards for Courses of Training in Occupational Therapy (Kidner, 1930). Once this was accomplished and the Minimum Standards were promulgated, the Board of Managers strongly recommended that a National Register or directory be established to ensure high standards for the profession (AOTA, 1924). Now, with the adoption of the Minimum Standards, there was a measure to determine the quality of training schools, and Mrs. Slagle, in her role as Secretary-Treasurer, was able to respond to requests to approve training schools. However, this was on a voluntary basis, and there was not a real mechanism to ensure adherence to standards. The move to establish a National Register would provide a more effective mechanism to enforce the Minimum Standards.

Everett S. Elwood, Managing Director of the National Board of Medical Examiners and later President of AOTA (1938 to 1947), was among those advocating for the profession to move toward a National Register. A member of AOTA since 1923, Elwood (1927) recommended that the Association:

> ...take advantage of your position by making certain the back door is carefully fastened against pretenders, that others do not crawl in under the fence, and that those who are permitted to enter the front door have the proper credentials for admission. (pp. 341-342)

The Committee on Teaching Methods recommended that the Association appoint a special committee to prepare and submit a proposal for a National Register. President Thomas Kidner did so, charging the special committee with the task of proposing a plan to establish a National Register and to rate and inspect training schools. Graduates of these approved schools would be qualified to be included in the Register (Kidner, 1925). In view of similar concerns to set standards and prevent unqualified people from practicing, the Massachusetts Society for Occupational Therapy had established a registration system in the early 1920s (Brackett, 1922). Now the national Association set out to establish a plan for a National Register. The purpose of the Register was to "protect patients from unqualified persons by maintaining high professional standards, while at the same time, safe-guarding properly qualified workers" (Kidner, 1930, p. 224) and "for the protection of hospitals and institutions from unqualified persons posing as occupational therapists" (AOTA, 1932, p. 7).

The appointed committee was slow to act. Kidner was anxious to move plans for a Register forward, so he and Mrs. Slagle gathered information about methods and procedures used by other organizations who had established registers. Although the intent of the Register was to require graduation from schools meeting Minimum Standards to be a main requirement of eligibility, it was acknowledged that, for a period of time, eligibility requirements should also include those with training and experience prior to establishment of the Minimum Standards. These workers would be grandfathered in if an application was submitted within 3 years of establishment of the National Register. Admission to the National Register based on successfully passing an examination was considered but deemed to be impractical at that time (Board of Management, 1927, 1928, 1929).

A plan for the National Register was finally approved by the Board of Management and by members at the 1930 annual meeting (Kidner, 1930). The register was started in 1931, funded in part by the efforts of a voluntary committee of AOTA that collected funds to pay for startup costs

(Board of Management, 1931b). There were two divisions to the Register: a main Register and a secondary Register. The qualifications for the Register were as follows:

1. Main Register (eligible to use the designation O.T. Reg.)

Three categories of personnel could qualify for the main register.

A. Category A—graduates of training schools that met the Minimum Standards of Training and have at least one year of successful work experience in occupational therapy.

B. Category B*—at least four years' successful work experience in occupational therapy work and high school education or equivalent.

C. Category C*—training and experience in application of specialty area as a curative treatment for sick and disabled, high school education or equivalent, and classes on theory and practice of occupational therapy, or submit short thesis on subject as deemed necessary.

*Admission to the register based on successful experience ceased to be in effect after December 31, 1933.

2. Secondary Register—(eligible to use the designation O. T. Asst. Reg.)—at least four years' successful work experience in occupational therapy and completed at least eighth grade public school education or equivalent. (AOTA, 1932)

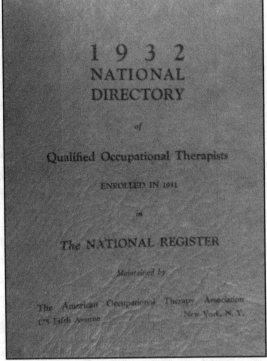

Figure 4-17. Photograph of the cover of the 1932 National Directory. The names of those admitted to the National Register were printed in the National Directory. The 1932 National Directory included such information as name of training school attended, experience, present position, and birth year. It was the only National Directory that included registrants' birth years. (Printed with permission from the Archive of the American Occupational Therapy Association, Inc.)

In 1931, an amendment to the constitution established the Committee on Registration to "carry out regulations for admission to the National Register … and to submit changes to the regulations from time to time" as deemed necessary (American Occupational Therapy Association, 1932, p. 5). The committee was also charged with the duty "to examine and pass all applications" for the Register (American Occupational Therapy Association, 1932, p. 5). The first Register, printed in 1932, contained the names of "three hundred and eighteen therapists … all qualified by a rigid set of standards." Thirteen names were also included in the secondary Register (AOTA, 1932, 1967a) (Figures 4-17 to 4-19). Initially, those admitted to the Register used the designation O.T. Reg. A vote of the membership at the 1940 business meeting officially changed the designation to O.T.R. (AOTA, 1940).

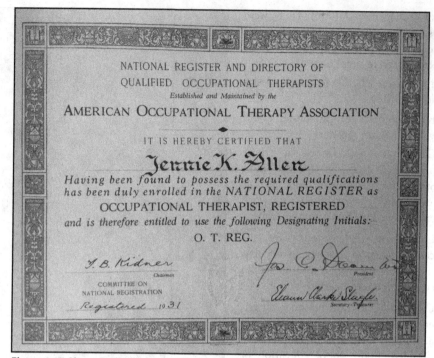

Figure 4-18. Photograph of Jennie K. Allen's Registration Certificate. Miss Allen served as Head of the Occupational Therapy Department of Cook County Hospital in Chicago and President of the Illinois Association of Occupational Therapy. (Printed with permission from the Archive of the American Occupational Therapy Association, Inc.)

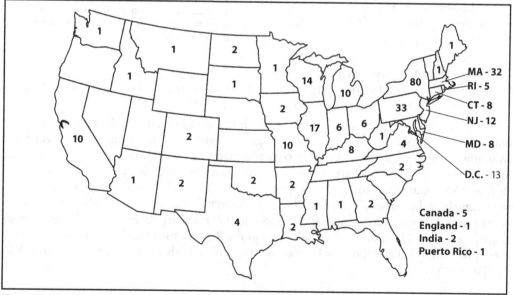

Figure 4-19. Map showing the distribution of the 318 occupational therapists listed in the 1932 National Directory by state.

ACCREDITATION OF TRAINING SCHOOLS THROUGH THE AMERICAN MEDICAL ASSOCIATION

With the National Register established, the Association took steps to develop a plan for the inspection of training schools. Mrs. Slagle was the sole person in charge of determining whether schools met Minimum Standards, the basis for allowing graduates to be admitted to the Register.

Slagle brought concerns or problems with specific schools to the attention of the Board of Management for further direction. However, to avoid the perception of a conflict of interest, the Association decided that an outside agency should take charge of the inspection program. In 1931, Thomas Kidner quietly approached the American Medical Association (AMA) to discuss the possibility of the AMA's Council on Medical Education and Hospitals (AMA-CMEH) taking responsibility for inspection of occupational training courses. The AMA had experience setting standards for medical education. The association also believed that this oversight by the AMA would bring increased legitimacy and status to the profession. Dr. Joseph C. Doane, President of AOTA (1930 to 1938), formally requested the AMA take responsibility for the inspection of occupational therapy training programs on March 10, 1931 (Figure 4-20).

In June 1933, recognizing that occupational therapists worked under the direction of the medical profession, the AMA agreed to this role. AOTA wanted the AMA-CMEH to use the Minimum Standards for Courses of Training in Occupational Therapy as the guide for inspections (Board of Management, 1931a). The AMA-CMEH began to survey occupational therapy training schools at the end of 1933 to consider Minimum Standards. Following this survey, the AMA-CMEH, in collaboration with AOTA, proposed new Mi nimum Standards. These standards were accepted in June 1935

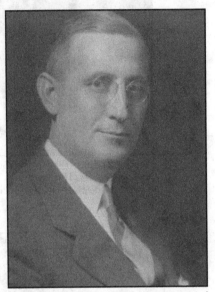

Figure 4-20. Dr. Joseph C. Doane served as president of the American Occupational Therapy Association from 1930 to 1938 during the time of the Great Depression. With his charming personality, Dr. Doane was skilled at presiding at meetings, and influencing ideas and opinions. (Printed with permission from the Archive of the American Occupational Therapy Association, Inc.)

as the "Essentials of an Acceptable School of Occupational Therapy" and published in the May 4, 1935; August 31, 1935; and August 29, 1936, editions of the Journal of the American Medical Association (Report of the Council on Medical Education and Hospitals, 1935). In addition to revision of admission and curricular requirements established by the Minimum Standards, the Essentials also set requirements for the program's organization, administration, resources, and faculty. It was recommended, but not required, that occupational therapy schools be affiliated with a college, university, or medical school. Faculty were required to be well trained and well qualified (Report of the Council on Medical Education and Hospitals, 1935, p. 1632). The AMA-CMEH wanted to publish a list of schools that met these standards by January 1939. Early publication of the Essentials provided time for schools to come into compliance with the new standards and allowed time to receive suggestions for any needed changes. The Essentials were revised in 1938, primarily for clarification and the addition of a section on clinical training standards (Board of Management, 1936b; Report on survey of occupational therapy schools, 1938).

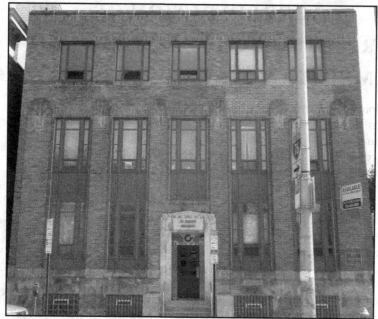

Figure 4-21. The old Philadelphia School of Occupational Therapy is listed on the U.S. National Register of Historic Places. Mrs. Pope Yeatman built the building specifically for the Philadelphia School in the early 1930s. The building was used until the late 1950s.

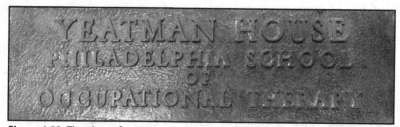

Figure 4-22. The plaque from Yeatman House. After completion of the new building for the Philadelphia School of Occupational Therapy, the old school building was used as a dormitory for the occupational therapy students. The dormitory was named the Yeatman House in honor of Mrs. Yeatman, a long-time supporter and President of the Board of Directors of the Philadelphia School. (Printed with permission from the Archive of the American Occupational Therapy Association, Inc.)

Five schools made the first list of approved schools published in the Journal of the American Medical Association in March 1938, including the Boston School of Occupational Therapy, the St. Louis School of Occupational and Recreational Therapy, the Philadelphia School of Occupational Therapy, the Department of Occupational Therapy at Milwaukee-Downer College, and the Department of University Extension at the University of Toronto. Kalamazoo State Hospital School of Occupational Therapy was given tentative approval (Report on survey of occupational therapy schools, 1938) and final approval in 1939 (Board of Management, 1939) (Figures 4-21 and 4-22).

Up until this time, graduation from a school that met the Minimum Standards for Courses of Training in Occupational Therapy was a requirement for admission to the National Register. With the move to accreditation of schools by the AMA-CMEH, graduation from an accredited school was now required for admission to the Register. To accommodate those who graduated prior to the

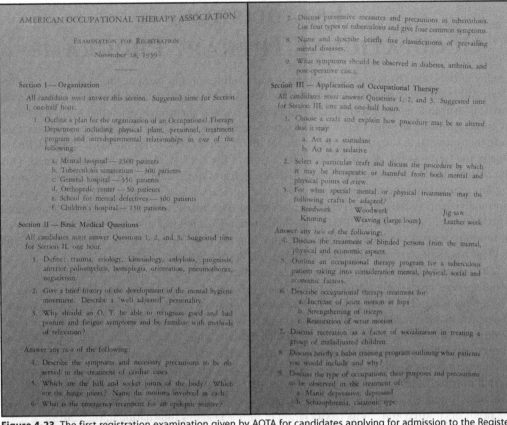

Figure 4-23. The first registration examination given by AOTA for candidates applying for admission to the Register based on training and experience. The application for registration was $10, and the examination fee was $10. Five dollars of the registration fee would be refunded if the candidate did not pass the examination. (Printed with permission from the Archive of the American Occupational Therapy Association, Inc.)

accreditation program, AOTA clarified that any occupational therapist in active in practice who graduated from a school that met the AOTA Minimum Standards at the time the student was in training was eligible for admission to the Register (Board of Management, 1936a).

The opportunity for occupational therapists to apply for admission to the Register based on training and experience ended on December 31, 1933. AOTA recognized that although many of these occupational therapists had missed the deadline, they were still qualified to practice. In this time of a manpower shortage, AOTA wanted to offer them one last chance to be admitted to the Register. A committee formed to devise a plan to allow admission to the Register recommended that these therapists take an examination to demonstrate their competence to engage in high standards of practice. A Board of Examiners was appointed to develop the examination (Admission to the Register by Examination, 1939; Lermit, Bartlett, & Naylor, 1938). More than 60 candidates applied to take this examination, which was given on November 18, 1939 (Board of Management, 1939) (Figure 4-23). Keeping in line with other medical and social professions, the planning committee also suggested that the Board of Examiners should, in the future, establish an examination that all candidates would be required to take to be admitted to the Register (Lermit et al., 1938).

ESTABLISHING
OCCUPATIONAL THERAPY PROGRAMS

One of the concerns of early practitioners was finding ways to fund occupational therapy services. Although the government covered the costs in military and veteran hospitals, there was no medical insurance to cover costs in civil hospitals. Hospitals themselves often had limited funding to cover operating expenses of occupational therapy services. Many community organizations were instrumental in the starting occupational therapy programs in hospitals and other facilities. One of the first was the Women's Auxiliary Board of the Presbyterian Hospital of Chicago. This Board provided the funds to hire Susan E. Tracy to travel to Chicago in 1917 to consult on starting an occupational therapy program. It was during Tracy's 5-month stay that the Presbyterian Hospital's occupational therapy program was started. The Board continued to fund the program as it grew (Bacon, 1932; Brainerd, 1932). The Presbyterian Hospital was just one example. A survey of community hospitals in New England indicated that many of the occupational therapy programs in those hospitals were also financed by ladies' auxiliaries (Adams, 1922).

The Junior League was another organization that helped to establish and maintain occupational therapy programs throughout the country. Inspired by the Settlement House movement, 19-year-old Mary Harriman, a New York debutante, founded the Junior League for the Promotion of Settlement Movements in 1901. Her goal was to organize an endless supply of volunteers from debutantes who would work to improve the social conditions in New York City, especially for immigrants. Her friend, a shy Eleanor Roosevelt, joined the New York Junior League as a volunteer in 1903, getting her first taste of public service by working for social justice. The Junior League idea started to spread throughout the United States, and in 1921, the Association of Junior Leagues of America was founded. Many of the Junior Leagues helped to establish health care facilities to meet the needs of children and adults (Association of Junior Leagues International, Inc., 2015).

The Junior League of the City of New York began doing occupational work with crippled children and other patients in hospitals including City Hospital, Bellevue Hospital, St. Luke's Hospital, and the Hospital for the Ruptured and Crippled starting in 1916. In 1917, the New York Junior League provided a course to train volunteers to help with occupation work in these hospitals. The Junior League funded salaries for two therapists in 1923 and for an additional therapist in 1929. A special committee, the Occupational Therapy Committee, was formed in 1931 to provide networking and educational opportunities for the occupational therapists and volunteers in New York City. The aim of this committee was to facilitate sharing of ideas and solving of common problems. From 1937 to 1940, the New York Junior League provided a training course to fill the need for trained volunteers in occupational therapy. In hard economic times and with limited budgets, these volunteers were trained to assist occupational therapists in their work. Volunteers participated in this course for 2 hours per week over the span of 3 months (Howard, 1939).

The Indianapolis Junior League provided funding to establish occupational therapy programs in the three Indiana University hospitals, including the general hospital, Coleman Hospital for Women, and Riley Hospital for Children in the 1920s. The Junior League earned the funds to support the occupational therapy programs through sales at gift shops, secondhand stores, and an annual entertainment event. The Indianapolis Junior League also facilitated and sponsored the first organizational meeting of the Indiana state society for occupational therapy (MacDonald, 1930).

There are many other examples of Junior Leagues helping to start occupational therapy programs. In addition to donating $5000 to help start the St. Louis School of Occupational Therapy (Medicine in St. Louis Hospital, 1919, p. 3), the Junior League of St. Louis started the Occupational Therapy Workshop in 1917 to help with the war relief effort (State Historical Society of Missouri, n.d.). In 1919, the Junior League of Milwaukee equipped and financed an occupational therapy department at Columbia Hospital in Milwaukee, which was directed by Hilda B. Goodman (Junior League of

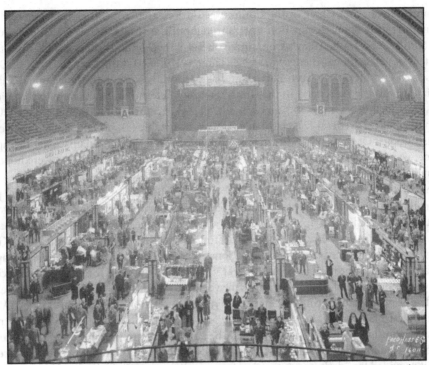

Figure 4-24. AOTA Exhibit Hall in 1932. The AHA played a significant role in encouraging hospitals to start occupational therapy programs. AOTA and AHA held joint conferences from 1922 through 1937. This arrangement allowed occupational therapists to exhibit photographs and provide live demonstrations at the conference so hospital administrators could see what occupational therapy did and discuss issues and concerns with therapists. (Printed with permission from the Archive of the American Occupational Therapy Association, Inc.)

Milwaukee, 1921; Phillips, 1928). The Junior League of Bridgeport, Connecticut, established an occupational therapy program at Bridgeport Hospital in the 1920s (Junior League of Eastern Fairfield County, 2015), and the Detroit Junior League started an occupational therapy program for those injured in the war. The goods made by disabled servicemen in Detroit were sold in the League shop (Gordon & Reische, 1982).

AOTA maintained a close relationship with the Junior Leagues. In the late 1920s, Junior Leagues in Albany, New York; Dayton, Ohio; Englewood, New Jersey; and Winnipeg, Canada, all requested information from AOTA on developing occupational therapy programs (Slagle, 1930). The support of the Junior League in developing, equipping, and funding occupational therapy programs throughout the United States has continued through the years (Figure 4-24).

PRACTICE AND RESEARCH

In pursuit of the Founding Vision, the Committee on Research and Efficiency was charged "to gather together information upon the subject of the effects of occupation upon the human being, and to keep in touch with the development of the work in the institutions in this country and abroad" (NSPOT, 1917). Despite the request of insurance companies for statistical evidence to justify payment, the lack of a sound scientific measure of improvement hindered research efforts (Editorial, 1923; House of Delegates, 1922). Much of the early research was exploratory and descriptive in nature.

George Barton, first Chair of the Committee on Research and Efficiency, collected information and literature about occupation work throughout the United States and the world (Barton, 1917). Similarly, Susan E. Tracy's Committee on Teaching Methods surveyed facilities to identify the extent of occupational therapy practice. Thomas Kidner, taking over as Chair of Committee on Research and Efficiency from Barton, and as part of his work with the National Tuberculosis Association, surveyed sanatoria in the United States to determine the extent of occupational therapy in these facilities. Of the 500 surveys sent, 122 were returned representing state (20), county (39), municipal (12), federal (7), charitable or semi-charitable (4), private (25), and miscellaneous (15) institutions. Of these, 37 indicated they provided some type of occupational therapy service (bedside, war, and/or classrooms/workshops). Many of the other institutions were hopeful about eventually providing occupational therapy (Kidner, 1920a).

In his role as Institutional Secretary of the National Tuberculosis Association, Kidner published a report that outlined plans for the building of modern sanatoria. In the report, he advocated for space to be allocated to occupational therapy activities, suggesting that an occupational therapy aide is needed for every 20 patients. In advocating for occupational therapy services, Kidner was among those who asserted that the prevocational services offered by occupational therapy should be covered under the provisions of the Federal Vocational Rehabilitation Act because occupational therapy was vital in preparing the patients for vocational education (Kidner, 1921, 1922a). Despite a number of people advocating for a more liberal interpretation, the Federal Board of Vocational Rehabilitation maintained the posture that vocational rehabilitation did not include mental or physical restoration "although such work may be a necessary preliminary to or accompaniment of vocational rehabilitation" (Cahn, 1924, p. 674) and occupational therapy was not a covered service except if provided for "definite preparation for a specific occupation" (Cahn, 1924, p. 673). Despite the fact that occupational therapy services were not covered under the Vocational Rehabilitation Act, Kidner was able to use his position with the National Tuberculosis Association to expand occupational therapy services in sanatoriums for those with tuberculosis.

The Association continued to gather information about the spread of occupational therapy to hospitals in the United States. In his 1931 Presidential Address, Dr. Joseph C. Doane provided statistics on the number of occupational therapists and the number of facilities providing occupational therapy services in the United States (Doane, 1931). Doane's report included numbers from 27 states. Doane indicated there were a total of 1287 occupational therapy workers (677 trained and 610 untrained) working in 383 hospitals, including 46 federal hospitals, 120 state hospitals, 48 county hospitals, 42 city hospitals, and 127 private hospitals. Included in these numbers were 163 mental hospitals, 72 facilities for tuberculous care, 90 general hospitals, 18 for orthopedic care, 16 for pediatric care, 13 for convalescent patients, and three correctional facilities (Doane, 1931). More than half of the hospitals in which occupational therapy services were provided were for mental health care and tuberculous care. Occupational therapists also worked with people with cardiac problems, industrial accident cases, children with cerebral palsy, the blind, crippled children, people with chronic diseases, and children with infantile paralysis (poliomyelitis).

The focus of Dr. Herbert Hall's research at his experimental workshop in Marblehead was on the design and use of wooden toy projects in the workshop. Hall was considering which wooden toy projects could be adapted to the needs of patients in various settings and would result in a product of such quality that it could be easily sold (Kidner, 1922b). This was in concert with Hall's belief that, although the process of participating in the project was important, the economic value obtained from selling a finished product was therapeutic.

Louis Haas, the Director of Men's Therapeutic Occupations at Bloomingdale's Hospital in White Plains, New York, also studied the adaptability of specific crafts such as basketry, chair caning, blacksmithing, cement work, weaving, jewelry making, and printing. Characteristics of these crafts, including the amount of physical exertion, coordination, and cognitive ability required, as well as the number of tools and precautions, were identified in the study. Haas also looked at the cost effectiveness of various crafts, considering such factors as the number of patients a therapist could supervise at one time when constructing projects, the cost of materials, and the value of the finished product. His department discontinued the use of certain crafts if they proved too difficult for patients, were not engaging, required excess staff time, or were too expensive (Haas, 1922). Dunton, in his series of articles on the economic study of crafts, provided a cost analysis as well as a description of characteristics of crafts (Dunton, 1925a, 1925b, 1926a, 1926b). The Committee on Installations and Advice followed with a series of articles that analyzed various craft activities (Robeson et al., 1928a, 1928b, 1928c). The research of Haas, Dunton, and the Committee on Installations and Advice formed the basis of what is now known as activity analysis.

RECONSTRUCTION AIDES AFTER WORLD WAR I

After World War I, in 1920, the reconstruction aides formed the World War Reconstruction Aides Association to maintain friendships made during their service, preserve the history of the reconstruction aides, and provide support (Figure 4-25). Many reconstruction aides continued in occupational therapy work and often attended the annual meetings. In 1925, two disabled reconstruction aides requested assistance to obtain hospitalization and compensation benefits from the federal government. In her role as Secretary-Treasurer, Mrs. Slagle wrote to the Surgeon General of the Army and the director of the Veterans' Bureau. Both responded, stating that the reconstruction aides in occupational therapy were hired by the Army as civilian employees and therefore were not covered by the War Risk Insurance Act. Only military employees were eligible for benefits (Board of Management, 1925). Through lobbying efforts of the reconstruction aides and other groups, the United States Congress amended the War Risk Insurance Act in 1926 to provide limited coverage for reconstruction aides who served in base hospitals overseas.

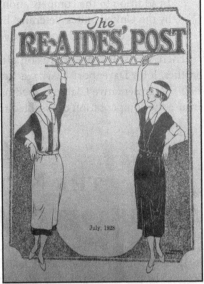

Figure 4-25. *Re-Aides' Post* was the official publication of the World War Reconstruction Aides Association. It was published from 1920 to 1950. The first issues from 1920 to 1926 were published as newspapers. Beginning in 1926, Re-Aides' Post was published as a small journal. On the cover were two figures dressed in working reconstruction aide uniforms: the one on the left represents occupational therapy and the one on the right represents physical therapy. The content addressed recollections of activities as reconstruction aides, updates on people's current lives, activities and meetings of the 14 units, and business activities of the Association. The journal was discontinued when the organization was disbanded in 1949. (Printed with permission from the Archive of the American Occupational Therapy Association, Inc.)

> For death or disability resulting from personal injury or disease contracted in the military or naval service on or after April 6, 1917, and before July 2, 1921, or for an aggravation or recurrence of a disability existing prior to examination, acceptance, and enrollment for service, when such aggravation was suffered or contracted in, or such recurrence was caused by, the military or naval service on or after April 6, 1917, and before July 2, 1921 … the United States shall pay to such commissioned officer or enlisted man, member of the Army Nurse Corps (female), or the Navy Nurse Corps (female), or women citizens of the United States who were taken … by the United States Government and who served in base hospitals overseas….

In addition to the compensation above provided, the injured person shall be provided by the United States Veterans' Bureau such reasonable governmental care or medical, surgical, dental and hospital services, etc. (Public Law 69-448)

There was still some confusion after this amendment passed, so Mrs. Slagle appealed to her brother, John Davenport Clarke, a Representative to the United States Congress (R-NY) (Slagle, 1929). Representative Clarke helped navigate through government channels to inquire about and ensure the compensation of disabled reconstruction aides (Clarke, 1929).

EFFECT OF THE NATIONAL ECONOMY ACT OF 1933 ON OCCUPATIONAL THERAPY

Franklin Delano Roosevelt, the Governor of New York, ran for President of the United States in 1932 with the promise to balance the federal budget. Shortly after taking office, he kept his promise by pushing legislation through Congress to slash the federal budget. This legislation, the National Economy Act, was passed on March 20, 1933. The purpose of this act was to reduce the federal deficit and maintain the credit of the United States. With passage of this act, government agencies were closed, and the salaries of civilian and federal workers were cut. Veterans' benefits, a significant part of the federal budget, were reduced by 50%. Specifically, Section 17 of the National Economy Act stated:

All public laws granting medical or hospital treatment, domiciliary care, compensation, and other allowances, pension, disability allowance, or retirement pay to veterans and the dependents of veterans of ... the World War ... are hereby repealed, and all laws granting or pertaining to yearly renewable term insurance are hereby repealed.

Effectively, the benefits provided by of the War Risk Insurance legislation were gutted. The services of occupational therapists, physical therapists, and dieticians were terminated when Veterans' Administration funds, authorized by the War Risk Insurance legislation, were no longer available.

In 1924, Walter Reed Hospital instituted a 6-month training course for occupational therapists to provide advanced training specific to military hospitals for graduates. The length of the program increased to 9 months in 1932. With the passage of the National Economy Act and severe budget cuts, the therapy departments and training programs at Walter Reed General Hospital closed (McDaniel, 1968, pp. 92-93). Robert Patterson, Surgeon General of the Army (1931 to 1935), spoke at the graduation of the last occupational therapy training class at Walter Reed, expressing "great regret at the temporary restrictions placed upon these courses of training at this hospital" (Patterson, 1933). The Act allowed the president to reestablish benefits at a later time through Executive Order. Courses resumed for physical therapists and dieticians in 1934, but not for occupational therapists (McDaniel, 1968, p. 93).

Some military programs had experienced severe cuts or had been closed due to economic reasons prior to the Great Depression. Fort Sam Houston and Brooke General Hospital discontinued their occupational therapy programs in 1926 because of financial concerns. The general and neuropsychiatric clinics at Fitzsimons General Hospital in Denver closed in June of 1933, reopening in 1934 on a very limited basis. The Army and Navy General Hospital occupational therapy programs in Hot Springs, Arkansas, noted for treatment of arthritis, closed in 1936. Also in 1936, Letterman General Hospital in San Francisco experienced severe cuts and reduced personnel and programs (McDaniel, 1968, pp. 95-96).

MILITARY STATUS FOR
OCCUPATIONAL THERAPISTS

In 1931, the supervisors of occupational therapists (Miss Alberta Montgomery), dieticians (Miss Grace H. Hunter), and physical therapists (Miss Emma Vogel) at Walter Reed General Hospital recommended to upgrade the professional status and increase salaries for the civilian Army personnel whom they supervised. The professional status and salaries of civilian Army personnel had not changed since World War I. Seeking the same professional status and benefits accorded to nurses, these three supervisors recommended the establishment of a Medical Auxiliary Corp, similar to the Army Nurse Corps (Vogel & Gearin, 1968, p. 3). The Army did not follow the recommendation, indicating that the economic conditions of the Great Depression would not allow it.

In 1937, United States Representative Carl Vinson (D-GA) requested the Surgeon General to consider commissioned military status for physical therapists. The Surgeon General indicated that military status would not be granted to physical therapists, nor to dieticians or occupational therapists with whom they were on par. The Surgeon General also indicated that these groups would not be afforded military status because they would not have to enter a war zone (Vogel & Gearin, 1968, pp. 4-5).

Senator Morris Sheppard (D-TX) introduced a bill in 1939 to afford military status to female occupational therapy aides, physical therapy aides, and dieticians. The Surgeon General supported military status for physical therapy aides and dieticians. The Secretary of War concurred. The bill did not pass because of economic reasons but was reintroduced excluding occupational therapy aides from the language of the bill. Undeterred, Senator Sheppard reintroduced the bill in 1940 and again 1941 (Vogel & Gearin, 1968, pp. 5-6). In an effort to include occupational therapy in these bills, AOTA President Everett S. Elwood (1939 to 1947) attempted to gain the support of the Surgeon General James C. Magee (1939 to 1943). Magee indicated that it was "undesirable" to include occupational therapy aides because just nine were employed in military hospitals. Of these, six served Veterans Administration patients, two served Civilian Conservation Corps patients, and only one served military patients (Magee, 1940).

Persisting in efforts to include occupational therapy in this legislation, the occupational therapy community mobilized. AOTA House of Delegates passed a resolution justifying military status for occupational therapy aides and requesting support. Marjorie Fish, Speaker of the House of Delegates, forwarded the resolution to the Chairman of the American Red Cross, the Secretary of War, the Surgeon General, and Senator Morris (Fish, 1940). State associations and individuals petitioned and wrote to the congressional committee members considering this legislation and to their U.S. Congressmen. Mrs. John Greene (Marjorie), Director of the Boston School of Occupational Therapy, called on personal contacts in power. She wrote to U.S. Representative Richard Wigglesworth, who had helped with the incorporation of the Boston School of Occupational Therapy years before (Greene, 1940). Representative Wigglesworth was the brother of Ruth Wigglesworth (Whitney), Mrs. Greene's former codirector at the Boston School. He forwarded her letter, which explained the development of occupational therapy as a profession since World War I, including increased educational standards and wider acceptance in civilian hospitals (Wigglesworth, 1940). Unfortunately, both attempts to pass Senator Sheppard's legislation to achieve military status for any of the groups was still unsuccessful (Vogel & Gearin, 1968, pp. 5-6).

TESTIMONIAL BANQUET
TO HONOR
ELEANOR CLARK SLAGLE

GIVEN BY THE AMERICAN OCCUPATIONAL THERAPY ASSOCIATION
AT THE HOTEL CHELSEA, ATLANTIC CITY, NEW JERSEY
TUESDAY, SEPTEMBER FOURTEENTH, NINETEEN HUNDRED AND THIRTY-SEVEN

SPEAKERS

JOSEPH C. DOANE, M. D.
PRESIDENT,
AMERICAN OCCUPATIONAL THERAPY ASSOCIATION
PRESIDING

ADOLPH MEYER, M. D.
DIRECTOR, HENRY PHIPPS CLINIC,
JOHN HOPKINS UNIVERSITY HOSPITAL

FREDERICK W. PARSONS, M. D.
COMMISSIONER OF MENTAL HYGIENE
STATE OF NEW YORK

MRS. FRANKLIN DELANO ROOSEVELT

Figure 4-26. (A-C) A testimonial banquet was held at the 1937 AOTA conference in Atlantic City, New Jersey, in honor of Eleanor Clarke Slagle's retirement. (Printed with permission from the Archive of the American Occupational Therapy Association, Inc.)

MENU

FRUIT CUP

QUEEN OLIVES   HEARTS OF CELERY   SWEET PICKLES

CREAM OF TOMATO SOUP

ROAST MARYLAND TURKEY
STUFFING   GIBLET GRAVY
CRANBERRY JELLY
VEGETABLES   CANDIED SWEETS

TOMATO AND LETTUCE SALAD
FRENCH DRESSING

LEMON PIE A LA CHELSEA

DEMI TASSE

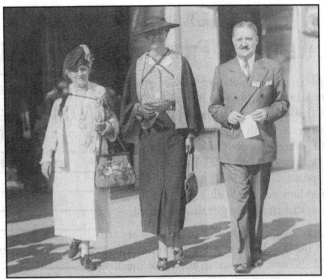

Figure 4-27. Eleanor Clarke Slagle, Eleanor Roosevelt, and Edgar C. Hayhow (a well-known health care administrator and 14th Chairman of the American College of Healthcare Executives) on the boardwalk at the Atlantic City conference in 1937. (Courtesy of the New York State Historical Association Library, Cooperstown, New York, John Davenport Clarke Papers, Coll. No. 12, Box 7.)

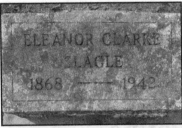

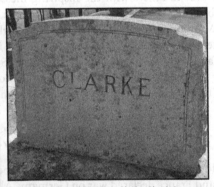

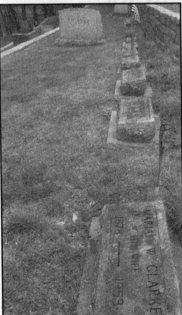

Figure 4-28. (A) Eleanor Clarke Slagle's gravestone in the family plot in Locust Hill Cemetery located in Hobart, New York. Note that the birthdate is inaccurate. Although documents such as census records, church records, and ship passenger lists are inconsistent identifying Slagle's birth year, she was most likely born in 1870. (B) The Clarke family main headstone. (C) The Clarke family plot. Eleanor Clarke Slagle's gravestone is third from the bottom. (Reprinted with permission from Lorna Puleo.)

SLAGLE RESIGNS AS SECRETARY-TREASURER OF AOTA

Slagle resigned from her position as Secretary-Treasurer of AOTA in 1937. She was honored by the Association later that year at the annual meeting in Atlantic City, New Jersey, with a testimonial banquet. Adolf Meyer and Eleanor Roosevelt paid tribute to her at the banquet (Figures 4-26 and 4-27). Having served in this volunteer position since 1921, her friends and AOTA membership honored her with a gift of $2000, a substantial sum at that time. The gift was inscribed:

Table 4-1 AOTA MEMBERSHIP DATA— 1920 TO 1940	
YEAR	NUMBER OF MEMBERS
1920	190
1925	749
1930	883
1935	831
1940	1,207

> Eleanor Clarke Slagle – She has been the corner stone in the development and promotion of occupational therapy. Now we in turn ask that she accept our gift as the corner stone of her new home which we hope will be the place of rest and happiness and release from the arduous duties. We offer it with deep affection and profound gratitude for her twenty-one years of untiring service in our behalf. (Pollock, 1942)

Proud of her service as a founder and officer who help to build the profession, Slagle turned the work over to others with the inspiring message, "The integrity of the profession is in your hands. I bid you Godspeed in your work" (Slagle, 1937). Slagle purchased her new country home, Philipse Manor, in Westchester County, New York. She continued to work for the New York State Department of Mental Hygiene until her death in 1942 (Editorial, 1942; Pollock, 1942) (Figure 4-28). Maud Plummer was named Executive Secretary, taking over many of Slagle's duties. Plummer resigned at the end of 1937. Meta R. Cobb was hired as the Executive Secretary, a paid position, to replace Miss Plummer (Board of Management, 1938).

WAR CLOUDS

War clouds were once again looming in Europe. In September 1939, Germany invaded Poland. England and France declared war on Germany. Although the United States maintained neutrality, President Roosevelt declared a limited national emergency on September 8, 1939. The decrease in funding post-World War I, the economic situation caused by the Great Depression, and the lull of peacetime made America ill prepared for war. Supplies, equipment, and facilities were limited, in poor condition, and outdated. The ranks of the civilian personnel serving in the military, including occupational therapists, physical therapists, and dieticians, were very limited (Table 4-1). AOTA began to organize to promote occupational therapy in the war effort.

REFLECTION

The dedicated and tireless efforts of the leaders of occupational therapy advanced the professional status of the profession. Over the decades of the 1920s and 1930s, Minimum Standards for Courses of Training in Occupational Therapy had been established and revised to continually advance high standards. Next, the National Register was established to provide for enforcement of standards, allowing admission only to those who met high standards of graduation from an approved school and 1 year of experience. Finally, at the request of AOTA, the AMA accepted responsibility for the inspection and accreditation of training schools to ensure the high standards of the profession. AOTA actively sought the sponsorship of the medical profession, a larger and more powerful organization, to obtain the benefits of their manpower and expertise and to gain recognition and status; however, this arrangement also allowed the medical profession more control of occupational therapy and further tied the profession to the medical model.

Whereas World War I had provided momentum for the growth of the profession, the end of the war brought a decreased need for occupational therapists in military hospitals. The poor economic situation in the late 1920s significantly reduced the number of occupational therapists working with military patients because the military looked to eliminate unnecessary expense. The military considered occupational therapists to be expendable. Lacking professional status and recognition, the role of occupational therapy in the military had been virtually eliminated by the start of World War II.

REFERENCES

Adams, J. D. (1922). The training of the occupational aide. *Archives of Occupational Therapy, 1*(3), 187-192.

Admission to the Register by Examination. (1939, February). *Occupational Therapy and Rehabilitation, 18*(1), 61-62.

American Occupational Therapy Association. (1924). Minimum standards for courses of training in occupational therapy. *Archives of Occupational Therapy, 3*(4), 295-298.

American Occupational Therapy Association. (1932). 1932 national directory of qualified occupational therapists enrolled in 1931 in the National Register. New York, NY: Author.

American Occupational Therapy Association. (1938). Constitution. *Occupational Therapy & Rehabilitation, 17*(6), 439-442.

American Occupational Therapy Association. (1940). Minutes of the business session, September 16, 1940. Archives of the American Occupational Therapy Association (Series 3, Box 13, Folder 84), Bethesda, MD.

American Occupational Therapy Association. (1967a). 50th Anniversary: Occupational therapy—Then...1917 and now...1967. New York, NY: Author.

American Occupational Therapy Association. (1967b). Presidents of the American Occupational Therapy Association. *American Journal of Occupational Therapy, 21*(5), 290-298.

American Occupational Therapy Association. (1921). American Occupational Therapy Association is New Name, *Modern Hospital, 17*(6), 554.

Association of Junior Leagues International, Inc. (2015). Founder Mary Harriman: A spirited reformer ahead of her time. Retrieved from https://www.ajli.org/

Bacon, A. S. (1932). The place of occupational therapy in the Presbyterian Hospital of Chicago, Illinois. *Occupational Therapy and Rehabilitation, 11*(1), 31.

Barton, G. E. (1917). Report of the Committee on Research and Efficiency. In Proceedings of the First Annual Meeting of the National Society for the Promotion of Occupational Therapy (pp. 24-27). Towson, MD: Spring Grove State Hospital and the Sheppard Hospital Press.

Bing, R. K. (1961). William Rush Dunton, Junior—American psychiatrist, a study in self (Doctoral dissertation). College, Park, MD: University of Maryland.

Board of Management. (1923, June 9). Minutes of the meeting of Board of Managers. Archives of the American Occupational Therapy Association (Series 3, Box 13, Folder 80), Bethesda, MD.

Board of Management. (1925). Disabled ex-service O.T. Aides. Minutes of the meeting of Board of Managers. Archives of the American Occupational Therapy Association (Series 3, Box 13, Folder 80), Bethesda, MD.

Board of Management. (1926a, September 26). Headquarters office. Minutes of the meeting of Board of Managers. Archives of the American Occupational Therapy Association (Series 3, Box 13, Folder 81), Bethesda, MD.

Board of Management. (1926b, September 26). Pledge and Creed. Minutes of the meeting of Board of Managers. Archives of the American Occupational Therapy Association (Series 3, Box 13, Folder 81), Bethesda, MD.

Board of Management. (1927, October 9). Minutes of the Board of Managers. Archives of the American Occupational Therapy Association (Series 3, Box 13, Folder 81), Bethesda, MD.

Board of Management. (1928, August 5). Minutes of the Board of Managers. Archives of the American Occupational Therapy Association (Series 3, Box 13, Folder 81), Bethesda, MD.

Board of Management. (1929, January 7). Minutes of the Board of Managers. Archives of the American Occupational Therapy Association (Series 3, Box 13, Folder 81), Bethesda, MD.

Board of Management. (1931a, January 3). Minutes of the Board of Management. Archives of the American Occupational Therapy Association (Series 3, Box 13, Folder 82), Bethesda, MD.

Board of Management. (1931b, September 28). Minutes of the Board of Managers. Archives of the American Occupational Therapy Association (Series 3, Box 13, Folder 82), Bethesda, MD.

Board of Management. (1936a, January 11). Minutes of the Board of Management. Archives of the American Occupational Therapy Association (Series 3, Box 13, Folder 83), Bethesda, MD.

Board of Management. (1936b, January 20). Minutes of the Board of Management. Archives of the American Occupational Therapy Association (Series 3, Box 13, Folder 83), Bethesda, MD.

Board of Management. (1938, January 3). Minutes of the Board of Managers. Archives of the American Occupational Therapy Association (Series 3, Box 13, Folder 84), Bethesda, MD.

Board of Management. (1939). Minutes of the Board of Managers. Occupational Therapy and Rehabilitation, 18(6), 399-410.

Brackett, E. G. (1922). Scope of occupational therapy and requirements for the training of occupational aides. *Archives of Occupational Therapy, 1*(3), 179-185.

Brainerd, W. (1932). The evolution of an occupational therapy department in a general hospital. *Occupational Therapy and Rehabilitation, 11*(1), 33-40.

Cahn, R. D. (1924, December). Civilian vocational rehabilitation. Journal of Political Economy, 32(6), 665-689.

Cameron, R. G. (1915, December). Occupational therapy. *Trained Nurse and Hospital Review, 55*(6), 342-345.

Cameron, R. G. (1917, January). An interview with Miss Susan Tracy. *Maryland Psychiatric Quarterly, 6*(3), 65-66.

Clarke, J. D. (1929). Personal correspondence to Eleanor Clarke Slagle on March 25, 1929. Archives of the American Occupational Therapy Association (Series 5, Box 24, Folder 161), Bethesda, MD.

Committee on Admissions and Positions. (1918). Report of the Committee on Admissions and Positions. In Proceedings of the Second Annual Meeting of the National Society for the Promotion of Occupational Therapy (pp. 18-19). Towson, MD: Sheppard and Enoch Pratt Hospital.

Committee on Admissions and Positions. (1919). Report of the Committee on Admissions and Positions. In Proceedings of the Third Annual Meeting of the National Society for the Promotion of Occupational Therapy (pp. 16-25). Towson, MD: Sheppard and Enoch Pratt Hospital.

Committee on Admissions and Positions. (1922). The Fifth Annual Meeting of the National Society for the Promotion of Occupational Therapy: Report of the Committee on Admissions and Positions. *Archives of Occupational Therapy, 1*(1), 74-76.

Committee on Publicity and Publications. (1922). Report of the Committee on Publicity and Publications: First Day—Morning Session. Proceedings of the Fifth Annual Meeting of AOTA. *Archives of Occupational Therapy, 1*(1), 64-66.

Committee on Publicity and Publications. (1925). Report of the Committee on Publicity and Publications in Minutes of the Ninth Annual Meeting of the American Occupational Therapy Association. *Occupational Therapy and Rehabilitation, 4*(6), 470-471.

Committee on Teaching Methods. (1917). Report of the Committee on Teaching Methods. In Proceedings of the First Annual Meeting of the National Society for the Promotion of Occupational Therapy (pp. 34-41). Towson, MD: Spring Grove State Hospital and Sheppard and Enoch Pratt Hospital.

Committee on Teaching Methods. (1918). Report of the Committee on Teaching Methods. In Proceedings of the Second Annual Meeting of the National Society for the Promotion of Occupational Therapy (pp. 20-25). Towson, MD: Sheppard and Enoch Pratt Hospital.

Committee on Teaching Methods. (1919). Report of the Committee on Teaching Methods. In Proceedings of the Third Annual Meeting of the National Society for the Promotion of Occupational Therapy (pp. 29-35). Towson, MD: Sheppard and Enoch Pratt Hospital.

Committee on Teaching Methods. (1922). The Sixth Annual Meeting of the National Society for the Promotion of Occupational Therapy: Report of Committee on Teaching Methods. *Archives of Occupational Therapy, 2*(1), 63-65.

Doane, J. C. (1931). Presidential address. *Occupational Therapy and Rehabilitation, 10*, 363-368.

Dunton, W. R. (1918). Principles of occupational therapy. In Proceedings of the Second Annual Meeting of the National Society for the Promotion of Occupational Therapy (pp. 26-30). Towson, MD: Spring Grove State Hospital and Sheppard and Enoch Pratt Hospital.

Dunton, W. R. (1919a). N.S.P.O.T. *Maryland Psychiatric Quarterly, 8*(3), 68-74.

Dunton, W. R. (1919b). *Reconstruction therapy.* Philadelphia, PA: W. B. Saunders Company.

Dunton, W. R. (1925a). Economic studies of crafts. I. Upholstery. *Occupational Therapy & Rehabilitation, 4*(3), 219-222.

Dunton, W. R. (1925b). Economic studies of crafts. II. Metal Work; III. Woodwork; IV. Toy making. *Occupational Therapy and Rehabilitation, 4*(6), 441-446.

Dunton, W. R. (1925c). Editorial. *Occupational Therapy and Rehabilitation, 4*(3), 227-228.

Dunton, W. R. (1926a). Economic studies of crafts, V. Chip Carving, VI. Domestic Crafts, VII. Crocheting, VIII. Miscellaneous (Women). IX Specials, X. Disturbed Women, XI. Basketry, XII. Pine Needle Basketry, XIII. Raffia Basketry. *Occupational Therapy and Rehabilitation, 5*(2), 135-142.

Dunton, W. R. (1926b). Economic studies of crafts: XIV. Weaving; XV, Leather; XVI Bookbinding; XVII. Batik; XVIII. Block Printing; XIX Miscellaneous (men); XX Painting; XXI. Sealing Wax. *Occupational Therapy and Rehabilitation, 5*(4), 293-308.

Dunton, W. R. (1955, June 2). [Letter to Mrs. Frances Shuff]. Archives of the American Occupational Therapy Association (Series 6, Box 47, Folder 320), Bethesda, MD.

Editor. (1922). Leisure and idleness. *Modern Hospital, 18*(2), 188.

Editorial. (1922a). *Archives of Occupational Therapy, 1*(1), 87.

Editorial. (1922b). The sixth annual meeting. *Archives of Occupational Therapy, 1*(5), 419-427.

Editorial. (1923). The need for research. *Archives of Occupational Therapy, 2*(3), 249-250.

Editorial. (1942). Eleanor Clarke Slagle memorial. *Occupational Therapy and Rehabilitation, 21*(5), 373-374.

Editorial. (1946). *Occupational Therapy and Rehabilitation, 25*(6), 267-268.

Elwood, E. S. (1927). The National Board of Medical Examiners and Medical Education, and the possible effect of the Board's program on the spread of occupational therapy. *Occupational Therapy and Rehabilitation, 6*(5), 341-348.

First Day—Afternoon Session. (1920). In Proceedings of the Fourth Annual Meeting of the National Society for the Promotion of Occupational Therapy (pp. 27-39). Towson, MD: Spring Grove State Hospital and Sheppard and Enoch Pratt Hospital.

First Day—Morning Session. (1922). Proceedings of the Fifth Annual Meeting of AOTA. *Archives of Occupational Therapy, 1*(1), 51-64.

Fish, M. (1940). Memo to Chairman of the American Red Cross Mr. Norman H. Davis, Secretary of War Henry L. Stimson, Surgeon General James C. Magee, Senator Morris Sheppard on December 12, 1940. Archives of the American Occupational Therapy Association (Series 4.1, Box 25, Folder 168), Bethesda, MD.

Forbush, B., & Forbush, B. (1986). *Gatehouse: The evolution of the Sheppard and Enoch Pratt Hospital, 1853-1986.* Baltimore, MD: J. B. Lippincott, Co.

Former Hobart Girl honored. (1931, January 8). *Stamford Mirror-Recorder* [New York]. Retrieved from http://www.fultonhistory.com/Fulton.html

Gordon, J., & Reische, D. (1982). *The volunteer powerhouse.* New York: The Rutledge Press.

Greene, M. B. (1924). Personal correspondence to Thomas B. Kidner on December 8, 1924 [Letter]. Archives of the American Occupational Therapy Association (Series 5, Box 23, Folder 155), Bethesda, MD.

Greene, M. A. (1940). Personal correspondence to Honorable Richard Wigglesworth on March 28, 1940 [Letter]. Archives of the American Occupational Therapy Association (Series 5, Box 25, Folder 168), Bethesda, MD.

Haas, L. J. (1920). Report of the secretary. In Proceedings of the Fourth Annual Meeting of the National Society for the Promotion of Occupational Therapy (pp. 3-4). Towson, MD: Spring Grove State Hospital and Sheppard and Enoch Pratt Hospital.

Haas, L. J. (1922). Crafts adaptable to occupational needs: Their relative importance. *Archives of Occupational Therapy, 1*(6), 443-455.

Hall, H. J. (1921, July). A remodeled constitution. *Maryland Psychiatric Quarterly, 11*(1), 18-19.

Hall, H. J. (1922). Editorial: The medical workshop. *Archives of Occupational Therapy, 1*(3), 243-246.

House of Delegates. (1922). Meeting of the Board Members and the House of Delegates of the American Occupational Therapy Association. *Archives of Occupational Therapy, 1*(4), 317-355.

Howard, F. M. (1939, December). Growth of the Occupational Therapy Committee of the Junior League of the City of New York. *Occupational Therapy and Rehabilitation, 18*(6), 395-398.

Johnson, S. C. (1917). The teacher in occupation therapy. In Proceedings of the First Annual Meeting of the National Society for the Promotion of Occupational Therapy (pp. 45-51). Towson, MD: Spring Grove State Hospital and Sheppard and Enoch Pratt Hospital.

Johnson, S. C. (1918). Educational Aspects of Occupation Therapy. In Proceedings of the Second Annual Meeting of the National Society for the Promotion of Occupational Therapy (pp. 44-49). Towson, MD: Spring Grove State Hospital and Sheppard and Enoch Pratt Hospital.

Jones, J. L. (1992). Therefore be it resolved: 25 years of delegate assembly/representative assembly legislation. *American Journal of Occupational Therapy, 46*(1), 72-78.

Junior League of Eastern Fairfield County. (2015). Our history: Serving the community for over 90 years. Retrieved from https://www.jlefc.org/?nd=history

Junior League of Milwaukee. (1921). Annual Report of the Junior League of Milwaukee 1917-1921. Milwaukee, WI: Junior League of Milwaukee.

Kelley, F. F. (1926, August 15). Busy hands help sickened minds: New therapy methods correct maladies by teaching patients to make things. *New York Times*, p. X6.

Kidner, T. B. (1920a). Report of the Committee on Research and Efficiency. In Proceedings of the Fourth Annual Meeting of the National Society for the Promotion of Occupational Therapy (pp. 5-9). Towson, MD: Spring Grove State Hospital and the Sheppard and Enoch Pratt Hospital.

Kidner, T. B. (1920b). Report of the Committee on the Revision of the Constitution. In Proceedings of the Fourth Annual Meeting of the National Society for the Promotion of Occupational Therapy (pp. 24-25). Towson, MD: Spring Grove State Hospital and Sheppard and Enoch Pratt Hospital.

Kidner, T. B. (1921, June 17). Notes on tuberculosis sanatorium planning. *Public Health Reports, 36*(24), 1371-1392.

Kidner, T. B. (1922a). Editorial: American Occupational Therapy Association. *Archives of Occupational Therapy, 1*(6), 499-502.

Kidner, T. B. (1922b). Report of the Committee on Research and Efficiency: The Fifth Annual Meeting of the National Society for the Promotion of Occupational Therapy. *Archives of Occupational Therapy, 1*(1), 76-78.

Kidner, T. B. (1925, November 14). Memo: The members of the Board of Management. Archives of the American Occupational Therapy Association (Series 3, Box 13, Folder 80), Bethesda, MD.

Kidner, T. B. (1928). Professional training in occupational therapy. *Psychiatric Quarterly, 2*(2), 184-188.

Kidner, T. B. (1930). The progress of occupational therapy. *Occupational Therapy and Rehabilitation, 9,* 221-224.

Lermit, G. R., Bartlett, K., & Naylor, C. (1938, June). Report of Committee for the study of plan for admission of therapists to the register by means of examination. *Occupational Therapy and Rehabilitation, 17*(3), 179-180.

MacDonald, J. H. (1930). Curative occupational therapy as conducted by the Junior League of Indianapolis in the Indiana University Hospitals. *Occupational Therapy and Rehabilitation, 10*(1), 39-44.

Magee, J. C. (1940). Personal correspondence to Everett S. Elwood on April 1, 1940. Archives of the American Occupational Therapy Association (Series 4.1, Box 25, Folder 168), Bethesda, MD.

McDaniel, M. L. (1968). Occupational therapists before World War II (1917-1940). In R. S. Anderson, H. S. Lee, & M. L. McDaniel (Eds.), *Army Medical Specialist Corps* (pp. 69-97). Washington, DC: Office of the Surgeon General, Department of the Army.

Medicine in St. Louis Hospital. (1919, February 16). *St. Louis Post-Dispatch,* pp. 3, 13.

National Society for the Promotion of Occupational Therapy. (1917). Constitution of the National Society for the Promotion of Occupational Therapy. Towson, MD: Sheppard Hospital Press.

National Society for the Promotion of Occupational Therapy. (1919). Report of the nominating committee. In Proceedings of the Third Annual Meeting of the National Society for the Promotion of Occupational Therapy (pp. 35-36). Towson, MD: Sheppard and Enoch Pratt Hospital.

National Society for the Promotion of Occupational Therapy. (1920a). Address by President-elect Dr. Herbert J. Hall. In Proceedings of the Fourth Annual Meeting of the National Society for the Promotion of Occupational Therapy (p. 39). Towson, MD: Spring Grove State Hospital and Sheppard and Enoch Pratt Hospital.

National Society for the Promotion of Occupational Therapy. (1920b). A general discussion on training of teachers. In Proceedings of the Fourth Annual Meeting of the National Society for the Promotion of Occupational Therapy (pp. 51-62). Towson, MD: Spring Grove State Hospital and Sheppard and Enoch Pratt Hospital.

National Society for the Promotion of Occupational Therapy. (1920c). Report of the nominating committee. In Proceedings of the Fourth Annual Meeting of the National Society for the Promotion of Occupational Therapy (pp. 25-26). Towson, MD: Spring Grove State Hospital and Sheppard and Enoch Pratt Hospital.

New Minimum Standards... (1930, October). New minimum Standards of Training for occupational therapists who desire to qualify for registration. Archives of the American Occupational Therapy Association (Series 3, Box 13, Folder 81), Bethesda, MD.

Occupational Therapy Notes. (1932, April). Obituary—Susan C. Johnson. Occupational Therapy and Rehabilitation, 11(2) 152-153.

Patterson, R. U. (1933, December). Remarks to the graduating classes of dieticians, physiotherapy aides, and occupational therapy aides at the Army Medical Center, June 29, 1933. *Occupational Therapy and Rehabilitation, 12*(6), 365-371.

Pattison, H. A. (1922). The trend of occupational therapy for the tuberculous. *Archives of Occupational Therapy, 1*(1), 19-24.

Phillips, R. F. (1928, August). The Junior League's occupational therapy work for children in Milwaukee: Organization and Financing. *Occupational Therapy & Rehabilitation, 7*(4), 261-266.

Pollock, H. M. (1942). In Memoriam: Eleanor Clarke Slagle—1876-1942. *American Journal of Psychiatry, 99*(3), 472-474.

Presbyterian Hospital of Chicago. (1929, June). Susan E. Tracy. In The Presbyterian Hospital Bulletin—No. 68 (pp. 4-6). Chicago, IL: The Presbyterian Hospital of Chicago.

Quiroga, V. A. M. (1995). *Occupational therapy: The first 30 years: 1900 to 1930.* Bethesda, MD: American Occupational Therapy Association.

Report of the Council on Medical Education and Hospitals. (1935). *Journal of the American Medical Association, 104,* 1631-1633.

Report of Secretary-Treasurer. (1922). Minutes of the Sixth Annual Meeting of the American Occupational Therapy Association. *Archives of Occupational Therapy, 2*(1), 49-59.

Report on survey of occupational therapy schools. (1938). *Journal of the American Medical Association, 110*, 979-981.

Robeson, H. A., Dunton, W. R., Haas, L. J., Kidner, T. B., Lindberg, B., Sample, G....Tompkins, A. B. (1928a). Analysis of crafts: Continuation of the report of Committee on Installations and Advice. *Occupational Therapy and Rehabilitation, 7*(2), 131-136.

Robeson, H. A., Dunton, W. R., Haas, L. J., Kidner, T. B., Lindberg, B., Sample, G.,...Tompkins, A. B. (1928b). Analysis of crafts: Continuation of the report of Committee on Installations and Advice. *Occupational Therapy and Rehabilitation, 7*(3), 211-216.

Robeson, H. A., Dunton, W. R., Haas, L. J., Kidner, T. B., Lindberg, B., Sample, G.,...Tompkins, A. B. (1928c). Report of Committee on Installations and Advice: Making a physical analysis of crafts. *Occupational Therapy and Rehabilitation, 7*(1), 29-43.

Round Table on Training Courses. (1923). Round table on training courses. *Archives of Occupational Therapy, 2*(2), 119 -132.

Second Day—Afternoon Session. (1922). Proceedings of the Fifth Annual Meeting of AOTA. *Archives of Occupational Therapy, 1*(3), 219-242.

Second Day—Morning Session. (1922). Proceedings of the Fifth Annual Meeting of AOTA. *Archives of Occupational Therapy, 1*(1), 153-162.

Slagle, E. C. (1918). Report of the Committee on Installations and Advice. In Proceedings of the First Annual Meeting of the National Society for the Promotion of Occupational Therapy (p. 28). Towson, MD: Spring Grove State Hospital and Sheppard and Enoch Pratt Hospital.

Slagle, E. C. (1919). Report of the Committee on Installations and Advice. In Proceedings of the Third Annual Meeting of the National Society for the Promotion of Occupational Therapy (pp. 26-28). Towson, MD: Spring Grove State Hospital and Sheppard and Enoch Pratt Hospital.

Slagle, E. C. (1920a). Report of the Committee on Installations and Advice. In Proceedings of the Fourth Annual Meeting of the National Society for the Promotion of Occupational Therapy (p. 22). Towson, MD: Spring Grove State Hospital and Sheppard and Enoch Pratt Hospital.

Slagle, E. C. (1920b). Report of the president. In Proceedings of the Fourth Annual Meeting of the National Society for the Promotion of Occupational Therapy (pp. 1-3). Towson, MD: Spring Grove State Hospital and Sheppard and Enoch Pratt Hospital.

Slagle, E. C. (1929). Personal correspondence to John D. Clarke on February 15, 1929. Archives of the American Occupational Therapy Association (Series 5, Box 24, Folder 161), Bethesda, MD.

Slagle, E. C. (1930). Report of the secretary-treasurer. *Occupational Therapy and Rehabilitation, 9*(6),379-393.

Slagle, E. C. (1937). Editorial: From the heart. Occupational Therapy and Rehabilitation, 16(5), 343-345.

State Historical Society of Missouri. (n.d.). The Junior League of St. Louis, Records, 1914-2000. Retrieved from http://shs.umsystem.edu/stlouis/manuscripts/s0628.pdf

Third Day—Morning Session. (1922). The Fifth Annual Meeting of the National Society for the Promotion of Occupational Therapy. *Archives of Occupational Therapy, 1*(3), 221-230.

Tracy, S. E. (1917). Personal correspondence to William Rush Dunton on April 22, 1917. Archives of the American Occupational Therapy Association (Series 1, Box 1, Folder 21b), Bethesda, MD.

United States Department of the Interior National Park Service. (2003). National register of historic places registration form: Philadelphia School of Occupational Therapy. Washington, DC: Author.

Vogel, E. E., & Gearin, H. B. (1968). Events leading to the formation of the Women's Medical Specialist Corps. In R. S. Anderson, H. S. Lee, & M. L. McDaniel (Eds.), Army Medical Specialist Corps (pp. 1-11). Washington, DC: Office of the Surgeon General, Department of the Army.

Wigglesworth, R. B. (1940). Personal correspondence to Mrs. John (Marjorie) A. Greene on March 29, 1940 [Letter]. Archives of the American Occupational Therapy Association (Series 5, Box 25, Folder 168), Bethesda, MD.

5

Rapid Growth and Expansion
1940s to 1960s

Key Points

- Occupational therapy needed to reestablish its role in the military after an economic decline and setbacks during the Depression years.
- The Women's Medical Specialist Corps, established in 1947, granted military status to occupational therapists.
- Manpower shortages spurred the increase in the number of occupational therapy schools, the start of war emergency courses, and the establishment of a curriculum for occupational therapy assistants.
- With the end of the Arts and Crafts Movement and medicine's focus on a biomedical model, occupational therapy shifted from a paradigm of occupation to reductionism

Highlighted Personalities

- Winifred Conrick Kahmann, OTR, President, 1947-1952
- Henrietta McNary, OTR, President, 1952-1955
- Ruth A. Robinson, OTR, President, 1955-1958
- Helen S. Willard, OTR, President, 1958-1961
- Wilma West, Executive Director, 1948-1951; President, 1961-1964
- Marjorie Fish, Executive Director, 1951-1963

Key Places

- Location of occupational therapy schools

Andersen, L. T., & Reed, K. L.
The History of Occupational Therapy: The First Century (pp. 125-160).
© 2017 Taylor & Francis Group.

Key Times/Events

- World War II
- War emergency courses, 1943-1945
- Conflict with physical medicine
- World Federation of Occupational Therapists organized in 1952

Political Events/Issues

- Federal Vocational Rehabilitation Act of 1943 (Public Law 78-113)
- Servicemen's Readjustment Act of 1944, also known as the GI Bill (Public Law 78-346)
- Hospital Survey and Construction Act of 1946 (Public Law 79-725), also known as the Hill-Burton Act
- National Mental Health Act of 1946 (Public Law 79-487)
- Army-Navy Nurses Act of 1947 (Public Law 80-36)
- Vocational Rehabilitation Act Amendment of 1954 (Public Law 83-565)
- Mental Health Study Act of 1955 (Public Law 84-182)

Educational Issues

- Increase in the number of schools
- Occupational therapy assistant education established in 1958
- First discussions of graduate-level education began in 1958

Sociocultural Events/Issues

- Women in the workforce
- The Rehabilitation Movement

Economic Events/Issues

- Economic boom and continued prosperity initiated by World War II

Technological Events/Issues

- Innovations in pharmacology
- Interstate highway system developed

Practice Issues

- Paradigm shift in practice from occupation to reductionism
- Tuberculosis now controlled by drugs; tuberculosis sanatoriums open
- Increased emphasis on rehabilitation including neurorehabilitation and activities of daily living training

Association Issues

- Passing the registration exam required for admission to the National Register—1945
- A Kellogg grant in 1944 funded the position of Educational Field Secretary
- Winifred Conrick Kahmann was the first OTR to be elected President—1947
- *American Journal of Occupational Therapy* first published in 1947—first official journal owned by the American Occupational Therapy Association

INTRODUCTION

"In these days ... the continuity of purpose seems overshadowed by doctrines of change...."

–Eleanor Clarke Slagle (1938, p. 14)

By the end of the 1930s, President Franklin Roosevelt was finishing his second term in office as the United States was still struggling to get out of the Great Depression. The United States maintained neutrality when the Nazi aggression in Europe started World War II. Roosevelt ran for an unprecedented third term. He believed that he was most qualified to govern during this difficult time of economic depression and the potential for another war. Finally, the attack on Pearl Harbor in 1941 drew the United States into the war. The war fueled an economic recovery with the increased need for manufacturing of goods and materials for war and the need for manpower to serve in and provide for the military. The country quickly went from significant unemployment to manpower shortages. With the men going off to war, women were needed to fill positions in shipyards and factories to manufacture ships, planes, tanks, and other military equipment, jobs traditionally filled by men (Figure 5-1). Roosevelt was elected to a fourth term in 1944 but died of a cerebral hemorrhage in April 1945. Germany surrendered in May 1945, but Japan continued to fight in the Pacific. Harry S. Truman, sworn in as president when Roosevelt died, made the difficult decision to end the war and save countless American lives by dropping atomic bombs on Hiroshima and Nagasaki. Japan surrendered a few days later, and the war was finally over.

The economic boom started by the war would last well beyond the war years. Truman was succeeded by the hero of World War II, Dwight D. Eisenhower. Eisenhower started the interstate highway system, improving transportation and commerce in the United States. The GI Bill made it possible for veterans to receive an education and to obtain loans to purchase homes and farms and start businesses.

Occupational therapy lost a founder and a foundation of the American Occupational Therapy Association (AOTA) when Eleanor Clarke Slagle passed away in 1942. Dr. William Rush Dunton Jr. was the only surviving founder. He continued to serve on various AOTA committees until he bid farewell in 1954 when he was 86 years old (Dunton, 1955). Dr. Dunton's lifetime of service was honored by the Association. He was named honorary board member and also given the right to use the designation OTR after his name.

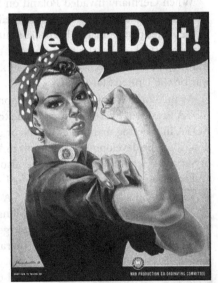

Figure 5-1. Rosie the Riveter represented the thousands of women who went to work in World War II. With the men off to war, there was a need for women to work in shipyards and factories to build ships, planes, and munitions needed for war. Traditionally men's work, women proved to be very capable of what was traditionally considered men's work. Some see this as the start of a huge influx of women into the workforce.

Everett S. Elwood, AOTA president from 1938 to 1947, guided the Association through the war years. The year 1947 brought a new era in the Association when the first registered occupational therapist and the first woman since Eleanor Clarke Slagle was elected president of AOTA. Winifred C. Kahmann, OTR (1947-1952), was followed by Henrietta W. McNary, OTR (1952-1955), Colonel Ruth Robinson, OTR (1955-1958), and Helen Willard, OTR (1958-1961). In the mid-1930s, during the Depression, the membership dipped to below 900. World War II jump-started the economy and spurred growth of the profession. The number of accredited professional training schools increased and the number of occupational therapists doubled in the 1940s. Membership continued to increase through the 1950s (Table 5-1). Despite the growing acceptance of occupational therapy, and despite the increase in the number of occupational therapy programs and occupational therapists, filling manpower needs became a major concern. In a predominantly female profession, marriage was seen as the greatest threat to manpower needs as women dropped out of the profession to get married and raise a family.

Table 5-1 AOTA MEMBERSHIP DATA— 1941 TO 1960	
YEAR	NUMBER OF MEMBERS
1941	1,326
1945	2,177
1950	2,967
1955	3,896
1960	4,938

UNITED STATES ENTRY INTO WORLD WAR II

When Germany invaded Poland on September 1, 1939, England and France declared war on Germany. The United States maintained a neutral stance for the most part, yet provided supplies to the Allies (England and France) as authorized by the Lend Lease Act. On December 7, 1941, the surprise attack at Pearl Harbor turned the tide of American opinion. Congress quickly declared war on Japan on December 8, 1941. Germany, who was in a pact with Japan, subsequently declared war on the United States.

As in World War I, with the war looming, many organizations had started to prepare for war. AOTA President Everett Elwood wrote to Surgeon General James C. Magee offering the services of AOTA in meeting manpower needs for the war effort should the need arise. In the letter, Elwood described the development of schools in World War I to train occupational therapists at the request of Surgeon General Gorgas. Elwood also discussed the growth and development of the profession and training schools since World War I (Elwood, 1939) (Figure 5-2).

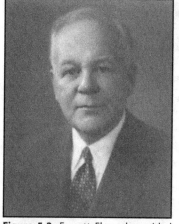

Figure 5-2. Everett Elwood provided wise and dignified leadership. With his calm personality he helped guide the association through the stressful war years. (Printed with permission from the Archive of the American Occupational Therapy Association, Inc.)

A report given by Harriet Robeson at the Board of Management in January 1940 informed the group that the Surgeon General was interested in the services of occupational therapy and had requested the Red Cross to establish a reserve of occupational therapists. To establish a reserve, the American Red Cross sent a survey to all occupational therapists inquiring about their willingness to serve in the medical departments of the Army and Navy should a war emergency occur (AOTA, 1940a). Robeson felt confident that AOTA requirements for registration would be met (Board of Management, 1940a). When the requirements were announced, the Surgeon General and the American Red Cross required an occupational therapist to be a graduate of an accredited training program, one that conformed to the American Medical Association's Council on Medical Education and Hospitals (AMA-CMEH) "Essentials of an Acceptable School of Occupational Therapy." Because the accreditation program had been in effect for a relatively short time, the Red Cross requirement for enrollment would essentially eliminate all occupational therapists except those graduates of the class of 1939, approximately 50 graduates (AOTA, 1940b; Board of Management, 1940b). AOTA's

House of Delegates and Board of Managers appealed to the American Red Cross and Surgeon General to change the requirements to also include those occupational therapists who were registered with AOTA, essentially grandfathering in those who had graduated from an approved school (Board of Management, 1940b; Fish, 1940) (Figure 5-3).

AOTA COMMITTEE ON NATIONAL DEFENSE

To help the association prepare for war, the AOTA formed a Committee on Occupational Therapy in National Defense in January 1941 with Helen S. Willard appointed chairperson. Throughout its existence, this committee was known by several names including the National Defense Committee, the Committee on Occupational Therapy and War Defense, the War Defense Committee. One of the many duties the committee undertook was to determine the occupational therapy manpower available should war break out. This was separate from the Red Cross Survey, completed in part because the committee had some doubts that the Red Cross information on available occupational therapists would be accurate (AOTA, 1941). The National Defense Committee survey found 504 active occupational therapists were available for Army service. The names of those available to serve were forwarded to the American Red Cross, the United States Civil Service, the Surgeon General's Office, and Veterans Administration in hopes of facilitating placement of therapists (Willard, 1941a).

The Surgeon General's Office planned to have 14 general hospitals and projected the need for 30 occupational therapists in these hospitals—a minimal number of therapists at best. The Surgeon General's Office plan was that:

> …men injured in the selective service camps who are disabled for further service will be transferred to veteran's facilities if their disability arises as a result of military service. Otherwise, in most instances, their discharge will take effect and they will be transferred to civilian institutions in their own communities. This applies especially to psychiatric cases. Very few cases will be held in Army hospitals for prolonged treatment. It has, therefore, seemed impractical to establish occupational therapy departments in the various military hospitals at the present time. (National Defense Committee, 1941)

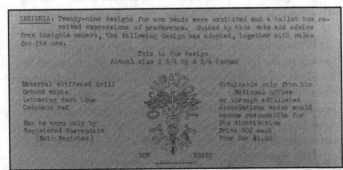

The Red Cross enrollment of 32 occupational therapists was deemed adequate to meet the needs of the military (National Defense Committee, 1941).

As Chair of the Committee on National Defense, Helen Willard was confronted by numerous issues. First, there was the issue of military status and subprofessional status for occupational therapists. Second, there was the issue of the military's misunderstanding of the professional standards and value of occupational therapy. Third, there was the infringement on occupational therapy from other agencies, such as the Gray Ladies, who worked with the American

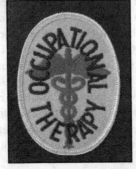

Figure 5-3. (A) AOTA chose an armband insignia from 29 designs submitted (AOTA, 1940c, November). (Printed with permission from the Archive of the American Occupational Therapy Association, Inc.) (B) The chosen insignia was used for arm bands/patches that could be worn by registered therapists. (Copyright © Dr. Lori T. Andersen. Reprinted with permission.)

Red Cross. And finally, there was the manpower shortage. It was estimated that 1,000 occupational therapists would be needed for military service (Kahmann & West, 1947, p. 335) with only 1,300 occupational therapists listed in the National Register nationwide. Solving the manpower shortage would help to stem the tide of encroachment by the Gray Ladies and others who lacked training because appropriately trained occupational therapists would then be available to fill positions (Sidebar 5-1).

SIDEBAR 5-1

White House Reception

The AOTA conference was held in Washington, DC, from August 31, 1941, through September 5, 1941. A special event awaited conference-goers that year:

> The Convention Committee has arranged a surprise for you. Mrs. Anna Eleanor Roosevelt has invited you to attend a reception at the White House, Washington, DC, on Tuesday afternoon, September second, nineteen hundred and forty-one, at four-thirty o'clock. (White House Reception, 1941, July)

MILITARY STATUS FOR OCCUPATIONAL THERAPISTS

Throughout the 1920s and 1930s, AOTA took great strides to increase the professional status of occupational therapy and promote the profession. Minimum Standards for Courses of Training of Occupational Therapists were set, a National Register was established, and the AMA started to accredit occupational therapy training schools. Despite these efforts, on the eve of World War II, top military leaders lacked an understanding of the complexity of occupational therapy, seeing it as little more than cheer-up work that could be done by volunteers.

Efforts to secure permanent military status for occupational therapists, physical therapists, and dieticians started in the late 1930s and continued into the 1940s. These groups argued that the requirement to serve as civilian employees in the military without the same protections and benefits of War Risk Insurance program and other benefits given to military personnel would impact the ability to recruit needed manpower. The military's position was that none of these civilian employees would be sent overseas; therefore, they would not be in harm's way, so the same protections were not necessary. Further, the Secretary of War indicated that occupational therapists were only needed in wartime, so permanent military status was not justified for them (Vogel & Gearin, 1968, pp. 1-5; Vogel, Manchester, Gearin, & West, 1968a, p. 102).

Military needs changed as the United States became involved in the war. Physical therapists and dieticians were sent overseas as early as 1942; therefore, Surgeon General James C. Magee (1939-1943) finally agreed that physical therapists and dieticians should have the same protections from risks and hazards as other military personnel. In 1942, a bill designed to improve the military status of the Army Nurse Corps was under consideration, so physical therapists and dieticians were simply added to the bill. The occupational therapy community mobilized to try to secure inclusion in this bill by writing to congressional representatives. AOTA leadership took steps to have occupational therapy included in the bill. On October 13, 1942, Helen S. Willard, Chairman of AOTA's War Service Committee, testified before the United States House Military Affairs Committee strongly recommending the inclusion of occupational therapy in the proposed legislation. Still, the military held fast to the position that occupational therapists would not be sent overseas; rather, disabled soldiers would be returned to the United States for occupational therapy treatment. Therefore, because occupational therapists would not be serving overseas, they did not need the protections of the War Risk Insurance Act (Vogel & Gearin, 1968, p. 7).

On December 22, 1942, with the passage of Public Law 77-828, physical therapists and dieticians were given military status, but only for the duration of the war and 6 months after. Occupational therapists were not included in the bill and therefore remained civilian employees. This adversely affected the military's ability to hire occupational therapists during the war. In an effort to secure the services of occupational therapists, the Surgeon General proposed to have them serve in the Women's Army Corps (WACs). Under this proposal, occupational therapists would be given military status in the WACs but would be assigned duty in the Medical Department. Occupational therapists did not consider this to be on par with the military status granted to physical therapists and dieticians. In the end, the War Department rejected this proposal also (Vogel et al., 1968b, p. 102). The military status of physical therapists and dieticians was upgraded again with the passing of Public Law 78-350 on June 22, 1944, giving them full commissioned status. Occupational therapists remained civilian employees.

Although not able to achieve military status, occupational therapists did achieve victory in upgrading their civil service status from subprofessional to professional. Because the Medical Department required occupational therapists to be graduates of an accredited program or registered with AOTA, Major Walter E. Barton was able to assist in pushing through a reclassification of occupational therapists from trades and industry to the medical section (Kahmann, 1943; Vogel et al., 1968b, pp. 106-117). This reclassification went into effect in September 1945 (Kahmann & West, 1947, p. 339).

By the end of the war, it became apparent that because of the exemplary service of occupational therapists, physical therapists, and dieticians in military service during wartime, their continued service would benefit the Army during peacetime. A permanent workforce would also eliminate future problems with the recruitment and mobilization of these personnel should the need arise again. Therefore, the Surgeon General of the Army, Major General Norman T. Kirk (1943-1947), recommended establishment of a Women's

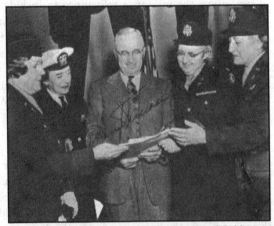

Figure 5-4. President Harry S. Truman signed Public Law 80-36 establishing the Women's Medical Specialist Corps and giving permanent commissioned status to dieticians, physical therapists, and occupational therapists.

Medical Specialist Corps, which would give permanent status for these groups. Legislation was drafted in accordance with the Surgeon General's recommendation, and on April 16, 1947, Public Law 80-36 (Army-Navy Nurses Act of 1947) was passed by Congress, authorizing the Women's Medical Specialist Corps and regular Army status for nurses, dietitians, physical therapists, and occupational therapists (Vogel & Gearin, 1968, p. 11) (Figure 5-4). The WMSC was overseen by a Chief and three Assistant Chiefs representing each of the professions. The first Chief of the WMSC was Colonel Emma E. Vogel, a physical therapist. Lieutenant Colonel Ruth A. Robinson, OTR, was appointed as assistant chief of the Occupational Therapist Section. Colonel Robinson later served as Chief of the Army Medical Specialist Corps (AMSC) from 1958 through 1962 (Figure 5-5).

In World War II, women who served as occupational therapists were civilian employees, compared with male occupational therapists, who were enlisted military personnel. In 1955, Public Law 84-294 was passed, amending the Army-Navy Nurses Act of 1947 to include male nurses and medical specialists as eligible for the same commissioned status as women. This affected six male occupational therapists serving at that time. With this change, the Corps was more appropriately renamed the Army Medical Specialist Corps (Hartwick, 1993, pp. 32-33) (Table 5-2).

OCCUPATIONAL THERAPY IN WORLD WAR II

On December 7, 1941, there were eight qualified occupational therapists and four occupational therapy assistants on duty in five Army hospitals (Vogel, Manchester, Gearin, & West, 1968b, p. 159). A number of factors contributed to the limited number of occupational therapists serving military hospitals, including the economic cutbacks in the military forced by the Great Depression; the lull of peacetime; the military's reluctance to include women in their ranks, including those from the predominantly female profession of occupational therapy; and the Surgeon General's misconception of occupational therapy as merely diversional. In addition, the lack of occupational therapy schools limited the number of graduates and therefore the number of occupational therapists available. With the resolute effort of leaders in AOTA, by V-J Day (Victory in Japan Day, August 14, 1945), there were 899 occupational therapists and apprentices working in 76 general, convalescent, regional, and station hospitals in the United

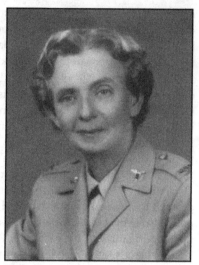

Figure 5-5. Colonel Ruth A. Robinson was the first occupational therapist to attain the permanent grade of Colonel in the United States Army. She served as Chief of the Army Medical Specialist Corps from 1958 to 1962. In addition to the many awards from AOTA, Colonel Robinson was awarded the Legion of Merit Award from the United States Army (AOTA, 1967b). Ruth Robinson maintains that her greatest contribution to the profession was helping to establish educational programs for certified occupational therapy assistants. (Printed with permission from the Archive of the American Occupational Therapy Association, Inc.)

States (Vogel et al., 1968a, p. 159). This included 452 apprentices and 447 graduate occupational therapists. Only 204 occupational therapists had volunteered service to the Army. The remainder were graduates of the war emergency courses, subsidized by the Army (West, 1947). In addition to the occupational therapists serving in the Army, 71 occupational therapists served in the Navy in World War II (Navy program, 1945) (Sidebar 5-2).

Occupational Therapy Branch—Surgeon General's Office

In May 1942, a conference on occupational therapy was convened by the National Research Council's Division of Medical Sciences. The conference, a series of four meetings that took place from May 15, 1942, through June 2, 1943, was held at the request of the Surgeon General of the Navy. The focus of these meetings was to develop recommendations on the organization of occupational therapy services in the military. Dr. Winfred Overholser, a psychiatrist and Superintendent of St. Elizabeth's Hospital in Washington, DC, was named Chairman, and Winifred C. Kahmann, OTR, who had replaced Helen Willard as Chairperson of AOTA on the War Service Committee, was named Secretary of the conference. The conference recommendations stated that each Army and Navy veteran should have an occupational therapy service under direct medical supervision, along with physical therapy (Vogel et al., 1968b, p. 104).

Two subcommittees were appointed by the President of AOTA to assist the conference in planning for occupational therapy services. One committee, whose members included Marjorie Greene, Director of the Boston School of Occupational Therapy; Helen S. Willard, Director of the

Table 5-2

TIMELINE FOR OBTAINING MILITARY STATUS FOR OCCUPATIONAL THERAPISTS AND DEVELOPING OCCUPATIONAL THERAPY SERVICES IN WWII

- April 1938 – Physical therapists seek to propose legislation to gain military status but were opposed by the Surgeon General's Office (Vogel & Gearin, 1968, p. 5).

- 1939 – Legislation first proposed in the US Congress to give military status to PT, OT, and dieticians. OT was dropped from language of the bill. This legislation did not pass (Vogel & Gearin, 1968, p. 5-6).

- December 7, 1941 - there were eight qualified OTs and 4 occupational therapy assistants on duty in five Army hospitals (Vogel, Manchester, Gearin, & West, 1968b, p. 159).

- October 13, 1942 - Helen Willard, Chairman of the War Service Committee of AOTA strongly recommended inclusion of OT in proposed legislation to give military status to PT and dieticians (McDaniel, 1968, p. 97).

- December 22, 1942 - P. L. 77- 828 was passed giving PTs and dieticians military status for duration of war and six months after (Vogel & Gearin, 1968, p. 7).

- April 1943 – A central organization for occupational therapy established in the Surgeon General's Office (Vogel, Manchester, Gearin, & West, 1968a, p. 106).

- August 19, 1943 – Reconditioning Division in the Surgeon General's Office (which included occupational therapy) was established with Major Walter E. Barton as director. (Vogel, Manchester, Gearin, & West, 1968a, p. 107).

- November 18, 1943 - Major Barton appointed Winifred Kahmann as chief of the newly established Occupational Therapy Branch (Vogel, Manchester, Gearin, & West, 1968a, p. 107).

- Sept 1, 1945 – The Surgeon General ordered all positions be reclassified from sub-professional to professional (Vogel, Manchester, Gearin, & West, 1968a, p. 118).

- June 2, 1944 – P. L. 78-350 passed giving full commissioned status to PTs and dieticians (Vogel & Gearin, 1968, p. 8).

- January 29, 1946 – The Surgeon General's Office recommends establishment of Women's Medical Specialist Corps. (Vogel & Gearin, 1968, p. 9-10)

- April 16, 1947 – Public Law 80-36 was signed by President Harry Truman establishing the Women's Medical Specialist Corps and giving permanent commissioned status to dieticians, physical therapists, and occupational therapists (Vogel & Gearin, 1968, p. 10-11).

SIDEBAR 5-2

Occupational Therapy Association of Hawaii, January 1942

About 6 weeks after the bombing of Pearl Harbor, AOTA headquarters received a letter from Mrs. Laura Nott Dowsett of Honolulu (President of the Occupational Therapy Association of Hawaii) dated January 16, 1942. The following excerpt was published in the *American Occupational Therapy Newsletter*:

> Just a line to let you know that we are all safe, well and very busy. Following the tragedy of Dec. 7, all accredited therapists in the islands were asked to sign up for volunteer service with the Nursing Service Bureau. A large number responded and I am particularly happy to report the splendid spirit of cooperation shown by the graduates of our training course. The work in the department at the moment relates closely to the emergency needs. Surgical dressings have become an interesting occupation for patients and volunteers alike. We have opened a Red Cross knitting unit for nurses, patients and technicians, which is an excellent service, as well as a treatment for war jitters. (Dowsett, 1942)

Philadelphia School of Occupational Therapy; and Marjorie Fish, Director of the Occupational Therapy Course at Columbia University, researched methods of recruitment and classification of personnel. The other committee, whose members included Winifred C. Kahmann; Charlotte Briggs, Director of Occupational Therapy at Niagara Tuberculosis Sanatorium; H. Elizabeth Messick, OTR, from the District of Columbia Health Department; Margaret S. Rood, Chief Occupational Therapist from the Cerebral Palsy Clinic at Indiana University Medical Center; and Virginia Scullin, Chief of Occupational Therapy at Pilgrim State Hospital in New York, considered other administrative aspects such as staff organization, equipment, and supplies. These two sub-committees recommended the following:

1. Appointment of a field director

2. Short course to orient occupational therapists to Army procedures

3. A medical officer to oversee occupational therapy treatment

4. Red Cross volunteers to provide recreational and diversional activities to patients under the supervision of occupational therapists

5. Establishing two occupational therapy units, neuropsychiatry and orthopedics, with five major types of treatment programs, to include physical injuries, neuropsychiatric conditions, tuberculosis, general medicine, and blindness

Establishment of occupational therapy in the military in World War II experienced a slow start, similar to that in World War I. A central organization for occupational therapy was established in April 1943, prompted by Colonel Roy D. Halloran, Director of the Neuropsychiatry Branch, Surgeon General's Office, and Major Walter E. Barton, a Halloran appointee. Colonel Halloran was a president of the Massachusetts Association for Occupational Therapy and a strong advocate for occupational therapy (Vogel et al., 1968b, pp. 104-105).

Colonel Halloran assigned Major Walter E. Barton to organize the occupational therapy services in the Neuropsychiatric Branch and subsequently, with reorganization of military units, a new Reconditioning Division. Winifred C. Kahmann was appointed chief of the newly established Occupational Therapy Branch in the Reconditioning Division on November 18, 1943. Two assistants for the Occupational Therapy Branch, Wilma L. West, OTR, and H. Elizabeth Messick, OTR, were appointed on June 6 and August 27, 1944, respectively (Vogel et al., 1968b, pp. 106-107).

Kahmann was an excellent choice to head the Occupational Therapy Branch, with her clinical and administrative experience as director of occupational therapy at the James Whitcomb Riley Hospital for Children and then as Director of Occupational Therapy and Physical Therapy at the Indiana University Medical Center, as well as her leadership roles in AOTA (Figure 5-6). Now with the structure established, the recruitment of occupational therapists began in earnest. An urgent call for occupational therapists to fulfill their patriotic duty and work for the Army was published in the occupational therapy newsletter

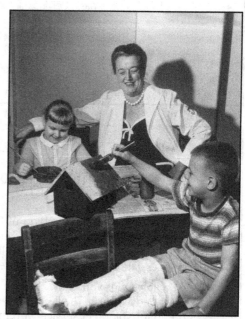

Figure 5-6. Winifred C. Kahmann OTR was the first registered occupational therapist elected president of the American Occupational Therapy Association. Mrs. Kahmann was described as a strong leader with excellent interpersonal relationships and a lively sense of humor. (Printed with permission from the Archive of the American Occupational Therapy Association, Inc.)

and journal (Barton, 1943a; Kahmann, 1944a). It gradually became more apparent that the decision of Major General James C. Magee, the Surgeon General of the Army, not to commission occupational therapists but to appoint them as civilian employees of the Medical Department was interfering with recruitment.

The need for occupational therapists was at first underestimated by the Surgeon General's Office at one occupational therapist per 1,000 beds. A survey by the AMA was more realistic, indicating a range from 400 to 660 therapists (Vogel et al., 1968b, p. 111). In early 1944, the projected need for occupational therapists was set at 1,000 (Kahmann & West, 1947, p. 335). It was unrealistic to assume that this need would be filled by the existing pool of trained occupational therapists because there were only 1,300 occupational therapists listed in AOTA's National Register (Vogel et al., 1968a, p. 159).

War Emergency Courses

Helen Willard, Chairperson of AOTA's National Defense Committee, was in receipt of numerous letters complaining about the American Red Cross Gray Ladies doing occupational therapy (Willard, 1942a). With a lack of appropriately trained manpower, the untrained American Red Cross Gray Ladies were filling the void. Helen S. Willard and the national office received numerous concerns from occupational therapists around the country about the work of the Gray Ladies, who were providing handicrafts to disabled soldiers. Helen S. Willard corresponded with Eleanor Vincent of the American Red Cross to express their concerns:

> Much of the work done by trained occupational therapists is largely diversional and
> has been recognized in our civilian hospitals as of medical value. There is, therefore,
> I am afraid, some danger of misunderstanding and damage to our profession in the
> giving of handicraft activities to men who are sick and disabled by persons who are not
> professionally accredited. (Willard, 1941c)

After dealing with the issue of military and professional status and encroachment by untrained people, Helen Willard recognized the need to increase manpower and called for the Education Committee to organize war emergency courses:

> I feel that it is urgently necessary that at the Education Committee on January 17th
> in Indianapolis, we should be prepared to set up the organization of war emergency
> courses and should probably plan for a Committee to proceed to Chicago on January
> 19th to confer with the American Medical Association in regard to these. The pressure is becoming terrific and I believe that our professional status is at stake. (Willard,
> 1941d)

The Association had just transitioned the educational standards from the Minimum Standards adopted in 1930, which required a total of 18 months of preparation, including 9 months of academic instruction and 9 months practical training to the new Essentials of an Approved Occupational Therapy School. These Essentials set by the AMA-CMEH in 1935 and implemented in 1939 required a total of 25 months of preparation, including 16 months of academic instruction and 9 months of practical training. To fill manpower needs as quickly as possible during the war emergency, the Occupational Therapy Branch of the Army Reconditioning Division and the AOTA Committee on Education outlined a compressed educational program. The proposed war emergency courses could be completed in 12 months. This new curriculum required 4 months of didactic coursework and 8 months of practical experience in selected Army hospitals under the supervision of an occupational therapist. During practical training period in an Army hospital, the student was considered an occupational therapy apprentice. In this way, the Army would have a person providing occupational therapy services, under supervision, in a relatively short period of time (Figures 5-7 and 5-8). On completion of a war emergency course, these students were allowed to sit for the national examination (AOTA, 1944). The curriculum for the war emergency courses

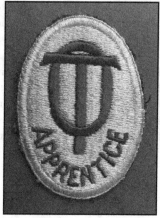

Figure 5-7. An occupational therapy apprentice patch worn by students enrolled in war emergency courses who were completing practical training. (Copyright © Dr. Lori T. Andersen. Reprinted with permission.)

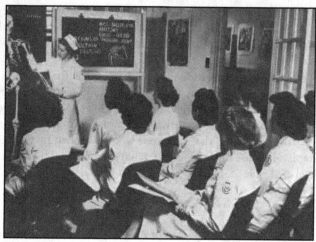

Figure 5-8. Occupational therapy apprentices participating in class at Battey General Hospital in Rome, Georgia.

was approved by the Occupational Therapy Branch, Surgeon General's Office; the AOTA War Manpower Commission; and the AOTA Committee on Education and was subsequently approved by the Surgeon General in May 1944 (Vogel et al., 1968a, p. 160). The Surgeon General's Office contracted with eight accredited civilian schools to provide these war emergency courses. The contract stipulated that the accredited programs provided the academic coursework under the direction of the Surgeon General's Office while 40 selected Army hospitals provided the apprenticeship opportunities. The federal government subsidized the war emergency courses (Sidebar 5-3).

The war emergency courses ran from July 1944 to June 1946. A total of 667 students enrolled in a war emergency course, and 545 completed the course by June 1946 (West, 1947). Upon completion of the academic phase of schoolwork and permission of the curriculum director, 55 students who had enrolled in regular occupational therapy training programs opted to complete the practical training portion of their education in the Army program (Army program, 1945).

The war emergency course curriculum was never formally approved by the AMA-CMEH. Although the courses did not meet the Essentials of an Acceptable School of Occupational Therapy with the requirement of 25 months of coursework, AOTA's Committee on Education took the position that higher prerequisite requirements qualified the war

---

SIDEBAR 5-3

Schools Providing War Emergency Courses

Eight accredited schools, in collaboration with the Surgeon General of the United States Army, provided war emergency courses from July 1, 1944, to June 30, 1944 (AOTA, 1944):

- Philadelphia School of Occupational Therapy
- University of Illinois, Urbana, Illinois
- Milwaukee-Downer College, Milwaukee, Wisconsin
- University of Southern California, Los Angeles, California
- Boston School of Occupational Therapy
- Richmond Professional Institute, Richmond, Virginia
- Mills College, Oakland, California
- Columbia University, New York, New York

emergency courses to meet the Minimum Standards. These higher prerequisites required students to have a college degree in a related field and coursework in the biological sciences, psychology, and sociology. In some cases, comparable experience could be substituted for a college degree. More than 90% of students had bachelor's degrees, and more than 3% had master's degrees (Vogel et al., 1968a, p. 160; West, 1947). After the war, the rigor and status of the war emergency courses became an issue. Some in the Association wanted to restrict the registration of war emergency graduates, whom they believed did not meet the same standards as regular school graduates. After discussion, AOTA granted full registration rights to graduates of war emergency courses (Education Committee, 1945).

OCCUPATIONAL THERAPY VOLUNTEER ASSISTANT TRAINING COURSES PROGRAM

Fiorello La Guardia, the flamboyant mayor of New York City, was appointed Director of the Office of Civilian Defense by President Roosevelt in 1941. One of the programs started by this office was an initiative to involve women and young people in the war effort through volunteering. The Junior League, well-known for organizing volunteer service programs, loaned Miss Wilmer Shields, a field social worker with the Association of Junior Leagues, to the Office of Civilian Defense to help. Eleanor Roosevelt also signed on to assist this initiative. La Guardia wanted to secure the assistance of national private social and health agencies, including AOTA, to work on a plan to recruit, train, and place volunteers. He invited AOTA Executive Secretary Meta Cobb to attend an organizational meeting for this national volunteer service program (La Guardia, 1941).

The AOTA Committee on National Defense was tasked to assist this effort of the Office of Civilian Defense. Chair of the committee, Helen Willard, concerned about encroachment from such groups as the Gray Ladies and determined to uphold the high standards of the profession, took steps to ensure that AOTA would have control of the training course for occupational therapy volunteers. She sought the support of Eleanor Roosevelt and was able to secure an appointment, writing to Meta Cobb, Executive Secretary, "I have just had word from Mrs. Roosevelt's secretary that she will see me in New York on the afternoon of Thursday, November 6th" (Willard, 1941a). In a memo to Roosevelt, Willard requested the Office of Civilian Defense channel applications for occupational therapy volunteer assistant courses through the AOTA- or AMA-approved occupational therapy schools to ensure training by qualified people (Willard, 1941b).

Helen Willard and her committee members, Marjorie Taylor, Winifred Kahmann, Marion Spear, Geraldine R. Lermit, and H. Elizabeth Messick, prepared outlines for the courses to train volunteer occupational therapy assistants. Sponsored by both the Office of Civilian Defense and the American Red Cross, the courses were given in various locations throughout the country (Willard, 1941e) (Figure 5-9). It was hoped that the Occupational Therapy Volunteer Assistant Training Course would help to meet the anticipated expanded need for occupational therapy services in the event of war. Volunteers were required to have a high school education, be between 18 to 50 years old, and pledge to volunteer services for a minimum of 150 hours. The syllabus for these courses included lectures on the occupational therapy history, the scope and practical application of occupational therapy, patient conditions, hospital organization, ethics and etiquette, craft instruction, and practical training. The course was designed to be a minimum of 58 hours over the span of 8 to 10 weeks—40 hours of lectures and 18 hours of practical training (AOTA, 1942a; U.S. Office of Civilian Defense, 1942).

On completion of the course, AOTA sent the volunteers a card certifying completion and an emblem to be worn on upper left sleeve of their uniform. Volunteers were responsible for purchasing the natural linen-color coat-smock–style uniform (Willard, 1942b) (Figure 5-10). Twenty-two courses were given, and 670 volunteer assistants trained between January 1943 and February 1944

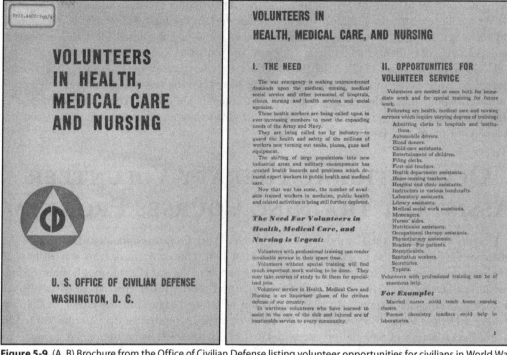

Figure 5-9. (A, B) Brochure from the Office of Civilian Defense listing volunteer opportunities for civilians in World War II. (Printed with permission from the Archive of the American Occupational Therapy Association, Inc.)

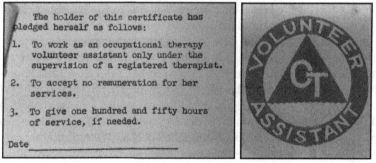

Figure 5-10. (A) Occupational therapy volunteer assistant card and (B) patch. (Printed with permission from the Archive of the American Occupational Therapy Association, Inc.)

(Willard, 1944, p. 5). The Occupational Therapy Volunteer Assistant courses continued to be given in some areas past the end of World War II because of manpower needs in civilian and military hospitals. By 1948, the New York State Occupational Therapy Association had provided nine courses, training a total of 469 volunteers (Oppenheimer, 1948).

LEGISLATION IMPACTING HEALTH CARE AND OCCUPATIONAL THERAPY

Social and economic influences in the 1940s and 1950s prompted passage of a number of laws that provided funding for rehabilitation services and facilities, research activities to improve and expand knowledge, and education and training for medical professionals. The Federal Vocational Rehabilitation Act of 1943, also known as the Barden–LaFollette Act (Public Law 78-113), amended the first Federal Vocational Rehabilitation Act of 1920, the Smith-Fess Act. Advances in medicine helped people survive illnesses and injuries that previously resulted in poor prognoses. These survivors needed continued care and rehabilitation. The rise in rehabilitation and the desire to return disabled soldiers and civilians to the workforce to help provide manpower for the war effort provided stimulus for this law. The Barden–LaFollette Act added coverage of medical and rehabilitative services to enable soldiers, sailors, and civilians with disabilities to participate in a remunerative occupation. In addition to vocational rehabilitation, this act allowed medical services, including "corrective surgery or therapeutic treatment necessary to correct or substantially modify a physical condition which ... constitutes a substantial handicap to employment" if the physical condition could be corrected or modified within a reasonable time frame. Prosthetic devices essential to employment were also covered, as were services for people with mental illness and intellectual disabilities. State vocational rehabilitation bureaus (Offices of Vocational Rehabilitation) were authorized by this act to administer vocational rehabilitation programs.

The National Mental Health Act of 1946 (Public Law 79-487) sought to develop and provide "the most effective methods of prevention, diagnosis, and treatment of psychiatric disorders." Grant funds were made available to aid research activities to improve health care for those with disabilities. Funds were also provided for education and training of mental health personnel and the establishment of the National Institute of Mental Health. The purpose of the Hospital Survey and Construction Act of 1946, also known as the Hill-Burton Act (Public Law 79-725), was to ensure adequate health care facilities for the public, including those in small communities and rural areas. To achieve this goal, funds were provided to plan, construct, or modify health care facilities and hospitals. Representative of the times, hospitals receiving grants were required to provide services to people in the area, regardless of creed or color or ability to pay, although providing separate but equal facilities would meet the requirements.

The Vocational Rehabilitation Act Amendment of 1954 (Public Law 83-565) authorized funding to provide, improve, and expand vocational rehabilitation programs and to significantly increase the number of people with disabilities served. Included in this initiative were funds to build and expand rehabilitation facilities, to conduct research and/or demonstration projects, and to educate and train rehabilitation specialists, including occupational therapists. This Act eventually led to the establishment of the National Institute for Disability and Rehabilitation Research (NIDRR). The Mental Health Study Act of 1955 called for "an objective, thorough, nationwide analysis and re-evaluation of the human and economic problems of mental health." The focus was on better utilization of resources to decrease the "incidence and duration of mental illness" and minimize the "emotional and financial drain on families ... and economic resources of the States and of the Nation." Funding was authorized for special projects to study the diagnostic and treatment practices and use of resources for rehabilitating those with mental illness (Table 5-3).

THE CHALLENGE BY PHYSICAL MEDICINE

The occupational therapy profession and the medical profession enjoyed an amicable relationship even before the time of the formal organization of the National Society for the Promotion of Occupational Therapy (NSPOT) and AOTA. Most of the early Presidents of the profession were physicians or men who held high positions in medical organizations. Many other physicians, strong supporters of occupational therapy, helped promote the profession. The relationship with medicine helped to secure occupational therapy's professional standing and was furthered when, in 1935, the AMA-CMEH agreed to assist with the accreditation of occupational therapy training programs. This amicable relationship was challenged in the late 1940s when the new medical

Table 5-3
LEGISLATION RELATED TO REHABILITATION SERVICES

YEAR	LEGISLATION	PURPOSE
1943	Vocational Rehabilitation Act Amendments of 1943 (Public Law 78-113); also known as the Barden-LaFollette Act	Provided funds for physical restoration services, including occupational therapy, as part of vocational rehabilitation programs. Helped create the Office of Vocational Rehabilitation.
1946	National Mental Health Act (Public Law 79-487)	Provided funds for research on the cause, diagnoses, and treatment of psychiatric disorders. Provided for training of personnel in mental health. Authorized establishment of the National Institute of Mental Health.
1946	Hospital Survey and Construction Act (Public Law 79-725); also known as the Hill-Burton Act	Authorized federal grants to states for the planning and construction and modernization of hospitals throughout the United States.
1954	Vocational Rehabilitation Act Amendment of 1954 (Public Law 83-565)	Authorized funds to expand vocational rehabilitation programs and services, to conduct research, and to educate and train rehabilitation specialists.
1955	The Mental Health Study Act of 1955 (Public Law 84-182)	Authorized funds to study the problems related to mental illness to better use resources.

specialty of physical medicine sought to secure their own professional standing within the medical profession.

In 1943, Bernard M. Baruch, a philanthropist, financed the Baruch Committee on Physical Medicine in memory of his father, Dr. Simon Baruch, a surgeon in the Confederate Army. He wanted to further his father's work in the practice of hydrotherapy. The committee undertook a study to determine ways to advance physical medicine as a medical specialty, the overall purpose of the committee (Folz, Opitz, Peters, & Gelfman, 1997).

Dr. Frank Krusen, initially a member of the Baruch Committee and later Chairperson, believed that physical medicine should include both physical therapy and occupational therapy. As defined in the Baruch Committee report, "physical medicine includes the employment of the physical and other effective properties of light, heat, cold, water, electricity, massage, manipulation, exercise, and mechanical devices for physical and occupational therapy, in the diagnosis or treatment of disease" (Krusen, 1944). Krusen had earlier suggested that physical therapy and occupational therapy training programs should be combined to enable technicians to practice both therapies (Krusen, 1934). Recommendations from the final report of the Baruch Committee published in April 1944 included the following:

1. Develop adequate programs to teach physical medicine to medical students as well as adequate programs to train occupational therapy technicians and physical therapy technicians

2. Establish more extensive programs in basic research and clinical research

3. Promote physical rehabilitation, including strategies to meet manpower needs for physiatrists, occupational therapy technicians, and physical therapy technicians

4. Provide medical direction in occupational therapy departments

5. Develop a program to teach occupational therapy as part of a physical medicine course in medical schools (Krusen, 1944)

In December 1944, the name of the AMA's Committee on Physical Therapy, a committee of physicians specializing in physical therapy, was changed to the Committee on Physical Medicine, thereby establishing the new medical specialty (Krusen, 1944).

Bernard M. Baruch gave more than $1 million to establish academic and clinical teaching and research centers in select universities to help implement the committee's recommendations (Krusen, 1944). The need to train physiatrists, occupational therapists, and physical therapists was a high priority during the war years. Additionally, the rise in the Rehabilitation Movement and increased emphasis on the "restoration of people handicapped by disease, injury, or malformation as nearly as possible to a normal physical and mental state" supported the need to train these medical professionals (Folz et al., 1997).

The funds to establish these academic, clinical, and research centers provided solutions to the problems of limited number of schools for training occupational therapists and limited research in occupational therapy. In World War II, as they had in World War I, occupational therapists worked closely with orthopedic physicians and neurosurgeons treating soldiers with fractures, amputations, and peripheral nerve injuries and central nervous system injuries (West, 1992). An increasing number of occupational therapists were working with patients with physical disabilities so a close relationship with physical medicine seemed a natural fit. The additional professional and financial support was very enticing for occupational therapy schools and practices desiring to develop further. Nevertheless, AOTA President Winifred Kahmann gave a cautious warning in her opening address at the AOTA annual conference in 1947:

> Occupational therapy is now on the threshold of an extensive and phenomenal development in physical medicine and medical rehabilitation. We must proceed cautiously and make no mistakes if we are to contribute treatment service of value within these organized groups. (Kahmann, 1947)

The new specialty area of physical medicine already had control of physical therapy education through the accreditation process, as well as control of the physical therapy registry. Unilaterally, physical medicine took steps to take occupational therapy into their fold by including occupational therapy as part of the physical medicine definition and promoting teaching occupational therapy in schools of physical medicine (Reggio, 1947). At the same time, physical medicine was fighting an internal battle with the medical profession to gain increased recognition and improve its own status by endeavoring to become a permanent committee in the AMA, a section on physical medicine. Some believed that claiming supervisory control of another profession, in this case occupational therapy, would justify their request. Physical medicine was granted permanent committee status in June 1949. Another internal dispute between the specialties of physical medicine and medical rehabilitation was resolved with the creation of the American Board of Physical Medicine and Rehabilitation in 1950 (Gelfman, Peters, Opitz, & Folz, 1997).

The Board of Trustees of the University of Illinois Medical School in Chicago referred members of the Baruch Committee, who wanted to discuss the establishment of a physical medicine division, to Beatrice Wade, who was Head of the Occupational Therapy Department, and to the Head of the Orthopedics Department. The physiatrists revealed their intent to take control of occupational therapy education and registry. Although enticed with grant support for a clinical director, Miss Wade was warned by some physical therapists about any arrangement with physical medicine. The physical therapists indicated that their relationship with physical medicine limited their ability to raise educational and practice standards (Colman, 1992).

Wade alerted Winifred Kahmann, President of AOTA, about the physiatrists' plan. In a meeting with Kahmann, Helen Willard, and Henrietta McNary, the physiatrists again presented their plan, which was summarily dismissed by the women. Among their concerns was the potential for the mental health component of occupational therapy to be lost (Colman, 1992). The physiatrists tried to circumvent the national organization by petitioning the administration of the University of Illinois to place the occupational therapy department under their control. In view of Wade's strong stand against this, the administration of the University of Illinois rejected the physiatrists' requests (Colman, 1992) (Figure 5-11).

In 1949, Helen Willard, Chair of the Education Committee, reported that "the relationship between occupational therapy and physical medicine had become a matter of great concern" (Willard, 1950, p. 36). The physiatrists pressed on through the AMA Council on Physical Medicine, recommending to the AMA-CMEH that "(1) occupational therapists should be known as occupational therapy technicians, and that (2) a physician or physiatrist should be medical director of a school of occupational therapy" (Willard, 1949, 1950, p. 36). AOTA countered that the term *technician* implied a subprofessional status at a time when many civil service agencies had just upgraded occupational therapy to professional status by virtue of education and training. Luckily, the AMA-CMEH supported AOTA's desire to retain the term occupational therapist (Willard, 1950). In a compromise, the 1949 revision of the Essentials of an Acceptable School of Occupational Therapy required:

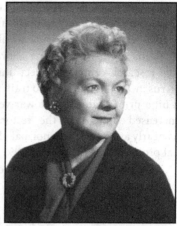

Figure 5-11. Bea Wade was appointed Head of the Occupational Therapy Department at the University of Illinois in 1951. (Printed with permission from the Archive of the American Occupational Therapy Association, Inc.)

1. Occupational therapy schools should be established only in medical schools approved by CMEH or accredited colleges or universities affiliated with acceptable hospitals.

2. The director of an occupational therapy program should be a qualified occupational therapist with an academic degree, registered or eligible for registration, and have a minimum of 3 years' clinical experience.

3. The clinical training portion of entry-level education should be directed by a physician or a committee of physicians whose qualifications are acceptable to CMEH. (Colman, 1992; Council on Medical Education and Hospitals, 1950)

The 1949 *Essentials* explicitly stated that therapists were being trained to work under the direction of qualified physicians (Council on Medical Education and Hospitals, 1950) (Table 5-4).

Wilma West (1992) credits Beatrice Wade with identifying the principles that outlined the relationships and responsibility of occupational therapists to medical specialties and physicians. These principles included the following:

1. Occupational therapy should be a service available to all medical specialties.

2. Occupational therapists are accountable to the physician who referred the patient for treatment.

3. Occupational therapy services are accountable to any intermediate service (e.g., physical medicine, psychiatry) under which it is organized.

In 1950, AOTA developed a key policy statement that reflected these principles, describing occupational therapy's "professional and allied relationships" (Kahmann, 1950) (Sidebar 5-4).

THE REHABILITATION MOVEMENT

The Rehabilitation Movement started in the early 1940s, prompted by a social movement and a concern to assist those disabled in World War II and civilians with disabilities to live productive lives. Other external forces furthering the Rehabilitation Movement included the rise of physical medicine and the efforts of Dr. Frank Krusen, the activities and advocacy of Dr. Howard A. Rusk, and federal legislation, specifically the Vocational Rehabilitation Act Amendments of 1943, the Hill-Burton Act of 1946, and the Vocational Rehabilitation Act Amendment of 1954.

Table 5-4
HISTORY OF EDUCATIONAL STANDARDS FOR OCCUPATIONAL THERAPISTS

YEAR	STANDARD	PURPOSE/REQUIREMENT
1923	Minimum Standards for Courses of Training in Occupational Therapy adopted	Candidates must have high school education or equivalent and be at least 20 years old. Total program must be at least 12 months in length: at least 8 months theoretical and practical and at least 3 months of supervised hospital practice training.
1927	Minimum Standards revised	Length of practice training increased from 3 to 6 months
1930	Minimum Standards revised	Total program length increased to at least 18 months, with 9 months of hospital practice training
1931	National Register established	To serve as an enforcement mechanism; only those graduating from schools meeting Minimum Standards plus 1 year of experience and/or grandfathered in, would be admitted to the Register and have right to use designation O.T. Reg.
1935	Essentials of an Acceptable School of Occupational Therapy adopted	AMA-CMEH designated to accredit schools. Minimum length of program should be 100 weeks, with at least 64 weeks of theoretical and technical instruction and 36 weeks of hospital practice. Established requirements for organization, administration, and physical resources for programs. Set qualifications for faculty.
1939	Essentials of an Acceptable School of Occupational Therapy now fully developed and enforced	Five schools inspected: four accredited and one given provisional accreditation.
1945	National examination started	Graduates of accredited schools required to successfully pass the national examination for admission to the National Registry. One-year experience requirement for admission to the Registry was eliminated.
1949	Essentials of an Acceptable School of Occupational Therapy revised	Occupational therapy schools to be established in medical schools of accredited universities. Occupational therapy school directors to have an academic degree and be a qualified OTR. Required clinical training in the areas of psychiatric conditions, physical disabilities, tuberculosis, pediatrics, and general medicine and surgery (other than physical disabilities).
1958	Essentials of an Acceptable School of Certified Occupational Therapy Assistants adopted	Length of program at least 12 weeks. Didactic instruction and supervised practical training to take place in AMA-approved hospitals.

Both Dr. Frank Krusen and Dr. Howard Rusk saw the need for medical treatment beyond the acute stage of illness or injury. The Baruch Committee, which included Dr. Krusen as a member, defined medical rehabilitation as restoration of people with disabilities "as nearly as possible to a normal physical and mental state" (Krusen, 1944, p. 1094). The committee explained that "medical rehabilitation fills the gap between the customary end point of medical attention and the real necessities of many patients" (Krusen, 1944, p. 1094). The need was significant. In 1940, four million people had permanent physical disabilities, with 800,000 more becoming permanently disabled each year. World War II greatly increased the number of those with disabilities (Krusen, 1944). Along with social responsibility for the care of those with disabilities, Krusen understood the economic benefit as well. He stated, "For every dollar spent for rehabilitation, $47 is returned to society" (Krusen, 1944, p. 1094).

Dr. Howard A. Rusk was known as the Father of Comprehensive Rehabilitation (Blum & Fee, 2008, p. 257). An internist in private practice, Rusk joined the U.S. Air Force when the United

---

SIDEBAR 5-4

Statement Policy on Occupational Therapy, 1950

Note: This policy statement was an attempt to state in positive language that occupational therapy worked with several types of physicians, not just physical medicine and rehabilitation specialists (physiatrists), and that direct contact with the referring physician was important.

OCCUPATIONAL THERAPY is a professional service which uses purposeful activities to aid the patient in recovery from and/or adjustment to disease or injury. It is prescribed by the patient's physician and administered by the occupational therapist with consideration not only of the specific disability but also of the patients' physical, mental, emotional, social and economic needs.

Relationship With the Physician
In the fields of psychiatry, pediatrics, tuberculosis and other medical specialties it is essential that the patient's physician prescribe occupational therapy in relation to the total treatment program. In order to insure continued guidance it is necessary that there be frequent contact between the therapist and the physician.

The Education of the Occupational Therapist
The education of the occupational therapist has been determined by the demand of the various fields of medicine in which the service is needed. Balance in emphasis on the medical specialties must therefore, be maintained.

The American Occupational Therapy Association Education Program
The American Occupational Therapy Association believes that its professional courses can be most effectively directed by qualified occupational therapists in accordance with the essentials established by the American Medical Association for acceptable schools of occupational Therapy. Advisory committees made up of representatives of the medical and allied professional fields are invaluable to the administration of the educational program.

Registration
Professional registration is an integral part of the educational program and as such has been established and is maintained under the jurisdiction of the American Occupational Therapy Association.

Prepared by the Education Committee, 1949 (Kahmann, 1950)

States entered World War II. Stationed at Jefferson Barracks in St. Louis, Rusk developed a comprehensive rehabilitation program after recognizing the need to provide activity for the convalescing patients (Blum & Fee, 2008; Gelfman et al., 1997). Rusk emphasized "integrated rehabilitation teams … focused on maximizing the psychological and social functioning of the disabled, in addition to maximizing their physical and vocational capabilities" (Gelfman et al., 1997, p. 558). After World War II, Rusk worked to develop a new specialty of medical rehabilitation and expand his comprehensive medical rehabilitation programs to the civilian population. Both physical medicine and medical rehabilitation were seeking recognition and improved status in the mid-1940s. Because of the similarities, medical rehabilitation merged with physical medicine to become a single specialty area of physical medicine and rehabilitation (Gelfman et al., 1997). Rusk went on to found the Institute of Physical Medicine and Rehabilitation at New York University in 1948, with

$1 million donated by Bernard Baruch (Pace, 1989). The Institute was renamed the Rusk Institute of Rehabilitation Medicine in 1984.

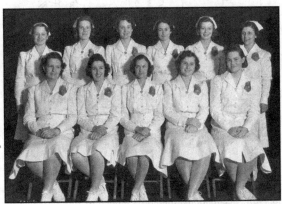

Figure 5-12. Boston School of Occupational therapy Class of 1941 included two leaders of the profession: Carlotta Welles and Wilma West. Assigned seats alphabetically, Welles and West sat next to each other in class (Peters, 2011, p. 209). Carlotta Welles is back row, fourth from left. Wilma West is front row, second from left. (Printed with permission from the Archive of the American Occupational Therapy Association, Inc.)

EXPANSION OF OCCUPATIONAL THERAPY SCHOOLS

By 1940, five schools had been accredited by the AMA-CMEH. In 1941, four more schools had started courses in occupational therapy: Columbia University and New York University, both in New York; Michigan State College in Ypsilanti, Michigan (later called Eastern Michigan University); and Mary Mount College in Milwaukee, Wisconsin (Board of Management, 1941). A total of 17 new courses in occupational therapy had been accredited and/or initiated between 1940 and 1945 (Figure 5-12). Fourteen more had been accredited and/or initiated between 1950 and 1967 (AOTA, 1967a) (Figures 5-13 to 5-16).

Just as World War I had, World War II spurred a manpower shortage, resulting in a number of new schools developing programs to fill manpower needs. In contrast to World War I, educational programs now had to meet specific standards. In spite of this, the Committee on Education expressed concerns with some of the new schools. The committee was specifically concerned about the limited importance placed on medical content and clinical practice in some schools' curriculums (Board of Management, 1944). The Association decided to create a series of guides to assist the increasing numbers of new schools with developing curriculums. Included were guides to help standardize curriculums and didactic course content, as well as guides to establish clinical training programs (West, 1951b). To have input into the accreditation process and to ensure schools' compliance with standards, the Committee on Education requested the AMA-CMEH to "designate

COLLEGES AND UNIVERSITIES OFFERING COURSES IN OCCUPATIONAL THERAPY
Accredited By The Council On Medical Education Of The American Medical Association, In Collaboration With The American Occupational Therapy Association

College or University	Curriculum Initiated	Curriculum Accredited
Boston University—Sargent College	1963	1965
Colorado State University	1946	1951
Columbia University	1941	1943
Florida, University of	1959	1961
Illinois, University of	1943	1944
Indiana University	1956	1960
Iowa, University of	1946	1948
Kansas, University of	1940	1944
Eastern Michigan University	1941	1944
Lawrence University (Milwaukee-Downer College)	1918	1938—Discontinued 1967
Loma Linda University (College of Medical Evangelists)	1959	1961
Mills College (no students accepted after 1959)	1944	1944
Minnesota, University of	1946	1948
Mount Mary College	1941	1943
New Hampshire, University of	1942	1945
New York, State University of, at Buffalo (Buffalo University)	1954	1958
New York University	1941	1943
North Dakota, University of	1954	1961
Ohio State University	1942	1944
Pennsylvania, University of (Philadelphia School of Occupational Therapy)	1918	1938
Puerto Rico, University of (Puerto Rico School of Occupational Therapy)	1951	1954
Puget Sound, University of (College of Pudget Sound)	1944	1947
Richmond Professional Institute	1942	1943
St. Catherine, College of	1945	1947
San Jose State College	1943	1944
Southern California, University of	1943	1944
*Temple University	1967	—
Texas Woman's University (Texas (State College for Women)	1944	1947
*Texas, University of, Medical Branch	1955	1959—Approval withdrawn
Tufts University, Boston School of Occupational Therapy	1918	1938
U.S. Army Med. Field Services School	1952	1955—Deactivated
Washington University School of Medicine (St. Louis School of Occupational Therapy)	1918	1938
Washington, University of	1959	1961
Wayne State University	1944	1948
Western Michigan University	1922	1938
Kalamazoo State Hospital School of Occupational Therapy (Western Michigan University)	1922	1936
Wisconsin, University of	1943	1947

*Awaiting Accreditation

Figure 5-13. Colleges and Universities offering courses, 1917-1967. (Printed with permission from the Archive of the American Occupational Therapy Association, Inc.)

a competent occupational therapist to accompany and assist the representative of the council in the inspection of schools and courses in occupational therapy" (Kahmann, 1944b, p. 37) (Sidebar 5-5; Figure 5-17).

The Association was also able to obtain funding from the Kellogg Foundation to establish an educational advisory service and to hire an Educational Field Secretary to assist new schools seeking accreditation. Initially the funding was for a period of 6 months; however, the Kellogg Foundation agreed

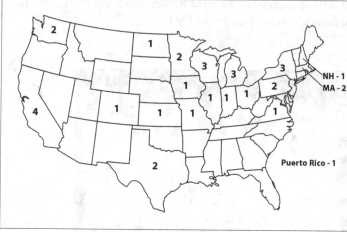

Figure 5-14. The number and location of occupational therapy educational programs offered by colleges and universities that were accredited and/or initiated between 1918 and 1967. Occupational therapists tended to stay and work in areas where they received their education. As a result, areas and states that did not have educational programs had a lack of occupational therapists.

to support and fund the Education Office through 1951 (Nationally speaking, 1949). Additionally, the Kellogg Foundation provided grants for student scholarships and loans helping to recruit students (Board of Management, 1944). Marjorie Fish, OTR, was appointed the first Educational Field Secretary. In her position, she established a close working relationship with the AMA-CMEH, completing supplementary inspection visits and sending reports to the CMEH (Fish, 1945) (Figure 5-18).

The idea of establishing graduate-level education started in the late 1940s. The University of Southern California started the first master's degree program in occupational therapy in 1947 (AOTA, 1977). In the mid-1950s, the Association formed a committee to consider the issue of graduate degrees in occupational therapy. In 1958, this committee prepared a "Guide for the Development of Graduate Education Leading to Higher Degrees in Occupational Therapy" (AOTA, 1958). This committee started the discussion on the mandate for an entry-level master's degree in occupational therapy, which would culminate 40 years later when the Representative Assembly of AOTA voted to mandate a master's entry level.

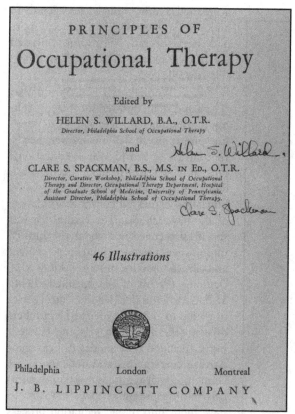

Figure 5-15. Signed first edition of Willard & Spackman's *Principles of Occupational Therapy,* the first occupational therapy text of modern times. (Copyright © Dr. Lori T. Andersen. Reprinted with permission.)

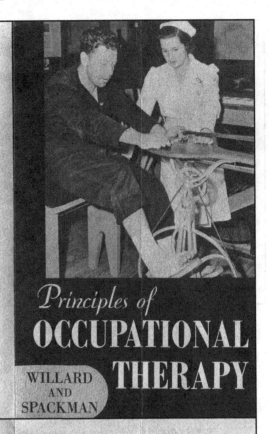

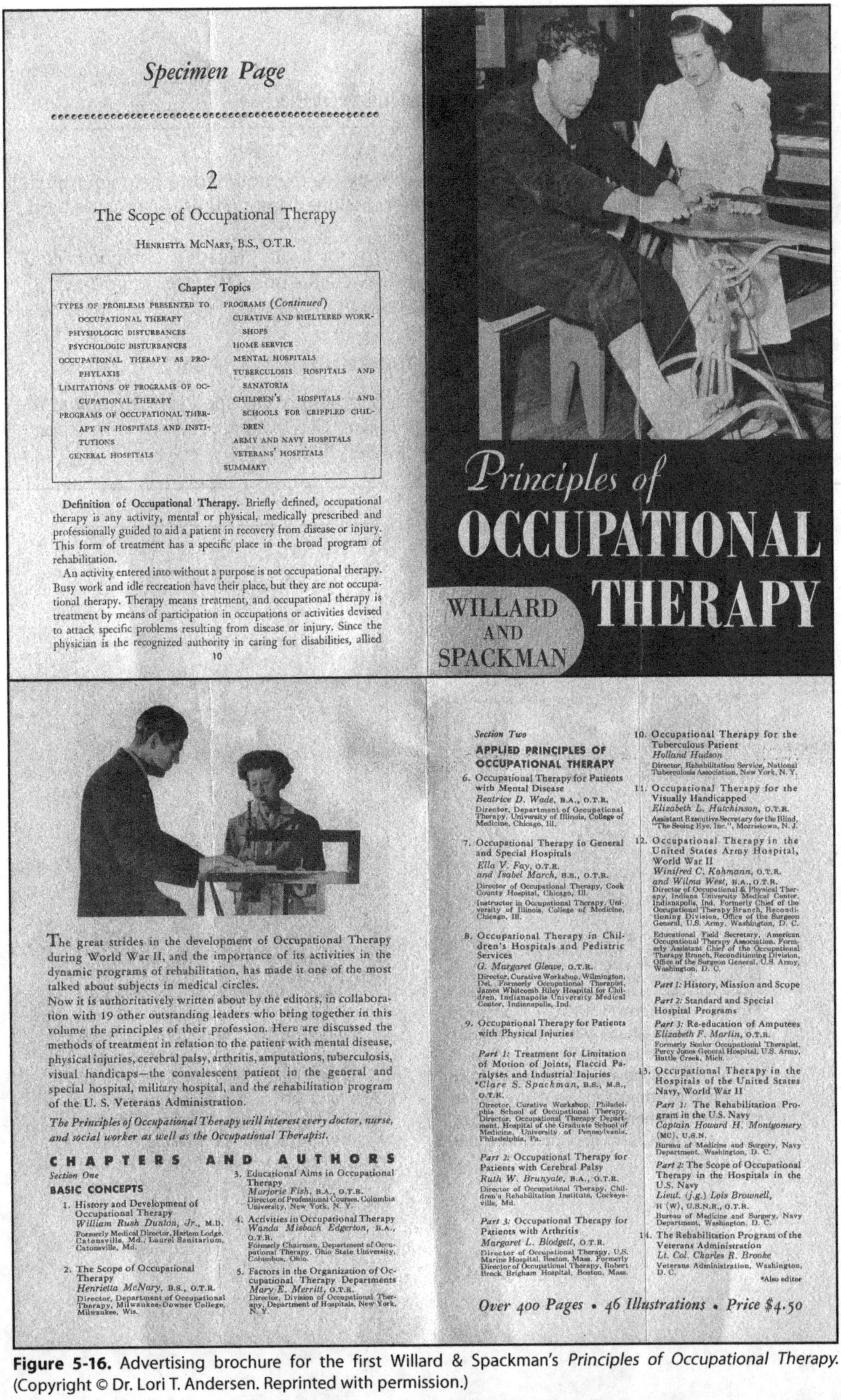

Specimen Page

eeeeeeeeeeeeeeeeeeeeeeeeeeeeeeeeeeeeeeeeeeeeeeeeeeeee

2

The Scope of Occupational Therapy

HENRIETTA MCNARY, B.S., O.T.R.

Chapter Topics	
TYPES OF PROBLEMS PRESENTED TO OCCUPATIONAL THERAPY	PROGRAMS (*Continued*) CURATIVE AND SHELTERED WORK-SHOPS
PHYSIOLOGIC DISTURBANCES	HOME SERVICE
PSYCHOLOGIC DISTURBANCES	MENTAL HOSPITALS
OCCUPATIONAL THERAPY AS PRO-PHYLAXIS	TUBERCULOSIS HOSPITALS AND SANATORIA
LIMITATIONS OF PROGRAMS OF OC-CUPATIONAL THERAPY	CHILDREN'S HOSPITALS AND SCHOOLS FOR CRIPPLED CHIL-DREN
PROGRAMS OF OCCUPATIONAL THER-APY IN HOSPITALS AND INSTI-TUTIONS	ARMY AND NAVY HOSPITALS VETERANS' HOSPITALS
GENERAL HOSPITALS	SUMMARY

Definition of Occupational Therapy. Briefly defined, occupational therapy is any activity, mental or physical, medically prescribed and professionally guided to aid a patient in recovery from disease or injury. This form of treatment has a specific place in the broad program of rehabilitation.

An activity entered into without a purpose is not occupational therapy. Busy work and idle recreation have their place, but they are not occupational therapy. Therapy means treatment, and occupational therapy is treatment by means of participation in occupations or activities devised to attack specific problems resulting from disease or injury. Since the physician is the recognized authority in caring for disabilities, allied

10

Principles of OCCUPATIONAL THERAPY

WILLARD AND SPACKMAN

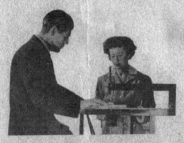

The great strides in the development of Occupational Therapy during World War II, and the importance of its activities in the dynamic programs of rehabilitation, has made it one of the most talked about subjects in medical circles.

Now it is authoritatively written about by the editors, in collaboration with 19 other outstanding leaders who bring together in this volume the principles of their profession. Here are discussed the methods of treatment in relation to the patient with mental disease, physical injuries, cerebral palsy, arthritis, amputations, tuberculosis, visual handicaps—the convalescent patient in the general and special hospital, military hospital, and the rehabilitation program of the U. S. Veterans Administration.

The Principles of Occupational Therapy will interest every doctor, nurse, and social worker as well as the Occupational Therapist.

CHAPTERS AND AUTHORS

Section One

BASIC CONCEPTS

1. History and Development of Occupational Therapy
   William Rush Dunton, Jr., M.D.
   Formerly Medical Director, Harlem Lodge, Catonsville, Md.; Laurel Sanitarium, Catonsville, Md.

2. The Scope of Occupational Therapy
   Henrietta McNary, B.S., O.T.R.
   Director, Department of Occupational Therapy, Milwaukee-Downer College, Milwaukee, Wis.

3. Educational Aims in Occupational Therapy
   Marjorie Fish, B.A., O.T.R.
   Director of Professional Courses, Columbia University, New York, N. Y.

4. Activities in Occupational Therapy
   Wanda Misbach Edgerton, B.A., O.T.R.
   Formerly Chairman, Department of Occupational Therapy, Ohio State University, Columbus, Ohio.

5. Factors in the Organization of Occupational Therapy Departments
   Mary E. Merritt, O.T.R.
   Director, Division of Occupational Therapy, Department of Hospitals, New York, N. Y.

Section Two

APPLIED PRINCIPLES OF OCCUPATIONAL THERAPY

6. Occupational Therapy for Patients with Mental Disease
   Beatrice D. Wade, B.A., O.T.R.
   Director, Department of Occupational Therapy, University of Illinois, College of Medicine, Chicago, Ill.

7. Occupational Therapy in General and Special Hospitals
   Ella V. Fay, O.T.R.
   and *Isabel March*, B.S., O.T.R.
   Director of Occupational Therapy, Cook County Hospital, Chicago, Ill.
   Instructor in Occupational Therapy, University of Illinois, College of Medicine, Chicago, Ill.

8. Occupational Therapy in Children's Hospitals and Pediatric Services
   G. Margaret Gleave, O.T.R.
   Director, Curative Workshop, Wilmington, Del. Formerly Occupational Therapist, James Whitcomb Riley Hospital for Children, Indianapolis University Medical Center, Indianapolis, Ind.

9. Occupational Therapy for Patients with Physical Injuries
   Part 1: Treatment for Limitation of Motion of Joints, Flaccid Paralyses and Industrial Injuries
   Clare S. Spackman, B.S., M.A., O.T.R.
   Director, Curative Workshop, Philadelphia School of Occupational Therapy. Director, Occupational Therapy Department, Hospital of the Graduate School of Medicine, University of Pennsylvania, Philadelphia, Pa.

   Part 2: Occupational Therapy for Patients with Cerebral Palsy
   Ruth W. Brunyate, B.A., O.T.R.
   Director of Occupational Therapy, Children's Rehabilitation Institute, Cockeysville, Md.

   Part 3: Occupational Therapy for Patients with Arthritis
   Margaret L. Blodgett, O.T.R.
   Director of Occupational Therapy, U.S. Marine Hospital, Boston, Mass. Formerly Director of Occupational Therapy, Robert Breck Brigham Hospital, Boston, Mass.

10. Occupational Therapy for the Tuberculous Patient
    Holland Hudson
    Director, Rehabilitation Service, National Tuberculosis Association, New York, N. Y.

11. Occupational Therapy for the Visually Handicapped
    Elizabeth L. Hutchinson, O.T.R.
    Assistant Executive Secretary for the Blind, The Seeing Eye, Inc., Morristown, N. J.

12. Occupational Therapy in the United States Army Hospital, World War II
    Winifred C. Kahmann, O.T.R.
    and *Wilma West*, B.A., O.T.R.
    Director of Occupational & Physical Therapy, Indiana University Medical Center, Indianapolis, Ind. Formerly Chief of the Occupational Therapy Branch, Reconditioning Division, Office of the Surgeon General, U.S. Army, Washington, D. C.
    Educational Field Secretary, American Occupational Therapy Association. Formerly Assistant Chief of the Occupational Therapy Branch, Reconditioning Division, Office of the Surgeon General, U.S. Army, Washington, D. C.

    Part 1: History, Mission and Scope
    Part 2: Standard and Special Programs
    Part 3: Re-education of Amputees
    Elizabeth F. Martin, O.T.R.
    Formerly Senior Occupational Therapist, Percy Jones General Hospital, U.S. Army, Battle Creek, Mich.

13. Occupational Therapy in the Hospitals of the United States Navy, World War II
    Part 1: The Rehabilitation Program in the U.S. Navy
    Captain Howard H. Montgomery (MC), U.S.N.
    Bureau of Medicine and Surgery, Navy Department, Washington, D. C.

    Part 2: The Scope of Occupational Therapy in the Hospitals in the U.S. Navy
    Lieut. (j.g.) Lois Brownell,
    H (W), U.S.N.R., O.T.R.
    Bureau of Medicine and Surgery, Navy Department, Washington, D. C.

14. The Rehabilitation Program of the Veterans Administration
    Lt. Col. Charles R. Brooke
    Veterans Administration, Washington, D. C.
    *Also editor

Over 400 Pages • 46 Illustrations • Price $4.50

Figure 5-16. Advertising brochure for the first Willard & Spackman's *Principles of Occupational Therapy.* (Copyright © Dr. Lori T. Andersen. Reprinted with permission.)

SIDEBAR 5-5
Career Romance Novels

In the 1940s and 1950s, a number of career books were published to help young girls learn about career opportunities available to them. Included among these were three books about the new profession of occupational therapy.

- *Betty Blake, OT: The Story of Occupational Therapy* (Dodd, Mead, & Company, 1940), written by Edith M. Stern in collaboration with Meta R. Cobb, OTR (see Figure 5-17)
- *Joan Chooses Occupational Therapy* (Dodd, Mead, & Company, 1944), written by Meta Cobb and Holland Hudson
- *Hillhaven* (Longmans, Green, and Co., 1949), written by Mary Wolfe Thompson

Dr. Joan Rogers, retired Chairperson of the Department of Occupational Therapy at the University of Pittsburgh, credits the book *Joan Chooses Occupational Therapy* with shaping her career in occupational therapy (Pitt's next chapter, 2015).

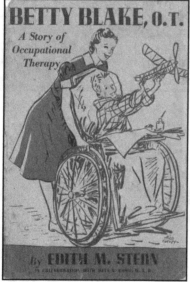

Figure 5-17. Betty Blake, OT: A Story of Occupational Therapy was written by Edith M. Stern in collaboration with Meta R. Cobb, OTR, Executive Secretary of AOTA, as a method to attract recruits to the profession of occupational therapy. (Copyright © Dr. Lori T. Andersen. Reprinted with permission.)

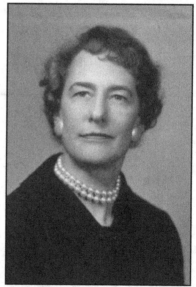

Figure 5-18. Marjorie Fish served as Speaker of the House of Delegates, first Educational Field Secretary, and Executive Director of AOTA from 1951 to 1963. Miss Fish also coauthored a book, *Occupational Therapy and Rehabilitation of the Tuberculous*, with Mr. Holland Hudson. (Printed with permission from the Archive of the American Occupational Therapy Association, Inc.)

EXAMINATION AND REGISTRATION

Membership in the Association had risen to 1,240 members by 1940. The Board of Management approved a motion to tie membership and registration together in August 1941. After October 1, 1941, only those who were AOTA members in good standing would be eligible for registration or re-registration. Those failing to re-register would need to pay lapse fees to be reinstated to the register. In 1941, the Board approved giving reciprocity to registered Canadian occupational therapists, granting them registration with AOTA (Board of Management, 1941) (Figure 5-19).

In October 1942, the Board of Management approved a motion to require graduates of approved schools to pass an examination for admission to the Register. Tentative plans were made to start administering an examination if war conditions permitted (AOTA, 1942b; Examination, 1943). Finally, on January 1, 1945, the Examination Committee had established a plan. The examination was to be administered twice per year, approximately 6 months apart. The examination was to be of 5 to 6 hours in length and consist of a section of true-false questions, a question on organization, essay questions, and a practical examination to be graded based

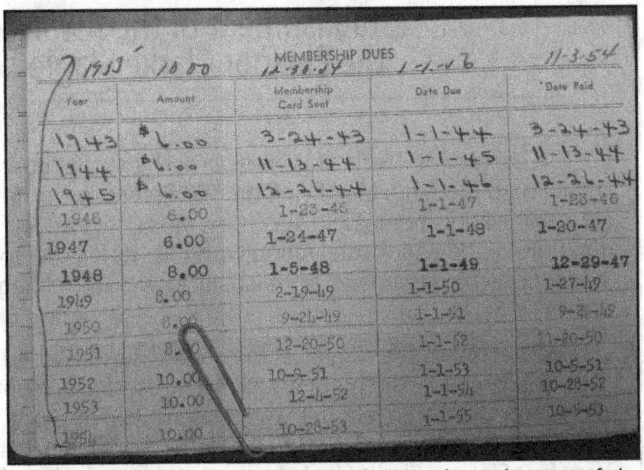

Figure 5-19. Record of membership dues. In the early years of the Association, membership records were kept on index cards. (Printed with permission from the Archive of the American Occupational Therapy Association, Inc.)

on reports from a hospital head therapist. A card file of questions was maintained from which questions were taken by a committee of three designated people to construct the examination. Students were charged a fee of $10 to take the examination. The first national examination was given on June 22, 1945 (Subcommittee on Examination, 1945). In 1947, the examination format changed to a two-part objective examination of 300 multiple-choice questions given in two separate sittings (Brandt, 1956; Otto, 1948).

A new policy requiring successful passage of the examination as one of the qualifications to be admitted to the National Register was approved in 1946. The policy stated:

> To become a Registered Occupational Therapist in the American Occupational Therapy Association a therapist must take and pass the Registration Examination. Anyone wishing to take the examination, may do so, only upon presentation of their certificate or diploma from a school whose course in Occupational Therapy is accredited by the American Medical Association. (Board of Management, 1946, p. 87)

Registered Canadian therapists, who had been given reciprocity, were now also required to pass the examination (Board of Management, 1946). In 1950, the University of Toronto and McGill University developed a combined occupational therapy/physical therapy curriculum. Expressing disapproval of this new combined curriculum, AOTA cancelled its reciprocity agreement with the Canadian Association of Occupational Therapy (Education Committee, 1951).

State licensure for occupational therapists became an issue in 1951 when some state legislatures considered introducing licensure bills. AOTA was not in support, deeming licensure "neither desirable nor practical at the present time" (West, 1951a, p. 63). The Association believed that the accreditation and registration processes already in place assured high professional standards, evidenced by the fact that there were no incidences of unqualified people compromising the high standards. The fear was that state licensure would give each individual state control of standard setting and a state may not recognize standards set by AOTA and the AMA-CMEH. Different standards in different states would restrict mobility and would have the potential to restrict otherwise qualified people from practicing. Additionally, licensing fees would be an additional expense for occupational therapists (West, 1951a) (Sidebar 5-6).

SIDEBAR 5-6

Establishment of the Award of Merit and the Eleanor Clarke Slagle Lectureship

---

The Award of Merit was established by the Board of Management at their April 1950 Board Meeting. Miss Eva Otto, the first recipient, was honored for her exemplary service as the Educational Field Secretary. Miss Otto had just submitted her resignation letter at the time of the Board vote. Along with this honor, the Board extended their best wishes for her approaching marriage, at which time her name changed to Mrs. Eva Otto Munzesheimer (AOTA, 1950, p. 236).

The Eleanor Clarke Slagle Lectureship was established by vote of the House of Delegates and Board of Management in 1953 to recognize meritorious service to the profession. Originally, the Slagle lecturer was chosen by a vote of the AOTA membership. Florence M. Stattel, OTR, from New Jersey was awarded the Slagle lectureship in 1954. She presented the very first Eleanor Clarke Slagle Lecture at the annual conference in 1955 (AOTA, 1954, p. 24).

PARADIGM SHIFT FROM OCCUPATION TO REDUCTIONISM

A confluence of events marked the shift of occupational therapy practice from a paradigm of occupation to a paradigm of reductionism. The professional image of occupational therapy that the early leaders had worked so hard to establish was in jeopardy in the early 1940s. The context in which the profession was founded had changed. Both the Arts and Crafts Movement and the Settlement House Movement had faded. The Progressive Era and hope of improving quality of life for society gave way to the Great Depression, creating severe economic difficulties and hardship for many. Occupational therapy was facing difficulty re-establishing its role in the military. Major Walter E. Barton, a psychiatrist, gave the profession a wake-up call when he questioned the value of occupational therapy in the Army. He pointed out that research efforts to "prove the value of occupational therapy in the recovery from disease and illness" were virtually nonexistent (Barton, 1943b, p. 264). Major Barton admonished the profession for failing "to adapt its therapeutic occupations to the changing demands of a new war" (Barton, 1943b, p. 264). The traditional crafts of weaving, basketry, reed work, rug hooking, knitting, and embroidery were not appropriate for men, the soldiers in World War II. He suggested that occupations such as more practical projects in woodworking, landscaping, and electrical work, would be more appropriate and interesting for men.

Advances in medicine, pharmacology, and technology helped to improve the survival rates of patients who suffered head injuries, strokes, and spinal cord injuries. Patients who would have succumbed to their injury or illness in a short time now survived but with limited physical abilities that required continued care and rehabilitation services. In contrast, tuberculosis, once a major disease affecting a significant percentage of the population, was now being treated effectively with drugs. With the declining number of people suffering from the disease, tuberculosis sanatoriums were slowly closing. The Salk vaccine against polio became available in the mid-1950s, halting the polio epidemic. Although those who were stricken with polio still required care and rehabilitation, there were no new victims of polio.

In the 1940s and 1950s, there was a push for medicine to be more scientific and evidence based. During that same time frame, physical medicine and rehabilitation adopted a biomedical model that focused on pathology and the disease process. Illness was viewed purely as a biological problem, not influenced by psychological, social, or environmental problems. To restore health, the pathological condition in the patient, specifically the diseased body part, needed to be fixed. With the shift to the biomedical model, the drive to be more scientific, and the impetus for more research, medicine became more reductionistic. The reductionistic philosophy looked at a person's ability to function in more easily measured, discrete parts.

During World War II and the start of the Rehabilitation Movement, occupational therapists started to work more closely with physiatrists and orthopedic physicians. As such, the number of occupational therapists practicing in physical disabilities settings and physical medicine and rehabilitation clinics increased. In such settings, occupational therapists accepted the reductionistic philosophy of medicine, a paradigm perceived as more scientific than the previously accepted paradigm of occupation. The paradigm of reductionism guided the profession through the 1950s and 1960s (Kielhofner & Burke, 1977; Gillette & Kielhofner, 1979).

In the changing sociocultural context, the waning of the Arts and Crafts Movement and the rise of the Rehabilitation Movement, occupational therapists wanted to dispel their image as crafts teachers (Editorial, 1951). Occupational therapy began to expand to include activities of daily living (ADL), work simplification, work tolerance, pre-vocational activities, progressive resistive exercises, adaptive equipment and aids, orthotic devices, and prosthetic training (Dirette, 2013; Kielhofner & Burke, 1977).

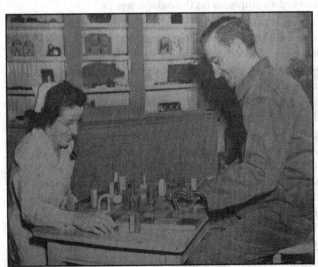

The concept of ADL was developed by Dr. George Deaver, Medical Director at the Institute for the Crippled and Disabled in New York City. Concerned that patients who came to the Institute for vocational training lacked the ability to perform simple self-care activities, Deaver, along with physical therapist Mary Eleanor Brown, developed a number of ADL assessments. Used to guide development of treatment plans to help patients become self-sufficient, these ADL assessments became the foundation of the rehabilitation services (Flanagan & Diller, 2013).

Figure 5-20. Wilma West playing chess with a soldier.

Whereas in the past carefully selected craft activities helped improve a patient's underlying abilities to enable participation in ADL, occupational therapists realized that teaching a specific ADL task would also help increase independence (Zimmerman, 1963, p. 320). With this new focus, occupational therapists incorporated new interventions into treatment programs, including training in the use of prosthetic devices, fabrication of splints, and construction of and education in the use of adaptive equipment to facilitate independence in ADL (Figure 5-20). Adaptations for

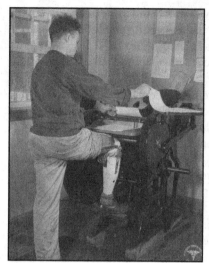

Figure 5-21. Soldier using a printing press as part of therapy program to strengthen lower extremity musculature, circa 1944. (Printed with permission from the Archive of the American Occupational Therapy Association, Inc.)

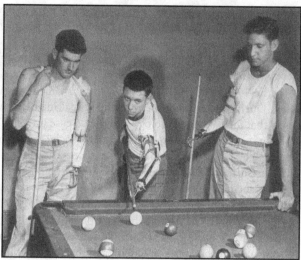

Figure 5-22. Soldiers using prostheses to play pool, circa 1945. (Printed with permission from the Archive of the American Occupational Therapy Association, Inc.)

homemaking and for self-help devices increased. Occupational therapy also focused on more mechanistic treatment, such as metric occupational therapy, which gradually increased activity to improve work tolerance, and kinetic occupational therapy, which was used to improve range of motion, muscle strength, and muscle control (Martella & Gibavic, 1949) (Figures 5-21 and 5-22). With these changes in philosophy and practice, occupational therapy education began to shift away from an emphasis on crafts and toward an emphasis on the basic sciences.

The intrapsychic pathology of mental illness was also reductionistic (Kielhofner & Burke, 1977). The psychodynamic theories initially developed by Sigmund Freud and furthered by Henry Stack Sullivan continued to inform mental health practice through the 1950s. Freud and Stack believed that the etiology of mental illness was within the person and caused by poor interpersonal relationships. Gail Fidler, a well-known occupational therapist, and her husband, Jay Fidler, a psychiatrist, interpreted the concepts of psychoanalytic theory and the psychodynamic frame of reference to occupational therapy practice. The Fidlers' use of crafts and activities allowed patients to nonverbally communicate feelings and thoughts. Puppetry, psychodrama, storytelling, and role-playing were used for this purpose (Moll & Cook, 1997; Phillips, 1996; Wade & Franciscus, 1954, p. 92). Occupational therapists also used groups and provided training to improve interpersonal relationships, communication skills, coping skills, social skills, and assertiveness (Moll & Cook, 1997; Wade & Franciscus, 1954, p. 77). Because poor interpersonal relationships were believed to be the root of the problem, the therapeutic relationship and the therapeutic use of self were of prime importance in treatment (Fidler & Fidler, 1954, p. 10).

With scientific advances in knowledge, specifically knowledge of the nervous system and motor control, new treatment models developed. Margaret Rood began developing her sensorimotor approach, Rood techniques, and Berta and Karel Bobath continued developing their neurodevelopment treatment approach with the focus of improving movement. Both of these neurophysiological treatment approaches posited that sensory input influenced motor output and incorporated the use of activities and adaptive equipment in treatment to improve skilled movement. Much of the focus of these treatment approaches is to use sensory input to facilitate and/or inhibit muscle tone and movement.

AMERICAN JOURNAL OF OCCUPATIONAL THERAPY INTRODUCED IN 1947

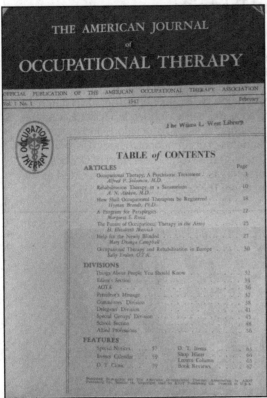

Figure 5-23. Cover of the first *American Journal of Occupational Therapy* (AJOT), published in February 1947. (Printed with permission from the Archive of the American Occupational Therapy Association, Inc.)

Charlotte Bone became the first editor of the *American Journal of Occupational Therapy* in 1947. Bone had voiced a number of concerns about the Association's official journal, *Occupational Therapy & Rehabilitation*. She was specifically concerned about the lack of timeliness of the journal, noting that dates of published events, such as the annual conference, had often passed before members even received the journal. Bone felt the journal should be edited by an occupational therapist and include articles more relevant to current practice. Plans to revive the current journal did not work out. Dr. William Rush Dunton owned the journal but the "name and contents were copyrighted ... and therefore owned by the publishers," Williams & Wilkins Company (Bone, 1971). The Board of Management decided to fund a new official publication of AOTA. Although she was not looking to take on the job as editor of a new journal, when AOTA asked, Bone agreed.

Initially, Bone was going to co-edit the new journal with Dr. Sidney Licht, who worked with Dr. Dunton on *Occupational Therapy & Rehabilitation*. After considering *Journal of the American Occupational Therapy Association* as the name for the new journal, they settled on *American Journal of Occupational Therapy* as the new name, believing that AJOT would be an easy acronym to remember. In a change of plans, Licht opted to stay on as editor of *Occupational Therapy & Rehabilitation*, covering content in all branches of medical rehabilitation. *Occupational Therapy & Rehabilitation* later changed its name to the *American Journal of Physical Medicine and Rehabilitation* (Bone, 1971) (Figures 5-23 and 5-24).

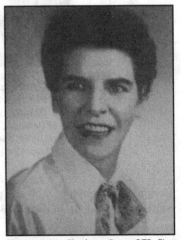

Figure 5-24. Charlotte Bone OTR, First Editor of AJOT. (Printed with permission from the Archive of the American Occupational Therapy Association, Inc.)

Charlotte Bone took on the job of editor of the new journal while she was teaching full time at the Boston School of Occupational Therapy. The editorial office was in her bedroom, and her living room served as "the mailing office." Charlotte Bone

---

Sidebar 5-7

World Federation of Occupational Therapists

Fifty-five occupational therapists from the United States attended the very first Congress of the World Federation of Occupational Therapists held in Edinburgh, Scotland, in August 1954. A total of 400 therapists representing 22 countries from around the world attended this first gathering (WFOT, 1954). The World Federation of Occupational Therapists aimed to promote occupational therapy practice and advance standards worldwide, facilitate cooperation and exchange of information among occupational therapy associations and other allied health groups, and advance the practice and standards of occupational therapy (History, 2015). Helen Willard and Clare Spackman helped to establish the World Federation of Occupational Therapists. Spackman served as the first Secretary-Treasurer and in 1956 was elected as the second President of World Federation of Occupational Therapists (see Figure 5-25).

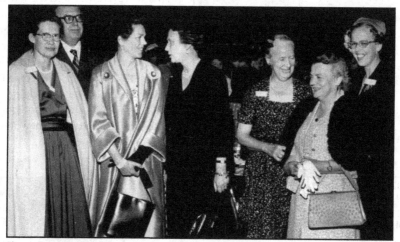

Figure 5-25. In 1958, the Congress of the World Federation of Occupational Therapists, the second WFOT Congress, was held in Copenhagen, Denmark. Attendees included (from left to right) Clare Spackman, OTR, President of the World Federation of Occupational Therapy; unknown gentleman; the Countess Bernadotte; HRH Princess Margaretha of Denmark; Helen Willard; Glyn Owens from England; and Ingrid Pahlsson from Denmark. (Printed with permission from the Archive of the American Occupational Therapy Association, Inc.)

was known as someone who was precise in speech and writing. She served as editor for two years taking great pride in her work (Bone, 1971, 1983).

CERTIFIED OCCUPATIONAL THERAPY ASSISTANTS

A number of other initiatives were undertaken to alleviate the shortage of occupational therapists nationwide during and after World War II. Although the Army's war emergency courses had started in mid-1944, it would be a full year before the first class would graduate. In December

1944, to fill immediate needs, the Army began providing a 1-month course for occupational therapy assistants. A total of 11 classes were given at Halloran General Hospital on Staten Island, New York. The program was discontinued in October 1945 after graduating a total of 278 students (Vogel et al., 1968a, pp. 181-182). In 1950, with the start of U.S. involvement in the Korean War, the Army initiated an occupational therapist's technician course, along with a course for occupational therapists. The 12-week technician's course, including 8 weeks of didactic coursework and 4 weeks of practical training, would prepare Army personnel to assist occupational therapists (McDaniel, 1968, pp. 503-506).

Significant shortages of occupational therapy personnel were also experienced in psychiatric facilities, and, in some cases, unqualified personnel were hired to fill these positions. The idea for a standardized course for training occupational therapy assistants was first proposed by Guy Morrow, an occupational therapist at Cleveland State Hospital. His proposal for a 1-year training program was referred to the AOTA Committee on Psychiatry of the Sub-Committee on Research and Services for study (Willard, 1949).

In March 1953, the AOTA Board of Management voted to appoint a committee "to make a study and report at the 1953 conference relative to recommendations for proposed standards of training, accreditation, and recognition of non-registered personnel (OT assistants and aides) in

the OT program. This study [was] to consider the re-establishment of an auxiliary registry" (New Business, 1953, p. 230). Florence Stattel, OTR, was appointed to chair the special committee charged to study the issue of nonregistered personnel (Recommendations of the Special Committee, 1953). Based on the report of this committee, the House of Delegates recommended the appointment of a committee to study and present a plan for developing a league of practical OT workers (Speaker of the House of Delegates, 1954). AOTA President Henrietta McNary appointed President-Elect Colonel Robinson to co-chair a committee with Gail Fidler to develop a plan for the implementation of recognition of nonprofessional personnel in occupational therapy (Johnson, 1988) (Figure 5-26).

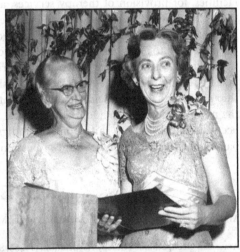

Figure 5-26. Helen S. Willard, President of AOTA, presenting the Award of Merit to Colonel Ruth A. Robinson in 1959. (Printed with permission from the Archive of the American Occupational Therapy Association, Inc.)

The committee submitted its recommendations to the Board in October 1955. A 12-week program conducted in AMA-approved hospitals under the supervision of an occupational therapist included didactic instruction, specialty skills, and supervised practical training. The plan also allowed for grandfathering of those who had worked in occupational therapy for at least 2 years and who submitted positive recommendations from a current supervisor and two other qualified people. The option to substitute experience for education for admission to the auxiliary registry would expire 3 years after implementation of training programs (Fidler & Robinson, 1956). On October 20, 1957, after much discussion and revision, the Board of Management approved the plan. The plan was implemented in October 1958 (Catteron et al., 1958; Cottrell, 2000).

The original plan provided for the training and certification of occupational therapy assistants only in the specialty area of psychiatry. The first two classes of certified occupational therapy assistants graduated from Westboro State Hospital in Massachusetts and Marcy State Hospital in New York in 1960 (Cottrell, 2000). In 1960, AOTA established a curriculum to qualify certified occupational therapy assistants for general practice (Cottrell, 2000; Johnson, 1988; Schwagmeyer, 1969).

REFLECTION

Despite efforts in the 1920s and 1930s to set professional standards to increase professional status and recognition, the poor economic conditions and misperception of the value of occupational therapy by military leaders at the start of World War II set the profession back. Occupational therapists walked a fine line between holding out for upgrades in military and professional status and doing one's patriotic duty by participating in the war effort under the status quo. The leaders recognized that efforts to upgrade military and professional status would have significant implications for occupational therapy in civilian hospitals after the war. The Association worked closely with the military to re-establish the role of occupational therapy in the military and to alleviate manpower shortages. War emergency courses, courses to train occupational therapy volunteer assistants, and the development of occupational therapy assistant programs were helpful in easing manpower shortages during and after the war.

Legislation spurred the Rehabilitation Movement, making funding available for rehabilitation facilities, for provision of therapy services, and for training of professionals, including occupational therapists. The role of women in society had an impact on the profession at a time when manpower needs increased. Women educated as occupational therapists usually dropped out of the profession to marry and raise a family, a societal role expectation. In spite of this, more women were entering the workforce with a greater variety of job opportunities available. Women started to take leadership roles in the Association, transitioning from the norm of men holding these leadership roles. A change in the sociocultural context, the end of the Arts and Crafts Movement, and the move of medicine to adopt a biomedical model and increase emphasis on science prompted occupational therapy to shift from a paradigm of occupation to a paradigm of reductionism—a paradigm that would dominate the profession for several years.

REFERENCES

American Occupational Therapy Association. (1940a, March). Notice—medical technologists. *American Occupational Therapy News Letter, 11*(1), 1.

American Occupational Therapy Association. (1940b, September 16). Minutes of the business session. Archives of the American Occupational Therapy Association (Series 3, Box 13, Folder 84), Bethesda, MD.

American Occupational Therapy Association. (1940c, November). Insignia. *News Letter, 11*(1), 3.

American Occupational Therapy Association. (1941, January 17). Proceedings of the American Occupational Therapy Association board meeting. Archives of the American Occupational Therapy Association (Series 3, Box 13, Folder 85), Bethesda, MD.

American Occupational Therapy Association. (1942a). *Guide for training course: Occupational therapy volunteer assistants.* New York: Author.

American Occupational Therapy Association. (1942b). Minutes of meeting of Board of Management—October 10, 1942. *Occupational Therapy & Rehabilitation, 21*(6), 363-368.

American Occupational Therapy Association. (1944). Announcement of emergency course in occupational therapy. *News Letter, 6*(3), 1-2.

American Occupational Therapy Association. (1950). Meetings of the Board of Management: Report of the Educational Field Secretary. *American Journal of Occupational Therapy, 5*(2), 235-238.

American Occupational Therapy Association. (1954). Annual reports: Meeting of the House of Delegates. *American Journal of Occupational Therapy, 8*(1), 24-35.

American Occupational Therapy Association. (1958). A guide for the development of graduate education leading to higher degrees in occupational therapy. *American Journal of Occupational Therapy, 12*(6), 334-335.

American Occupational Therapy Association. (1967a). *50th anniversary: Occupational therapy—Then...1917 and now...1967.* New York, NY: Author.

American Occupational Therapy Association. (1967b). Presidents of the American Occupational Therapy Association. *American Journal of Occupational Therapy, 21*(5), 290-298.

American Occupational Therapy Association. (1977). *60th anniversary 1917-1977.* Rockville, MD: Author.

Army-Navy Nurses Act of 1947 (Public Law 80-36) (1947).

Army program. (1945, September). *American Occupational Therapy Association News Letter, 5*(2), 1.

Barton, W. E. (1943a). The army expands its occupational therapy program. *Occupational Therapy & Rehabilitation, 22*(5), 247-248.

Barton, W. E. (1943b). The challenge to occupational therapy. *Occupational Therapy & Rehabilitation, 22*(6), 262-269.

Blum, N., & Fee, E. (2008). Howard A. Rusk (1901-1989): From military medicine to comprehensive rehabilitation. *American Journal of Public Health, 98*(2), 256-257.

Board of Management. (1940a, January 3). Minutes of the meeting of Board of Managers. Archives of the American Occupational Therapy Association (Series 3, Box 13, Folder 84), Bethesda, MD.

Board of Management. (1940b, March 19). Memorandum for the Surgeon General. Archives of the American Occupational Therapy Association (Series 5, Box 25, Folder 168), Bethesda, MD.

Board of Management. (1941, August 31). Minutes of the Board of Managers. Archives of the American Occupational Therapy Association (Series 3, Box 13, Folder 85), Bethesda, MD.

Board of Management. (1944, March 21). Minutes of the Board of Managers. Archives of the American Occupational Therapy Association, Bethesda, MD. Unpublished document.

Board of Management. (1946). Minutes of the meeting of the Board of Management, May 10, 1946, and committee reports. *Occupational Therapy & Rehabilitation, 25*(3), 80-88.

Bone, C. D. (1971). Origin of the American Journal of Occupational Therapy. *American Journal of Occupational Therapy, 25*(1), 48-52.

Bone, C. D. (1983). Interview transcript. Archives of the American Occupational Therapy Association: Bethesda, MD.

Brandt, H. (1956). The AOTA registration examination. *American Journal of Occupational Therapy, 10*(6), 281-287, 309.

Catteron, M., Dobranske, V. C., Messick, H. E., Peoples, M. W., Piper, B., Robinson, R. A. & Crampton, M. W. (1958). The recognition of occupational therapy assistants. *American Journal of Occupational Therapy, 7*(5), 221.

Colman, W. (1992). Maintaining autonomy: the struggle between occupational therapy and physical medicine. *American Journal of Occupational Therapy, 46*(1), 63-70.

Cottrell, R. P. (2000). COTA education and professional development: a historical review. *American Journal of Occupational Therapy, 54*(4), 407-412.

Council on Medical Education and Hospitals. (1950). Essentials of an acceptable school of occupational therapy. *American Journal of Occupational Therapy, 4*(3), 125-128.

Dirette, D. P. (2013). Trading in our paradigm shifts for a staircase. *Open Journal of Occupational Therapy, 1*(4), 1-7.

Dowsett, L. N. (1942, January). News from Hawaii [Letter]. *American Occupational Therapy Newsletter, 3*(2), 2.

Dunton, W. R. (1955, June 2). [Letter to Mrs. Frances Shuff]. Archives of the American Occupational Therapy Association (Series 6, Box 47, Folder 320), Bethesda, MD.

Editorial. (1951). Disemphasizing crafts. *American Journal of Occupational Therapy, 4*(1), 39.

Education Committee. (1945). Excerpts from the minutes of meeting, Education Committee, AOTA. *Occupational Therapy and Rehabilitation, 24*(2), 109-118.

Education Committee. (1951). Meetings of the Board of Management—Monday, October 16 and Thursday, October 19, 1950. *American Journal of Occupational Therapy, 5*(2), 72-73.

Eleanor Clarke Slagle. (1938). *Psychiatric Quarterly, 12*(1), 8-15.

Elwood, E. S. (1939, October 12). [Letter to Major General James C. Magee, Surgeon General]. Archives of the American Occupational Therapy Association (Series 5, Box 29, Folder 168), Bethesda, MD.

Examination. (1943, July). *News Letter, 5*(2), 2.

Federal Vocational Rehabilitation Act of 1943 (Public Law 78-113) (1943).

Fidler, G. S., & Fidler, J. W. (1954) *Introduction to psychiatric occupational therapy.* New York, NY: Macmillan Company.

Fidler, G. S., & Robinson, R. A. (1956). Report of the Committee to Plan Implementation of Recognition of Non-professional Personnel in the field of occupational therapy. *American Journal of Occupational Therapy, 10*(1), 27-28.

Fish, M. (1940, December 12). [Memo to Chairman of the American Red Cross Mr. Norman H. Davis, Secretary of War Henry L. Stimson, Surgeon General James C. Magee, and Senator Morris Sheppard]. Archives of the American Occupational Therapy Association (Series 4.1, Box 25, Folder 168), Bethesda, MD.

Fish, M. (1945). Report of the Educational Field Secretary. *Occupational Therapy & Rehabilitation, 24*(1), 44-63.

Flanagan, S. R., & Diller, L. (2013). Dr. George Deaver: The grandfather of rehabilitation medicine. *Physical Medicine and Rehabilitation, 5*(5), 355-359.

Folz, T. J., Opitz, J. L., Peters, J., & Gelfman, R. (1997). The history of physical medicine and rehabilitation as recorded in the diary of Dr. Frank Krusen: Part 2. Forging ahead (1943-1947). *Archives of Physical Medicine and Rehabilitation, 78*, 446-450.

Gelfman, R., Peters, J., Opitz, J. L., & Folz, T. J. (1997). The history of physical medicine and rehabilitation as recorded in the diary of Dr. Frank Krusen: Part 3. Consolidating the position (1948-1953). *Archives of Physical Medicine and Rehabilitation, 78*, 556-561.

Gillette, N., & Kielhofner, G. (1979). The impact of specialization on the professionalization and survival of occupational therapy. *American Journal of Occupational Therapy, 33*(1), 20-28.

Hartwick, A. M. R. (1993). *Army medical specialist corps: The 45th anniversary.* Washington, DC: Center of Military History, United States Army.

History. (2015). World Federation of Occupational Therapy history. Retrieved from http://www.wfot.org/AboutUs/History.aspx

Hospital Survey and Construction Act of 1946 (Public Law 79-725) (1946).

Johnson, J. A. (1988). Certified occupational therapy assistants: reflections on their thirtieth anniversary. *Occupational Therapy in Health Care, 5*(2/3), 213-220.

Kahmann, W. C. (1943). War service report. *American Occupational Therapy News Letter, 5*(2), 1.

Kahmann, W. C. (1944a). Demand urgent for occupational therapists. *American Occupational Therapy News Letter, 6*(1), 1.

Kahmann, W. C. (1944b). Report of the Committee on Education. *Occupational Therapy & Rehabilitation, 23*(6), 36-38.

Kahmann, W. C. (1947). President's opening address at the twenty-seventh annual convention. *American Journal of Occupational Therapy, 1*(6), 379-380.

Kahmann, W. C. (1950). Nationally speaking. *American Journal of Occupational Therapy, 4*(3), 111-112.

Kahmann, W. C., & West, W. A. (1947). Occupational therapy in the United States Army Hospitals, World War II. In H. S. Willard & C. S. Spackman (Eds.), *Principles of Occupational Therapy* (pp. 329-384). Philadelphia, PA: J. B. Lippincott Company.

Kielhofner, G., & Burke, J. P. (1977). Occupational therapy after 60 years: An account of changing identity and knowledge. *American Journal of Occupational Therapy, 31*(10), 675-689.

Krusen, F. H. (1944). The future of physical medicine with special reference to the recommendations of the Baruch Committee on physical medicine. *Journal of the American Medical Association, 125*(16), 1093-1097.

Krusen, F. M. (1934). The relationship of physical therapy and occupational therapy. *Occupational Therapy & Rehabilitation, 13*(2), 69-77.

La Guardia, F. H. (1941, September 2). [Letter to Meta R. Cobb]. Archives of the American Occupational Therapy Association (Series 5, Box 25, Folder 169), Bethesda, MD.

Martella, J., & Gibavic, A. N. (1949). A rehabilitation program for the tuberculous through occupational therapy. *American Journal of Occupational Therapy, 3*(5), 232-237.

McDaniel, M. L. (1968). Occupational therapy educational programs, April 1947 to January 1961. In R. S. Anderson, H. S. Lee, & M. L. McDaniel (Eds.), *Army Medical Specialist Corps* (pp. 481-509). Washington, DC: Office of the Surgeon General, Department of the Army.

McDaniel, M. L. (1968). Occupational therapists before World War II (1917-40). In R. S. Anderson, H. S. Lee, & M. L. McDaniel (Eds.), *Army Medical Specialist Corps* (pp. 69-97). Washington, DC: Office of the Surgeon General, Department of the Army.

Mental Health Study Act of 1955 (Public Law 84-182) (1955).

Moll, S., & Cook, J. V. (1997). "Doing" in mental health practice: Therapists' beliefs about why it works. *American Journal of Occupational Therapy, 51*(8), 662-670.

National Defense Committee. (1941, August 31). Minutes of the meeting of the National Defense Committee of the AOTA, August 31, 1941. Archives of the American Occupational Therapy Association (Series 5, Box 25, Folder 169), Bethesda, MD.

National Mental Health Act of 1946 (Public Law 79-487) (1946).

Nationally speaking. (1949). Kellogg Foundation Grant. *American Journal of Occupational Therapy, 3*(1), 31.

Navy program. (1945, September). *American Occupational Therapy Association News Letter, 5*(2), 1.

New business. (1953). Committee reports: Meeting of the Board of Management, March 15, 1953. *American Journal of Occupational Therapy, 7*(5), 227-230.

Oppenheimer, E. D. (1948, May 14). Report for the annual meeting of the NYSOTA of the OTVATC—May 14, 1948. Archives of the American Occupational Therapy Association (Series 5, Box 24, Folder 166), Bethesda, MD.

Otto, E. M. (1948). Committee reports: Registration Committee report September 1948. *American Journal of Occupational Therapy, 2*(5), 310-311.

Pace, E. (1989, November 5). Howard Rusk, 88, dies; Medical pioneer. *The New York Times.*

Peters, C. O. (2011). Powerful occupational therapists: A community of professionals, 1950-1980. *Occupational Therapy in Mental Health, 27,* 199-410.

Phillips, M. E. (1996). The use of drama and puppetry in occupational therapy during the 1920s and 1930s. *American Journal of Occupational Therapy, 50*(3), 229-233.

Pitt's next chapter. (2015, Spring). *Occupational Therapy Newslink, 4*(3), 1.

Recommendations of the Special Committee. (1953). Recommendations of the Special Committee of the American Occupational Therapy Association. Bethesda, MD: Archives of the American Occupational Therapy Association (Series 6, Box 50, Folder 340).

Reggio, A. W. (1947). Federal security agency, U.S. Public Health Service. *American Journal of Occupational Therapy, 1*(6), 390.

Schwagmeyer, M. (1969). The certified occupational therapy assistant today. *American Journal of Occupational Therapy, 23*(1), 69-74.

Servicemen's Readjustment Act of 1944 (Public Law 78-346) (1944).

Speaker of the House of Delegates. (1954). Report of the Speaker of the House of Delegates: Minutes of the mid-year meeting of the Board of Management, March 28, 1954. *American Journal of Occupational Therapy, 8*(5), 221.

Subcommittee on Examination. (1945, October). Minutes of the meeting of the Board of Management, June 27, 1945, and committee reports. *Occupational Therapy & Rehabilitation, 24*(5), 212-217.

U.S. Office of Civilian Defense. (1942). *Volunteers in health, medical care and nursing.* Washington, DC: Author.

Vocational Rehabilitation Act Amendment of 1954 (Public Law 83-565) (1954).

Vogel, E. E., & Gearin, H. B. (1968). Events leading to the formation of the Women's Medical Specialist Corps. In R. S. Anderson, H. S. Lee, & M. L. McDaniel (Eds.), *Army Medical Specialist Corps* (pp. 1-11). Washington, DC: Office of the Surgeon General, Department of the Army.

Vogel, E. E., Manchester, K. E., Gearin, H. B., & West, W. L. (1968a). Training in World War II. In R. S. Anderson, H. S. Lee, & M. L. McDaniel (Eds.), *Army Medical Specialist Corps* (pp. 137-182). Washington, DC: Office of the Surgeon General, Department of the Army.

Vogel, E. E., Manchester, K. E., Gearin, H. B., & West, W. L. (1968b). Wartime organization and administration. In R. S. Anderson, H. S. Lee, & M. L. McDaniel (Eds.), *Army Medical Specialist Corps* (pp. 101-136). Washington, DC: Office of the Surgeon General, Department of the Army.

Wade, B. D., & Franciscus, M. L. (1954). Occupational therapy for the mentally ill. In H. S. Willard & C. S. Spackman (Eds.), *Principles of occupational therapy* (2nd ed., pp. 76-116). Philadelphia, PA: J. B. Lippincott Company.

West, W. L. (1947). The future of occupational therapy in the army. *American Journal of Occupational Therapy, 1*(2), 89-91.

West, W. L. (1951a). From the executive director. *American Journal of Occupational Therapy, 5*(2), 60-63.

West, W. L. (1951b). From the executive director. *American Journal of Occupational Therapy, 5*(4), 164-165.

West, W. L. (1989). Ruth A. Robinson. *American Journal of Occupational Therapy, 43*(7), 481-482.

West, W. L. (1992). Ten milestone issues in AOTA history. *American Journal of Occupational Therapy, 46*(12), 1066-1074.

WFOT. (1945). *American Occupational Therapy Association News Letter, 13*(10), 1.

White House reception. (1954). *American Occupational Therapy News Letter, 2*(3), 1.

Willard, H. S. (1941a, October 21). [Letter to Meta R. Cobb]. Archives of the American Occupational Therapy Association (Series 5, Box 25, Folder 169), Bethesda, MD.

Willard, H. S. (1941b, November 5). [Memo to Mrs. Roosevelt]. Archives of the American Occupational Therapy Association (Series 5, Box 25, Folder 169), Bethesda, MD.

Willard, H. S. (1941c, December 20). [Letter to Miss Eleanor Vincent]. Archives of the American Occupational Therapy Association (Series 5, Box 25, Folder 169), Bethesda, MD.

Willard, H. S. (1941d, December 22). [Letter to Marjorie Fish]. Archives of the American Occupational Therapy Association (Series 5, Box 25, Folder 169), Bethesda, MD.

Willard, H. S. (1941e). Occupational therapy and defense. *American Occupational Therapy Newsletter, 3*(1), 3.

Willard, H. S. (1942a, February 21). [Letter to Meta R. Cobb]. Archives of the American Occupational Therapy Association (Series 5, Box 24, Folder 165), Bethesda, MD.

Willard, H. S. (1942b, June). [Letter to Presidents of State Associations re: uniforms and emblems]. Archives of the American Occupational Therapy Association (Series 5, Box 24, Folder 165), Bethesda, MD.

Willard, H. S. (1944). Meeting of the Board of Management: Volunteer courses. *American Occupational Therapy News Letter, 6*(2), 1-8.

Willard, H. S. (1949). Committee reports: Education committee. *American Journal of Occupational Therapy, 3*(4), 221.

Willard, H. S. (1950). Committee reports: Report of the education committee. *American Journal of Occupational Therapy, 4*(1), 35-36.

Zimmerman, M. E. (1963). Occupational therapy in the A.D.L. program. In H. S. Willard & C. S. Spackman (Eds.), *Principles of occupational therapy* (3rd ed., pp. 320-357). Philadelphia, PA: J. B. Lippincott Company.

6

Turning Points
1960s to 1970s

Key Points

- The professional Association celebrated 50 years as an organization in 1967.
- American Occupational Therapy Association (AOTA) bylaws were revised in 1964 to accommodate the increased activities of the Association.
- The recruitment of students to address manpower shortages continued to be a major focus of concern.
- The American Occupational Therapy Foundation was created in 1965 to house entities that could be tax exempt.
- The concept of working under a prescription was changed to a referral as occupational therapy continued the process of decreasing control of occupational therapy services by medicine and physicians.

Highlighted Personalities

- A. Jean Ayres, theorist
- Gail S. Fidler, theorist
- Mary P. Reilly, theorist
- Wilma L. West, AOTA Executive Director, 1950-1951, and President, 1961-1964
- Ruth Brunyate (Wiemer), AOTA President, 1964-1967
- Florence S. Cromwell, AOTA President, 1967-1970 (first term)
- Marjorie (Marj) Fish, AOTA Executive Director, 1952-1963
- P. Francis Helmig, AOTA Executive Director, 1964-1968
- Harriett J. Tiebel, AOTA Executive Director, 1968-1971

Andersen, L. T., & Reed, K. L.
The History of Occupational Therapy: The First Century (pp. 161-194).
© 2017 Taylor & Francis Group.

Key Places

- Clifton Springs, New York—Site of 50th anniversary celebration

Political Events/Issues

- Community Mental Health Act, 1963
- Medicare, Title 18, Social Security Act, 1965
- Medicaid, Title 19, Social Security Act, 1966
- Allied Health Act, 1966

Economic Events/Issues

- Grant monies, especially from the Vocational Rehabilitation Agency (VRA), became a major source of funding for the Association.
- VRA grants supported two field consultants: one in rehabilitation and one in psychiatry.

Educational Issues

- *Essentials of an Accredited Program in Occupational Therapy* revised in 1965. Affiliations divided into physical and psychosocial disabilities totally 6 months and there was a de-emphasis on crafts.
- Master's degree programs started
- Increased focus on continuing education to update knowledge and skills

Technological Events/Issues

- Rapid increase in the use of pharmacologic agents to treat a variety of health conditions
- Development of new splinting materials expanded the use of splints

Key Times/Events

- Plaque placed on Consolation House in Clifton Springs, New York, where founding meeting of the Association was held

Sociocultural Events/Issues

- Deinstitutionalization started in California when Ronald Reagan was governor
- Community-based practice for mental health and intellectual disabilities (mental retardation) was promoted to reduce the cost of institutional care in state budgets
- Paradigm shift occurred in psychiatry to psychoanalytic and psychodynamic theories (talking cures) in mental health
- Increased interest nationally and worldwide in physical rehabilitation

Practice Issues

- Physical disabilities overtook mental health/psychiatric occupational therapy as the major area of practice
- Practice shifted to biomedical models as opposed to social and temporal aspects of arts and crafts models used in mental health and tuberculosis settings
- Practice in tuberculosis and poliomyelitis decreased; practice in neurological disorders such as stroke and spinal cord injury increased
- Practice in pediatrics expanded with the development of perceptual and sensory motor theories
- Manpower shortages limited expansion of occupational therapy services
- Increased focus on continuing competency to practice beyond initial certification

Association Issues

- Major reorganization of the Association, 1964
- Last meeting of House of Delegates, 1964
- First meeting of Delegate Assembly, 1965
- Statement on Referral adopted, 1969
- Standards for Occupational Therapy Service Programs adopted, 1969
- Guide for the Development and Use of Personnel Policies adopted in 1967 and revised in 1969
- Statement of Basic Philosophy Principles and Policy adopted, 1969

Foundation Issues

- Authorization to form the Foundation established at annual conference in 1964
- The Foundation was incorporated in the state of Delaware in 1965 for charitable, scientific, literary, and education purposes
- Two percent of Association dues forwarded to the Foundation approved in 1969

INTRODUCTION

"Occupational therapy can be one of the great ideas of the 20th century medicine."

–Mary Reilly (1962)

John F. Kennedy became President of the United States in 1961. The Cuban missile crisis occurred in 1962 as the specter of nuclear war arose after photographs confirmed the presence of Soviet missiles in Cuba. On November 22, 1963, Kennedy was assassinated in Dallas, Texas. Lyndon B. Johnson became President during a swearing-in ceremony aboard Air Force One during the flight back to Washington, DC, and served from 1963 to 1969. The 1963 March on Washington included more than 200,000 people gathered for a peaceful demonstration calling for more action on civil rights. The marchers were addressed by Rev. Martin Luther King Jr., who gave his "I Have a Dream" speech. King would be assassinated in 1968. During the 1968 Democratic National Convention in Chicago, there was a youthful rebellion and social uprising of anti-Vietnam War protesters. In 1968, *Sesame Street* started on the Public Broadcasting System as a series designed to teach educational and social concepts to preschoolers. In July 1969, astronauts Neil Armstrong and Buzz Aldrin became the first humans to set foot on the moon.

In the 1960s, occupational therapy practice in physical disabilities overtook mental health (psychiatric occupational therapy) as the dominant area of practice. In a 1968 article, the percentage of graduates working in psychiatric settings is given as 25% (Howe & Dippy, 1968, p. 524). Many changes were occurring in the practice of physical disabilities, including the development of physical medicine and rehabilitation departments and clinics as a result of success during World War II in treating physical injuries. At the same time, changes in mental health (neuropsychiatry, mental illness) moved practice from a chronic setting (government-run hospital) to a short-term community center or supportive outpatient service. The changing practice patterns in mental health often did not include occupational therapy services.

During the same time period, models of practice were being developed by occupational therapists, and some were based on core occupational therapy philosophy and concepts, increasing the potential for professional autonomy and decreased reliance on sponsorship by other health-related professions. Examples include the communication process (Fidler & Fidler, 1963), occupational behavior (Reilly, 1966), and sensory integration (Ayres, 1968).

The 1960s marked the era of the New Frontier and the Great Society envisioned by President Johnson. The torch had been passed, as the nation's new President proclaimed, to a new generation, one with new ideas and a renewed drive to move toward a progressive future. It was an age of limitless possibilities and growing social consciousness. Medicare exemplified the changing contract between the government and American society. The Association and the profession of occupational therapy stood on the threshold of a half-century of growth and service. But more action was needed. The Association needed to respond to external factors such as the ideas that lead to the passage of the Medicare and Medicaid. Occupational therapy practitioners needed to influence government policy, not just respond to it. Changes in the Association's structure would be needed to permit lobbying on behalf of ideas important to occupational therapy as a profession and organization.

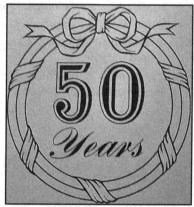

Figure 6-1. Symbol celebrating the 50-year anniversary of the founding of the professional Association: 1917-1967. (Reprinted with permission from the American Occupational Therapy Association.)

Theory and practice were also evolving. Psychiatric occupational therapy was transforming from psychoanalytic theory based on insight to community psychiatry designed to address community living problems. Theory and practice in physical rehabilitation was rapidly expanding as ideas developed during and after World War II become commonly accepted and facilities were built to accommodate rehabilitation services and clinics. Occupational therapy education shifted from diagnosis-based lectures and student training to focusing on the person with a disability who needed to function in the community and society.

The Association celebrated 50 years since its founding by placing a marker on the house in Clifton Springs, New York, where the founding meeting was held in March 1917 (Figure 6-1). New bylaws adopted in 1964 changed the organization structure to permit the Association to address external issues affecting the practice of occupational therapy, specifically federal legislation. The Association hired a paid lobbyist for the first time in 1968 to represent the Association and occupational therapy to Congress. Tax law required that to maintain aspects of tax-exempt status, two organizations would be needed, and thus a foundation was formed to carry on certain activities related to education, scholarship, and research.

EDUCATION

Revision of the Essentials

In December 1965, the Essentials of an Accredited Curriculum for Occupational Therapists were approved (AOTA, 1965b). However, the document was never published in the *American Journal of Occupational Therapy*. The official publication was the *Guidebook for an Accredited Curriculum in Occupational Therapy* (AOTA, 1965b). Several important changes were incorporated. Under the 1949 Essentials, students completed 8 to 12 months of clinical affiliations in five different specialty areas: psychiatric conditions, physical disabilities, tuberculosis, pediatrics, and general medicine and surgery. Under the 1965 Essentials, the number of months of clinical experience (hospital affiliation, clinical experience, field work) were reduced from 8 to 10 months to 6 months (24 weeks). The clinical affiliation in tuberculosis was dropped completely, and the 6 months were divided in two major categories: psychosocial dysfunction and physical dysfunction. Experience in working with tuberculosis was dropped because many hospitals and sanitariums that treated persons with tuberculosis had closed as treatment using sulfa drugs became more effective. The change in labeling the clinical affiliations (fieldwork) was a deliberate attempt to view clients' problems broadly or generically rather than based on diagnostic specific criteria. The change also provided more flexibility for educational program faculty to place students in a variety of settings rather than being restricted to specific diagnostic categories.

Another major change in the Essentials statement is that the section on occupational therapy skills does not mention handicrafts or any specific art or craft by name, although there is a list in the explanatory paragraph that woodwork, weaving, ceramics, fine art, and leather are frequently used. The actual requirement of nine semester credits lists creative and manual skills, vocational and avocational activities, daily living skills, and teaching methods. Dropping specific references to crafts by name began the process of reducing the focus on handicrafts as therapeutic occupations and increasing the focus on activities of daily living, productive occupations, and play-leisure pursuits. The change also allowed educational programs more flexibility in organizing course content in skill acquisition and therapeutic application. Craft content could be offered within the occupational therapy curriculum rather than using established courses in the art, fine arts, education, or home economics departments that taught skills such as weaving, ceramics, or woodworking but not therapeutic application to occupational therapy practice.

Overall, the concept of pathology was changed to six semester credits in physical and psychosocial dysfunction. The concept of evaluation and treatment procedures for problems of psychosocial and physical dysfunction was introduced. These changes are in agreement with the concepts of the basic approach discussed under the section on education in which the focus is on the individual as a person, not on the disease entity. Finally, another important change is that the Council of Physical Medicine and Rehabilitation is no longer listed as a partner with the American Medical Association (AMA) and the AOTA in setting the standards for education. The Association had won the dispute to avoid control by physiatrists over the educational standards.

Number and Distribution of Educational Programs

The number of educational programs in occupational therapy did not change significantly despite the documented need for more practitioners. In 1960, there were 31 programs, and in 1969, there were 32. Twenty-one states had an occupational therapy education program, but 29 did not. Most of the programs were in Eastern or Midwestern states. Only five were located in Western states. Most of the programs were not filled to capacity. Total capacity as listed by the AMA was 835 slots, but only 726 were filled. The need for better recruitment techniques and better knowledge about occupational therapy was evident.

One solution to increase the number of educational programs was to provide grant funds to colleges and universities. In 1966, the Allied Health Professions Act was passed by Congress to increase the number of support personnel available to help physicians provide better health care (Mase, 1968). This Act provided the funds to establish allied health departments to provide education in fields associated with medicine, including occupational therapy, physical therapy, medical technology, medical record library science, radiological technology, inhalation (respiratory) therapy, and cytotechnology. The funding allowed programs to develop in colleges and universities instead of in hospitals or as subspecialties under nursing (Mase, 1968). Although occupational therapy education already required a college or university degree, the increased funding would increase the number of programs available in the coming years.

Curriculum Study

The Association formally began the Curriculum Study in 1958, but most of the work was done in during the 1960s. In 1958, the Association was awarded a grant from the National Foundation for Infantile Paralysis (AOTA, 1958b). This project was the first comprehensive self-study of the profession of occupational therapy. The project was designed to provide:

- A job analysis of occupational therapy performance in selected departments to ascertain and define current job requirements to answer the question: "What is the job required of the graduate occupational therapist?"

- A curriculum survey of all occupational therapy schools and selected student affiliation centers to delineate the specific knowledge and techniques acquired by students in their professional education to answer the question: "What knowledge and skills are the schools teaching the student occupational therapist?"

- A matching of the instructional pattern against job demands to determine the functional status of the current curriculum to answer the questions: "What is the functional status of the curriculum?" or "How should education be revised to better equip us for function?" (AOTA, 1958a)

Personnel hired to complete the grant's activities included Wilma West, who initiated the project, and Marguerite Abbott, who served as the Project Director the first year but was unable to continue due to health reasons. Ms. West took over as Project Director. Carlotta Welles completed the job analysis phase, and Mary Booth completed the academic survey phase. All 31 schools were evaluated, as were numerous student affiliation sites. The project was designed for 3 years but took 5 years to complete. Ultimately, 16 reports were written and released from the original study ending in 1963.

The second part of the Curriculum Study was funded by Vocational Rehabilitation Administration (VRA) grant 123-T-66 (AOTA, 1966a). Generally, the purpose was to explore the implications of the original study in five areas: patient evaluation in physical and psychosocial dysfunction, treatment planning in physical and psychosocial dysfunction, treatment methods and activities in physical and psychosocial dysfunction, supervision, and administration. The participants were to consider four points:

- The individual occupational therapy student's need for a curriculum in which his or her best potential can grow and develop, rather than one which fits him or her into a rigid pattern

- The individual school's need for a curriculum and curriculum guidelines that not only provide minimal essentials but foster maximal efforts

- The need of the individual practicing therapist to be taught in the schools and encouraged in the clinics so that he or she will develop and not simply adjust to practices

- The patient's need for primary consideration in the setting up of his or her treatment goals and plans

At the same time, participants were warned that (1) the period of preparation always will be limited, (2) increasing knowledge always will necessitate establishing a cutoff point, (3) this cutoff point may fall short of what is desirable knowledge, (4) each new occupational therapist must take a personal responsibility for continuing his or her own education, and (5) the experienced therapist must find ways to help him- or herself continue his or her education. The results of the study group's efforts are a list of objectives divided into those considered common to health-related professions and a second list of objectives specific to occupational therapy published in AJOT (Kilburn, 1966). A total of 92 objectives are listed in the two large categories: 19 health-related objectives and 73 specific to occupational therapy. Each is subdivided into three subgroups: (1) to acquire knowledge and understanding, (2) to develop skills and abilities and (3) to cultivate attitudes and interests. For the health-related objectives, the numbers for the three subgroups were 9, 4, and 6. For the specific occupational therapy objectives, the numbers for the three subgroups were 23, 27, and 23. Thus, a relative balance of objectives per subgroup was obtained.

In a second article, there are 96 recommendations and ideas listed. The number for each entity is as follows: the Council on Standards (16 objectives), Committee on Basic Professional Education (24 objectives), Council on Practice (17 objectives), the Association (8 objectives), individual members (27 objectives), and the planning committee in charge of the VRA grant (3 objectives) (AOTA, 1967a). A more complete list of educational objectives appeared the following year and marked the first time a list of educational objectives was made available to all practitioners and anyone else interested in occupational therapy education (AJOT, 1968). The objectives are organized into six categories: normal growth and development, pathology, basic concepts in the theory and practice of occupational therapy, evaluation, treatment planning and treatment procedures, and supervision and administration. The objectives for normal growth and development and for pathology list only those related to knowledge and understanding. No objectives for developing skill and ability or for cultivating attitudes are listed because those sections were not formulated. The sections on basic concepts, evaluation, treatment planning, and supervision and administration are more completely developed into the three subcategories. Although the labels have changed over the years, the general categories of objectives remain identifiable in the format of the standards in force. These objectives also permit evaluation of course content as opposed to the Essentials document, which primarily lists resources that are available for occupational therapy students and faculty but do not state how the resources are to be used or evaluated.

An important note is that none of the objectives are about the philosophy, assumptions, or theoretical rationale of occupation as a unique concept or as the principal medium for intervention. The focus is on principles borrowed from psychology, sociology, and medicine, but not on the theoretical base of occupation. One objective does address the theoretical basis for the practice of occupational therapy, but none of the objectives address the philosophical and theoretical rationale for the use of occupation as a therapeutic or intervention approach, nor the role of occupation in maintaining health and wellness or in reducing dysfunction.

Adoption of the Basic (General) Approach to Education

The discussion of a basic or general approach to occupational therapy education grew out of an idea expressed at the 1955 Regional Institute. The statement was made that "the general occupational therapy approach be referred to the Educational and Clinical Procedures Committee and their component parts for further study, evaluation, mechanics, and implementation" (AOTA, 1955, p. 73). The idea was to shift the "emphasis from the use of diagnostic categories to the concept of treatment of patients in terms of their basic needs" (AOTA, 1968b, p. 540).

In October 1958, a report to the Medical Advisory Council meeting stated the "association has officially endorsed the basic approach in the practice of occupational therapy, i.e., treatment of the patient as a whole [person], rather than in relation to a particular disease entity" (AOTA, 1958c, p. 1). The following points were added related to educating occupational therapy students:

- That emphasis should be placed on commalities [sic (commonalities)] rather than disease entities
- That consideration should be given to patients as predominantly psychiatric or predominantly physical problems; that studies should include all age groups, all disease entities, stages of illness, varieties of treatment situations and availability of, and type of, facilities
- That developmental opportunities for the therapist should be provided, and full cognizance given to the importance of the therapist's personality in relation to her function (AOTA, 1958c, p. 1)

After 2 years of study by three subgroups across the country, three recommendations were stated in the final report: (1) the subject of the basic approach should be discussed more extensively so that all therapists could participate in the thinking, (2) the use of diagnosis should be discarded as the basis of assigning clinical affiliations, and (3) schools should teach theory on the basis of commonalities and differences rather than by diagnosis (Matthews, 1959). As noted in the discussion of the 1965 Essentials, recommendations 2 and 3 were adopted in the revision. The first recommendation was not followed specifically, although its concepts were inherent in the revision of the Essentials.

Part of the participants' concern was directed at the list of clinical training requirements and the need in the educational programs to have course content designed to prepare the student for each of the different clinical training diagnostic categories. The Essentials of an Acceptable School of Occupational Therapy (American Medical Association–Council on Medical Education and Hospitals [AMA-CMEH], 1949) required the student to complete clinical training in five diagnostic areas—orthopedics or physical disabilities, psychiatry, pediatrics, general medicine and surgery, and tuberculosis—for a total of not less than 9 months. Anderson (1959) calls the problem the five-disability approach to professional education. As the number of students increased, finding placements for all the students became difficult, and there was a certain number of repetitive work assignments the students were required to complete. Reducing the diagnoses to two primary areas, physical and psychiatric, reduced the number of training sites needed for each student and the amount of overlap in student assignments. Related, although not cited in the literature, was the closure of many tuberculosis sanatoriums as the treatment of tuberculosis became more manageable on an outpatient basis, making student placement in tuberculosis facilities increasing difficult to accomplish.

A second concern was teaching theory and application based on commonalities rather than differences. This issue could be called the 40-diagnosis approach to teaching students about applying occupational therapy to specific diagnoses. Forty is the number of diagnoses described in the manual *The Objectives and Functions of Occupational Therapy*, published in 1958. Students were expected to know the specifics of treating each of the difference diagnoses listed in the manual. The proponents of the basic approach suggested teaching the commonalities of media, methods, and techniques used in the application of occupational therapy rather than teaching the application to each different diagnosis. The rationale was that understanding the principles of occupational therapy was more important than memorizing details related to a diagnosis. The underlying philosophy was to treat the person, not the diagnosis.

The impact of the basic approach is seen in the 1965 revision of the Essentials, when the clinical experience was changed to "one three-month period or an equivalent amount of time must be in the area of psychosocial dysfunction … and one three-month period … in the area of physical dysfunction" (AMA-CMEH, n.p.). Course preparation was changed to six semester credits in physical and psychosocial dysfunction. Gone were the references to specific diagnostic categories in both the course preparation and clinical training.

PRACTICE

The Changing Role and Function of Occupational Therapy

As Chair of the Legislative Committee under the Council on Development, Ruth Brunyate prepared a report to review the status of occupational therapy (AOTA, n.d.). She outlined changes that had occurred over time in the role, focus, objectives, relationship to the patient, relationship to medicine, and function of the occupational therapist, assistant, and aide. She stated that the traditional role of occupational therapy had been treatment of the ill or handicapped and/or support of patients receiving other forms of treatment, such as surgery or psychotherapy, but that the new role included screening evaluation, programming consulting, and health planning. The traditional focus of occupational therapy had been on the ill and disabled, but the new focus was on health needs as scientific and technological advances increased both leisure hours and degree of stress. The objectives of intervention traditionally had been to correct mental or physical illness in individual patients or hospital populations. The new objectives included prevention and correction of deficits, disease, and disability; case finding; and the improvement of individual and social health.

The traditional relationship to the patient was in a hospital with one-to-one coverage in physical disabilities and ward coverage in psychiatry. The new relationship to patient included hospitals and one-to-one relationships but had expanded to include clinics, home or community, and group or consultancy. The traditional relationship to medicine had been based on prescription, through which the physician specified objectives, techniques, and procedures to be used and determined admission to and discharge from occupational therapy. The new relationship was one of collaboration, in which occupational therapy practitioners worked jointly with the physician and other professional personnel and either party could initiate the contact.

In direct service for a specific pathology, the occupational therapist determines the suitability of services for the patient, evaluates patient performance, and selects occupational therapy goals, treatment plan and techniques, and discharge. The therapist "contributes to the physician's diagnostic armamentarium, to patient management and health planning decisions, all with discrete clear recognition that the physician holds ultimate authority and responsibility for medical management" (Brunyate, n.d., p. 2). In consultant service, the therapist (1) functions upon a request from other professors, (2) initiates contribution when those components of professional knowledge, judgment, and skill unique to occupational therapy are not otherwise available, or (3) initiates contributions when the knowledge, judgment, and skills the individual therapist holds are unavailable to the patient or for society's benefit. The function of the occupational therapist was traditionally that of a clinician. New functions included educator, administrator, researcher, academician, and consultant, with supervision occurring at all levels appropriate to experience and personal and professional skills. The function of the assistant was traditionally that of a craftsman prior to certification. The new functions included clinician, administrator, and participant in research, education, and consultation, all at the technical level of competency with professional supervision appropriate to experience and personal and professional skills. The function of an occupational therapy aide was traditionally that of a handyman or orderly. The new functions included supporting the mechanics of the therapy program, transporting patients, and ensuring patient safety and order in the department. The aide does not provide treatment, even under professional supervision.

Defining Occupational Therapy

Although occupational therapy practitioners had been describing occupational therapy for many years, no official statement had been adopted by the Association that could be used as a general statement. Pattison's definition from 1922 had often been used as the default statement, but by the 1960s, it was not an accurate description or definition of current practice. A series of semiofficial definitions appears beginning in 1960 (Table 6-1). A manual designed to guide physicians in the use of occupational therapy published in 1960 focused on the concept of selected activity for physical and psychological problems and emphasized that therapists are "professionally skilled: to administer programs in occupational therapy". A fact sheet describing occupational therapy published in 1961 listed the types of activities and stated the objective or outcome expected from occupational therapy. In 1963, a description of occupational therapy practice appeared as part of the document on philosophy, principle, and policy (AOTA, 1963). However, the description was not designed as a standalone statement. In 1965, the Delegate Assembly adopted the definition prepared by the World Federation of Occupational Therapists for the 1958 meeting (AOTA, 1966b). This definition was comprehensive but still did not meet the needs of the Association for a short, formal definition.

At the urging of Ruth Brunyate, a formal, but short, definition of occupational therapy was adopted by the Executive Board and published in 1968 (AOTA, 1968a) (see Table 6-1). This definition would be revised and expanded many times over the coming years to meet the needs for legislation, especially state licensure laws. Common themes covered in the definition of occupational therapy are the unique features of the profession (activity or occupation), statement of the major

	Table 6-1
	DEFINITIONS OF OCCUPATIONAL THERAPY
1960	Occupational therapy is a program of selected activity conducted as treatment under medical direction for physical and psychological problems. The activity undertaken by the patient, the atmosphere in which he performs, and his relationships with the professional staff are the dynamic factors in occupational therapy. (AOTA, 1960b, p. 3)
1961	Occupational therapy is treatment of a patient by a registered occupational therapist through individual or group participation in restorative activity. The therapy may be needed because the patient has been disabled by an accident or disease, is physically or mentally ill; handicapped by a birth defect or the infirmities of age. The treatment program may include the use of creative and manual arts, recreation, education and social activities; prevocational testing and training; or training in everyday activities such as personal care and homemaking. The objective of occupational therapy is to make the patient as independent and well-adjusted as possible, through improving or restoring emotional, physical or vocational capacities and promoting and sustaining social and psychological function. (AOTA, 1961)
1963	The unique contribution of occupational therapy is that it uses a program of normal activity to aid in the psychosocial adjustment of the patient, as specific treatment or as a simulated work situation. Thus it relates to the patient's everyday life and provides the link between hospitalization and return to the community. (Spackman, 1963)
1963	Occupational therapy is particularly concerned with man and his ability to meet the demands of his environment. The therapist administered treatment for the patient designed to: (1) evaluate and increase his physical function in relation to activities of daily living, the needs of his family, and the requirements of his job; (2) improve his self-understanding and psychosocial function as a total human being. Treatment involves the scientific use of activity process and/or controlled social relationship to meet the specific needs of the individual patient. (AOTA, 1963, p. 159)
1965	Occupational therapy is a rehabilitative procedure guided by a qualified occupational therapist who, under medical prescription, uses self-help, manual, creative, reactional and social, educational, prevocational, and industrial activities to gain from the patient the desired physical function and/or mental response. (AOTA, 1966b)
1968	Occupational therapy is a professional health service that is a vital part of the rehabilitative team. It is concerned with the use of purposeful activity in the medical–psychological treatment of persons disabled from physical or emotional disability. (Franciscus & Abbott, 1968, p. 13)
1968	Occupational therapy is the art and science of directing man's response to selected activity to promote and maintain health, to prevent disability, to evaluate behavior and to treat or train patients with physical or psychosocial dysfunction. (AOTA, 1969a, p. 1)

outcomes (objectives, goals, purposes), description of the population of clients served (age, type of disability, disorders), a summary of the service programs offered through occupational therapy (individual, group, consultation), the process model used to deliver services (evaluation, planning, intervention, re-evaluation, discharge), and the means through which the results are achieved (media, modalities, methods, techniques) (Reed & Sanderson, 1980). Other useful descriptors are the type of profession occupational therapy is assumed to be (medical subspecialty, independent health, health related, rehabilitation), educational criteria (bachelor's degree required in the 1960s; now master's or doctorate degree required) and credentialing process (registration required in the 1960s; now state licensure required).

Medical Diagnoses and Treatment

During the 1960s, changes in medical practice resulted in changes in occupational therapy practice. For example, tuberculosis was successfully treated with the drug isoniazid and led to a significant decrease in the need to hospitalize people for treatment. As a result, sanatoriums closed because more patients could be treated by short-term hospitalization or as outpatients. The practice of occupational therapy in tuberculosis decreased. The last article in AJOT on tuberculosis appeared in 1960 (Appleby, Morton, Lawson, Loudon, & Brown, 1960). Editions of Willard & Spackman's textbook on occupational therapy covered tuberculosis through the first three editions but did not include a chapter in the fourth edition. As noted previously, the clinical affiliation (fieldwork) assignment in tuberculosis was discontinued with the implementation of the 1965 Essentials. Another diagnosis that was successfully treated was poliomyelitis (polio), with a vaccine available beginning in 1955. The last article in AJOT on treating acute polio appeared in 1957 and was a personal account rather than a description of a treatment program (Halford, 1957). Likewise, vaccination decreased the incidence of rheumatic fever, reducing the number of children often called "cardiac cripples" as a result of rheumatic fever. The last article in AJOT on rheumatic fever appeared in 1953 (Yasumarua & Baldwin, 1953).

Psychiatric occupational therapy (mental health practice) was also changing. Government-funded institutions designed for long-term care were closing in favor of community mental health centers and outpatient clinics. Insurance carriers reduced coverage and put lifetime limits on total number of days to be paid under the insurance policy. Use of drug treatment and behavioral therapy approaches increased. Ideas about mental problems as myth, faulty learning, or diagnostic condition were discussed. Psychologists took over treatment formerly controlled by physicians (Albee, 1969; Grinker, 1969; Sloane, 1969).

In contrast to the loss of practice areas, there was an increase in articles on stroke and the treatment of hemiplegia, spinal cord injuries (especially quadriplegia), and other neuromuscular disorders as drug

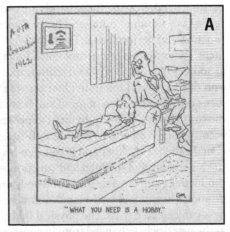

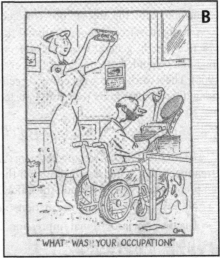

Figure 6-2. (A, B) Napkins from the 1962 AOTA convention printed with occupational therapy cartoons. (Copyright © Dr. Lori T. Andersen. Reprinted with permission.)

treatments improved, including the wide use of antibiotics that reduced the incidence of infection. Cerebrovascular disease, including stroke and hemiplegia due to a stroke, would become the major disorder seen by occupational therapy practitioners (Figure 6-2).

Current Practice as Seen in Slagle Lectures

Owen (1968) began the study of why and how occupational therapy works in practice. She analyzed eight Eleanor Clarke Slagle lectures presented in the 1960s using three philosophical questions: What is real? What is true? What is good? The analysis suggested that answers are derived from three schools of philosophical thought: Realism, Existentialism, and Pragmatism. Reality for occupational therapy is based in socioeconomic, cultural, and biological forces, according to West (1968). For Ayres (1963b), reality is based in neurology and perceptual-motor abilities. For Yerxa (1967), reality is an authentic existence. For Fidler (1966), reality is based on experience and meaning derived from that experience. Wegg (1960) has a similar view based on employment as a learning experience. Reilly (1962) suggests reality occurs or is achieved through the use of a person's hands because those hands are energized by the person's mind and will. Ackley (1962) sees reality as a union of mind and body. Zimmerman (1960) adds the concept of observation to note function and performance. Truth for West is based in normal and abnormal growth and development. Ayres focused on neurological function and dysfunction. Both respected the laws of nature as sources of truth. For Yerxa, truth is individually determined. For Fidler and Wegg, the interaction of society and the individual provide the consensual validation for truth. Reilly and Ackley focus on the interaction of mind and body to achieve truth. Zimmerman suggests that the concept of truth changes as an individual experiences struggles, necessities, and tragedies in life. Good, according to West and Ayres, is a well-functioning body. For Yerxa, good is the attainment of self-actualization. For Fidler and Wegg, good is awareness of society and the individual's attainment of the highest level of independent functioning. The concept of good for Reilly and Ackley is tied to productivity activated by mind and body and modulated by purposefulness and symbolism, which promotes health and well-being. Zimmerman adds the concept of beauty and the idea that goodness can extend beyond the physical body. The philosophy of occupational therapy has expanded as the practice has changed from occupying the sick to retard dysfunction (regression and atrophy) to encompassing the ideas of preventing disability and promoting health and well-being.

A study of Wisconsin occupational therapists in 1967 showed that the most common areas of practice were in general hospitals (44), special hospitals for the emotionally disturbed (39), nursing home/extended care facilities (24), and outpatient rehabilitation clinics (19) (Poole & Kassalow, 1968). Their work titles were either director, chief, or staff therapist. The work settings for occupational therapy assistants were not reported.

Prescription Versus Referral

The *Occupational Therapy Reference Manual for Physicians* (AOTA, 1960e) stated that the "treatment plan is the responsibility of the attending physician or the physiatrist" and that a written prescription should include the following information:

- Necessary identifying information, including the patient's name, age, ward, and chart number
- Diagnosis or provisional impression, including pertinent history and physical findings
- Treatment objectives
- Frequency and length of treatment
- Precautions and/or limitations to be observed
- Signature of referring physician (pp. 7-8)

These variations in type of prescription presented a problem of consistency among occupational therapy practitioners, which led to an ongoing discussion about the communication process between physicians and therapists. Barton agreed that the preparation of many physicians did not fit them for an understanding of occupational therapy. Physicians were known to let the nursing supervisors select patients. Some physicians saw occupational or recreational therapy as diversional, and hence a luxury and not essential. Being unaware of the treatment potential, the physicians' instruction was to "keep them busy." Barton stated that it was difficult to interest physicians in learning more about the contribution that occupation therapy could make and, as a consequence, occupational therapy received a very low priority in physician thinking.

The communication gap between physician and therapist led to a discussion as to whether there was any value in writing a prescription. Mazer and Goodrich (1958) described the use of the prescription as an outdated and essentially useless procedure that hindered communication, fostered an authoritative-dependent relationship, oversimplified the occupational therapy experience, and had a tendency to confine the role of occupational therapy to that of a "technical assistant" rather than a collegial relationship. Nichols (1960) agreed, stating that prescriptions in the classical sense did a great deal of harm because they wasted valuable time while the physician wrote the prescription and because "the system foster[ed] a lack of initiative on the part of the occupational therapist"

(p. 4). According to Nichols (1960), when the therapist was "allowed a great deal of professional leeway," the therapist almost always rose to the challenge, had a good knowledge of the patient, and became "truly a member of the treatment team" (p. 4).

Conte (1960) reemphasized the problem of the prescription, stating that the "occupational therapy prescription must go, because it serves as a device which keeps us apart" (p. 3). Instead, colleagues had to work together to develop a therapeutic team. Fidler (1963) summarized the issue of why the mechanism of a medical prescription and the concept of medical supervision were undergoing revision by stating that the "treatment planning is too complex to be specifically prescribed and strict adherence to the medical prescription inhibits therapeutic potential because of the limitations it places upon the therapist's on-going decision making and on patient-therapist interaction and response" (pp. 122-123). In place of the prescription, she suggested "active participation clinical conferences, face to face discussion with the physician and others, and review of the medical record" (Fidler, 1963, p. 123). The transfer of a diagnosis into occupational therapy goals and processes is the responsibility of the occupational therapist, according to Fidler.

The shift in thinking as to who is responsible for what aspects of the therapeutic process set in motion the shift from the concept of a prescription as an authoritative relationship between physician and therapist to that of a referral as a reciprocal, collaborative relationship with all members of the therapeutic team. Therefore, during the 1950s, the terms *prescription* and *referral* are both used (Spackman, 1952, p. 169). However, the description of information to be included on the form as described by Spackman is consistent with the concept of prescription, not referral.

To refer is "to direct for information or anything required" (Barnes & Noble, 1996, p. 1620). Referral is "the act of directing a patient to a therapist, physician, agency, or institution for evaluation, consultation, or treatment" (VanderBos, 2007). Referral as defined in occupational therapy literature is "the practice of requesting occupational therapy services and delegating the responsibility for, or the application of the practice of Occupational Therapy to a qualified occupational therapists and subsequent staff" (AOTA, 1986).

Although the process of transitioning from prescription to referral was in place, the process of fully moving to the thinking of a referral took some time. For example, Spackman (1963) states:

> The occupational therapist may accept patients for treatment only upon a written referral from a physician. The physician in referring a patient should state the diagnosis, if known, the present condition of the patient, the limitations or the precautions to be observed, the prognosis, the results to be achieved and the frequency and the length of treatment. It is the occupational therapist's responsibility to select suitable activities which should serve to attain the physician's treatment objectives. (p. 8)

She further states that the "physician, in referring patients for occupational therapy, should select only those who are in need of a medically directed, planned program of activity" (Spackman, 1963b, p. 116). Examples are those needing long-term care; those with psychological problems or with illness of psychosomatic origin; those needing special services, such as activities of daily living or adapted equipment; and sometimes those with a terminal diagnosis. Spackman continues this line of thinking in the 1971 edition of Willard & Spackman's textbook, stating that "the occupational therapist's responsibility is to select suitable activities which should serve to attain the physician's treatment objectives" (p. 7). Spackman restricts the referral process to the physician and therapist to develop a therapeutic rationale to the exclusion of other team members and continues to view the physician as the only controlling authority for the initiation of a therapeutic program. The mixed messages practitioners were receiving regarding the referral as a substitute for a physician's prescription vs. referral as a mechanism for decision making among colleagues probably did not help the profession move forward on a smooth track.

In June 1969, the Association adopted the first of three statements on referral "to clarify publicly the position of the profession relative to referral for occupational therapy service and responsibility to the medical management plan of the patients treated" (AOTA, 1969e, p. 530). For the first time, a statement was made that implied that occupational therapy practitioners may accept a referral from other professionals. The statement was that occupational therapy practitioners "respond to a request for service whatsoever the source" and that the practitioner "enters a case at his own professional discretion and on his own cognizance" (AOTA, 1969e, p. 531). The statement also implied that in certain situations, such as activity programs for diversional, social, or recreation purposes, the practitioner did not need a referral but only the "physician's knowledge" (AOTA, 1969e, p. 531). Three issues would dominate the discussion of referral in the coming years: who can refer to occupational therapy, how much information is needed from the referring source, and when or under what circumstances (diagnoses, disorders, injuries, conditions) is a referral needed or not needed.

Practice Models

The practice models in physical disabilities began to be focused more on perceptual motor (development of the sensorimotor systems) and neurorehabilitation (based on neurophysiology and facilitation) as opposed to the social or temporal aspects of arts and crafts. A third focus was on the use of activities of daily living. Ayres (1963a) outlined the development of perceptual-motor abilities in her Slagle lecture. Her work on perceptual-motor abilities would evolve into her theory of sensory integration (Ayres, 1968) (Figure 6-3; Table 6-2). Ayres also wrote three chapters on neuromuscular integration in the third edition of Willard & Spackman's textbook (1963b). Zimmerman (1963) wrote on developing programs using activities of daily living, also in Willard & Spackman.

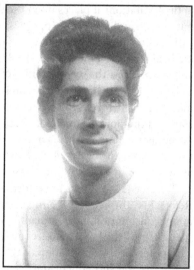

Figure 6-3. A. Jean Ayres, PhD, OTR. (Printed with permission from the Archive of the American Occupational Therapy Association, Inc.)

The emphasis in psychiatric occupational therapy was still primarily on psychoanalytical practice based on Freud (Diasio, 1967). Fidler began a trend toward including media and methods of occupational therapy with her book on communication in occupational therapy (Fidler & Fidler, 1963) (Table 6-3; Figure 6-4). Other influences were learning theory based on operant conditioning and behavior modification (Smith & Tempone, 1967) and developmental theories (Llorens et al., 1964; Mosey, 1967).

Mary Reilly began a new trend in thinking about theory in the 1960s, from following theories developed in other professions to creating theory based on assumptions and concepts from the practice of occupational therapy. In 1966, she published an article on her theory of occupational behavior based on the concept that occupational therapy should be concerned with the concept of such occupational roles as student, homemaker, worker, and hobbyist, to name a few (Reilly, 1966). Her theory was the first to focus on the unique role of occupational therapy in supporting occupational performance as the primary outcome of occupational therapy practice (Figure 6-5; Sidebars 6-1 and 6-2; see Table 6-2).

LEGISLATION

Medicare and Occupational Therapy

The Social Security Act of 1935 was amended by the addition of Title 18 (Public Law 89-97) in July 1965, otherwise known as Medicare. The purpose was to provide health care coverage to persons aged 65 years and older. There were originally two sections. Part A was called Hospital

Table 6-2
PRESIDENTIAL BIOGRAPHIES

A. (ANNA) JEAN AYRES

January 18, 1920–December 16, 1988

Born in Visalia, California. She received her bachelor's degree in occupational therapy from the University of Southern California (USC) in 1946 and her master's degree from USC in 1954. Her doctorate degree is from USC in educational psychology in 1961. From 1964 to 1966, she did postdoctoral study at the Brain Research Institute at the University of California, Los Angeles (UCLA). In addition to her degree in occupational therapy, she was also a licensed psychologist. She worked at the Birmingham Veterans' Administration Hospital in Van Nuys, California, from 1946 to 1947; at the Pasadena (name changed to Braewood) Sanitarium in Pasadena, California, from 1947 to 1948; at Kabat-Kraiser Institute (named changed to California Rehabilitation Center), Santa Monica, California, from 1948 to 1953; and at United Cerebral Palsy, Los Angeles, California, from 1954 to 1955. She was Assistant Professor, Occupational Therapy Department, USC, from 1955 to 1964; Special Education, USC, from 1966 to 1973; and Visiting Associate (Adjunct) Professor, Occupational Therapy, from 1976 to 1988. She was in private practice from 1977 to her retirement.

Ayres began publishing in 1949, with an article on the analysis of crafts for electroshock patients and then on work behavior and habits. She began her study on perceptual-motor behavior during her postdoctoral studies and developed her theory of sensory integration in the late 1960s and early 1970s. She published many articles and two books: *Sensory Integration and Learning Disorders* (1973, Western Psychological Services, Los Angeles, CA) and *Sensory Integration and the Child* (1970, Western Psychological Services, Los Angeles, CA). She also published several assessments that were grouped together in the Southern California Sensory Integration Tests (1980, Western Psychological Services, Los Angeles, CA) and a revised version called the Sensory Integration and Praxis Tests (1989, Western Psychological Services, Los Angeles, CA).

She was awarded the Eleanor Clarke Slagle lectureship in 1963, was named to the Roster of Fellows in 1973, and was a charter member of the Academy of Research in 1983.

GAIL MAXINE SPANGLER FIDLER

September 18, 1916–April 26, 2005

Born in Lebanon, Pennsylvania. She received a Bachelor of Arts degree in 1938 from Lebanon Valley College in Annville, Pennsylvania, and her certificate in occupational therapy in 1942 from the Philadelphia School of Occupational Therapy. While attending occupational therapy classes, she worked at the Smith Memorial Playground in Philadelphia. After graduation, she worked at the state hospital in Norristown, Pennsylvania, from 1942 to 1943 and at Walter Reed General Hospital in Washington, DC, from 1943 to 1944; was Chief Occupational Therapist at the Convalescence Hospital at Fort Story, Virginia, from 1944 to 1946; and was Chief of the Occupational Therapy Service at the Veterans Hospital in Lyons, New Jersey, from 1946 to 1950. She was a special consultant to the Pennsylvania Department of Welfare from 1952 to 1953 and special instructor at the Philadelphia School of Occupational Therapy. She was Coordinator of the Office of Vocational Rehabilitation Institute grant in 1955 and the project in psychiatry at AOTA from 1955 to 1956

In 1959, she accepted a position at Columbia University College of Physicians and Surgeons, and at the New York State Psychiatric Institute where she worked until 1968. From 1964 to 1967, she was Clinical Director of the master's program at New York University. She served on the Executive Board of the Association from 1969 to 1971; as Associate Executive Director for Practice, Education, and Research from 1971 to 1975; and as Interim Executive Director for 8 months in 1975. In 1990, she was the interim Director of the Occupational Therapy Program at College Misericordia in Pennsylvania. She received the Eleanor Clarke Slagle lectureship in 1965, was named to the Roster of Fellows in 1973, was given the Award of Merit in 1980, and received the President's Commendation in 2012.

She is best known for her work in psychiatric occupational therapy and her mentorship. With her husband, Jay W. Fidler, she published two books: *Introduction to Psychiatric Occupational Therapy* (1954, Macmillan, New York, New York) and *Occupational Therapy: A Communication Process in Psychiatry* (1963, Macmillan, New York, New York). In 2002, she authored *Lifestyle Performance: A Model for Engaging the Power of Occupational Therapy* (SLACK Incorporated, Thorofare, New Jersey) with Beth Velde (Figure 6-17).

(continued)

Table 6-2 (continued)
PRESIDENTIAL BIOGRAPHIES

MARY REILLY

October 11, 1916–February 28, 2012

Born in Boston, Massachusetts. She received a certificate in occupational therapy from the Boston School of Occupational Therapy in 1940. She later received a Bachelor of Science degree in occupational therapy from the University of Southern California in 1951, a master's degree from San Francisco State College, and a degree in education from the University of California, Los Angeles, in 1959. Her dissertation was entitled "A Theoretical Basis for Planned Change in Professional Education," which would set the course for her later ideas about professional education and theory of practice.

She was named a charter member of the American Occupational Therapy Foundation Academy of Research and was also named to the Roster of Fellows in 1973. Her Eleanor Clarke Slagle lecture delivered in 1961 is one of most cited in the occupational therapy literature. She served on various Committee on Education subcommittees during the 1950s. Her first job was at the Sigma Gamma Hospital School in Detroit, Michigan, where she worked with children with cerebral palsy. She then served in the U.S. Army and as a civilian therapist in the program that would become the United States Army Medical Specialists, was eventually promoted to the rank of Captain, and earned the Army Meritorious Serve Award and Letterman Army Certificate of Achievement. She was an occupational therapy consultant for the Service Command Surgeon's Office, Fourth Service Command, Atlanta, Georgia, from 1944 to 1945. Her work included supervising occupational therapy programs in 11 general, two convalescent, and six regional station hospitals. She was Professor and Graduate Coordinator of the Occupational Therapy Program at the University of Southern California in Los Angeles from 1955 to 1978. She first published on the theory of Occupational Behavior in 1966.

WILMA (WILLIE) LOUISE WEST

November 16, 1916–December 17, 1996

Born in Rochester, New York. In 1939, she graduated from Mount Holyoke College with a major in economics and sociology. After attending a lecture by Marjorie Fish on occupational therapy, she applied to the Boston School of Occupational Therapy in the advanced standing course and graduated in 1941. One of her classmates was Carlotta Wells. From 1941 to 1943, she was employed at the Robert Brigham Hospital in Boston, where she worked with clients with arthritis, cardiac conditions, and rheumatic fever. She next joined the staff of the Walter Reed General Hospital as an assistant and then Head of the Orthopedic Section. From June 1944 to August 1946, she worked as an assistant to Mrs. Kahmann in the Occupational Therapy Branch of the Surgeon General's Office doing recruiting, processing, selecting and assigning to schools the students selected for training in the war emergency courses, visiting occupational therapy schools that were giving the Army courses and consulting with them about the program, directing student training in Army hospitals, inspecting Army hospital occupational therapy departments, compiling a standard equipment and supply list, and writing in collaboration with others the War Department Technical Manual of Occupational Therapy.

She received the Meritorious Civilian Service Award from the War Department for her service and was Commissioned as Captain in the Women's Medical Specialist Corps, United State Army Reserve. She served as the Educational Field Secretary in the National Office of the Association beginning in July 1947. Soon after, she was asked to assume the duties of Executive Director, a position she held until 1951. A scholarship by the Baruch Committee on Physical Medicine allowed her to attend the University of Southern California to complete the master's program as the first graduate of the program started in 1946. In 1953, she returned to the Army during the Korean War and served as Director of Occupational Therapy at Fort Sam Houston, Texas. For several years she worked part-time, including chairing the Curriculum Study from 1960 to 1964. In 1964, she became a consultant in occupational therapy for the Office of Maternal and Child Health, Department of Health, Education, and Welfare until her retirement in 1977.

From 1961 to 1964, she served as president of AOTA. From 1972 to 1982, she served as President of the AOTF. She received the Award of Merit in 1951, was the Eleanor Clarke Slagle lecturer in 1967, was a charter member of the Roster of Fellows in 1973, and received the first AOTA/AOTF Presidents' Commendation for a lifetime of service to the profession in 1990. Other awards included a HEW Superior Service Award in 1972 and a Certificate of Appreciation from the U.S. Army Surgeon General in 1981.

(continued)

Table 6-2 (continued)
PRESIDENTIAL BIOGRAPHIES

RUTH W. BRUNYATE WEIMER

April 11, 1916–October 14, 2008

Born in Orange, New Jersey. She graduated from Hollins College, Roanoke, Virginia, in 1938 with a degree in psychology. She received her certificate in occupational therapy from the Philadelphia School of Occupational Therapy in 1940. Her master's degree in education was from Johns Hopkins University in Baltimore, and she was awarded an Honorary Doctor of Letters from Towson University in 1980. She worked as an occupational therapist at the Seashore House in Atlantic City, New Jersey. From 1943 to 1961, she served as Director of Occupational Therapy at the Children's Rehabilitation Institute in Reisterstown, Maryland, which became the Kennedy-Kreiger Institute of Johns Hopkins Hospital. In 1962, she became an Assistant Professor of Occupational Therapy at the Milwaukee-Downer College in Milwaukee. In the same year, she was employed as a consultant in occupational therapy by the State of Maryland. In 1966, she became Chief of the Division of Occupational Therapy for the Maryland Department of Health, until her retirement in 1980.

She presented the Eleanor Clarke Slagle lectureship in 1957, was named as a charter member to the Roster of Fellows in 1973, and was given the Award of Merit in 1968, the Lindy Boggs Award in 1983, and the AOTA/AOTF Wilma West award for lifetime of service. Other awards were the establishment of the Ruth W. Brunyate Lectureship by the community College of Baltimore, a Presidential Commendation in 1979, and an Honorary Doctor of Humane Letters by Towson University. She was a member of the National Health Council Board. She was President of AOTA from 1964 to 1967. Weimer knew Dr. Dunton because she worked in the state of Maryland and was a member of the Maryland Occupational Therapy Association.

FLORENCE STUART CROMWELL

May 14, 1922–November 5, 2016

Born in Pennsylvania and raised in Ohio. She attended Miami University, where she received a bachelor's degree in education before receiving a second bachelor's degree in occupational therapy from Washington University in St. Louis in 1949 and a master's degree in occupational therapy from the University of Southern California in 1952. Cromwell served in the Navy from 1943 to 1946. Some of her leadership experiences in the Navy provided her with skills that were useful when she served two terms as President of AOTA, from 1967 to 1970 and 1970 to 1973. She served as Acting Chair at USC from 1973 to 1976. She worked at Los Angeles County General Hospital; Goodwill Industries of Southern California; Vising Nurse Association of Philadelphia; Research Therapists, OVR Project, United Cerebral Palsy Association of Los Angeles County; part-time instructor, Occupational Therapy Department, USC; and Consultant, Master's Degree Pilot Program. She was named as a charter member to the Roster of Fellows in 1973 and was given the Award of Merit in 1974. She was editor of the journal *Occupational Therapy in Health Care*. She was interested in interprofessional relationships.

MARJORIE FISH

October 20, 1905–November 27, 1994

Born in St. Louis, Missouri. She received a degree from Swarthmore College in Swarthmore, Pennsylvania, and her diploma in occupational therapy from the Boston School of Occupational Therapy. She worked at Danvers State Hospital in Massachusetts, then returned to the Boston School to serve as Assistant Director and Field Secretary. She became the Director of the Occupational Therapy Education Program at Columbia University starting in 1941. She went to Sydney, Australia, to start another education program. She was the first Educational Field Secretary of the Association and then served as Executive Director from 1951 to 1963, when it was headquartered in New York City. West said of Fish upon her retirement: "Your tireless efforts and unending interest in executing the myriad responsibilities inherent in your position are the hallmark of your devotion." Later, Fish worked as a training consultant in rehabilitation for the U.S. Department of Health, Education, and Welfare. She was also active in the World Federation of Occupational Therapists.

(continued)

Table 6-2 (continued)
PRESIDENTIAL BIOGRAPHIES

P. (PALENIA) FRANCES HELMIG

May 9, 1911–July 21, 1980

Born in Atlantic City, New Jersey. She received her Bachelor of Arts degree from the New Jersey State Teachers College in Upper Montclair and became a mathematics teacher. She received a master's degree from the University of Southern California in 1952. She graduated from the Advanced Standing Course at the Philadelphia School of Occupational Therapy in 1941 and stayed there a year as Assistant Director of the Curative Workshop. She joined the Navy in October 1942 and was the first WAVE officer assigned in the U.S. Naval Hospital in Philadelphia, where she headed the hospital's Occupational Therapy Department from 1942 to 1946. She held the rank of Commander in the U.S. Naval Reserve, Medical Service Corps. From 1949 to 1950, she was a consultant in Chicago to the National Society for Crippled Children and Adults. From 1952 to 1953, she was a consultant in rehabilitation to the Health and Welfare Council in Philadelphia. From 1946 to 1949 and 1953 to 1959, she was director of the Rochester Rehabilitation Center. From 1959 to 1961, she was Director of Occupational Therapy at the Emily P. Bissell Hospital in Wilmington, Delaware. During her tenure as Executive Director of AOTA, she was severely injured in an automobile accident in California. Although she resumed her duties after her recovery, she resigned 3 years later.

HARRIET JONES TIEBEL

May 6, 1915–September 15, 2006

Born in Berwyn, Illinois. She attended Barnard College and received a diploma from the Philadelphia School of Occupational Therapy. She worked at the Payne Whitney Clinic and Goldwater Memorial Hospital in New York City. She became a WAVES officer and served at the United States Naval Hospital in St. Albans, New York. An interest in American history led to further study at Columbia University, where she received a master's degree. She served as the New York State Delegate to the House of Delegates from 1946 to 1948 and was Speaker of the House of Delegates in 1958. She was Executive Director of AOTA from 1968 to 1972.

SIDNEY LICHT

April 18, 1907–March 1, 1979

Born in New York City. He graduated from New York university in 1931. Dr. Licht's career in physical medicine included employment in Boston, and New Haven, Connecticut. He became Editor of *Occupational Therapy and Rehabilitation* in 1951 upon Dr. Dunton's retirement and changed the name to the *American Journal of Physical Medicine* because the journal was no longer primarily devoted to occupational therapy. Dr. Licht severed on the Board of Management as a Board Fellow and severed as a consultant in medical journalism to AJOT from 1969 to 1979. He edited the monograph entitled *Occupational Therapy Source Book* (1948, Williams & Wilkins, Philadelphia, PA), a collection of early articles on occupational therapy, and co-edited with Dr. Dunton two editions of the textbook *Occupational Therapy: Principles and Practices* (1950, 1957, Charles C. Thomas, Springfield, IL). He was the guest lecturer at the luncheon in Clifton Springs to celebrate the 50th year of the Association.

Adapted from:

American Occupational Therapy Association (1967). Presidents of the American Occupational Therapy Association (1917-1967). *American Journal of Occupational Therapy, 21*(5), 290-298.

American Occupational Therapy Association (1979). Sidney Licht – 1907-1979. *American Journal of Occupational Therapy, 33*(12), 762.

American Occupational Therapy Association (1968). Mrs. Tiebel assumes duties of executive director. *American Journal of Occupational Therapy, 22*(2), 65.

Cromwell, F.S. (1968). Nationally speaking. *American Journal of Occupational Therapy, 22*(3), 155-159.

American Occupational Therapy Association (1947). Meritorious civilian service awards. *American Journal of Occupational Therapy, 1*(1), 33.

In memoriam, Sidney Licht—1907-1979. (1979). *American Journal of Occupational Therapy, 33*(12), 762.

Marjorie Fish, O.T.R. (1947). *American Journal of Occupational Therapy, 1*(2), 101.

Meet our headquarters: New Executive Director. (1964). *American Journal of Occupational Therapy, 18*(4), 164.

People you should know (1950). *American Journal of Occupational Therapy, 4*(5), 228.

Remembering former executive director Marjorie Fish. (1994). *OT Week, 9*(2), 62.

Table 6-3
STATEMENT OF POLICY
1. Maintain and control the voluntary registration of its practitioners
2. Regulate, in conjunction with the Council on Medical Education and Hospitals of the American Medical Association, the education of occupational therapists to prepare them for their treatment function
3. Establish and maintain standards of clinical practice in occupational therapy which will improve patient treatment
4. Foster continuing growth in the professional competence of occupational therapists
5. Encourage and facilitate increase in the body of specific occupational therapy knowledge available to physicians
6. Protect the standards of occupational therapy and the environment in which the occupational therapist functions
7. Strongly oppose and protest any administrative policy or structure which ignores or weakens the treatment function of occupational therapy.
(First statement adopted by Board of Management in 1949, published in AJOT in 1950 and revised in 1960.)
AOTA Board of Management. (1961). Statement of policy. *American Journal of Occupational Therapy, 15*(1), 24.

Insurance, and Part B was called Medical Insurance. An information insert to AOTA's newsletter was called Notes on Medicare for the Occupational Therapist. The insert stated that for inpatient hospital services, occupational therapy was not a required service, but if such a service was "ordinarily furnished by such hospital for the care and treatment of inpatients," the reasonable cost of the services was covered (AOTA, 1966c). For post-hospital extended care, the insert quoted a passage from the law: "occupational therapy furnished by the extended care facility or by others under arrangement with them made by the facility" was covered. Home health services were stated as specified in the definition of home health services. Occupational therapy in outpatient diagnostic services was to be covered if it was one of diagnostic services "ordinarily furnished" by the hospital to outpatients.

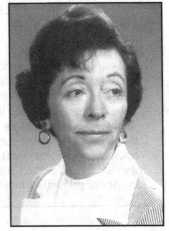

Figure 6-4. Gail S. Fidler, OTR. (Printed with permission from the Archive of the American Occupational Therapy Association, Inc.)

Although the initial assessment of occupational therapy coverage appeared satisfactory, problems were soon identified as the Social Security Administration began interpreting the law differently from the Association. A report entitled "Statement of Position on Medicare Legislation" and dated September 12, 1968, was prepared by the Legislative Committee and identified the Association's policy regarding Medicare. The Council on Development minutes report that there was no provision of services without a physician referral or by qualified occupational therapists in independent or private practice. Recommended additions to the policy were that:

Figure 6-5. Mary P. Reilly, EdD, OTR. (Printed with permission from the Archive of the American Occupational Therapy Association, Inc.)

Sidebar 6-1

Mary Reilly—Slagle Lecturer

"That man, through the use of his hands as they are energized by mind and will, can influence the state of his own health."

—Mary Reilly (1962, p. 2)

In an oral history interview with Chris Peters, Bob Bing related a story about Mary Reilly's selection as a Slagle lecturer.

> The story is that Willard and Spackman took Mary for a walk around the hotel after she had been selected and before it was announced. They tried to talk her out of it because they felt she was far too controversial. Good old Mary held her ground and delivered probably the most quoted lecture of all. (Peters, 2011, p. 262)

Sidebar 6-2

Lela Llorens—Slagle Lecturer

Llorens relates a story in which she, as a Black woman, was not able to attend meetings or stay in the conference hotel at the 1961 AOTA conference in (segregated) New Orleans because a state statute prohibited Blacks and Whites to associate in this way. This prompted AOTA to establish an anti-discrimination policy, refusing to hold Association meetings at facilities that discriminated (Peters, 2011, p. 379).

Eight years later, Llorens delivered her Slagle Lecture at the 1969 AOTA conference in Dallas, Texas. The auditorium was filled by the attendees and the balcony was filled with "cooks, bellhops, and maids, Black people who worked in the hotel" (Peters, 2011, p. 380). They came to offer their support to the Black woman who was delivering a lecture to an audience of primarily White women.

- The services of qualified occupational therapists be provided to those in need of that service, directly without the requirements of a physician's referral
- Qualified occupational therapists as independent practitioners be included under the supplementary medical insurance program (Part B) and thus be eligible to receive direct payment for services (AOTA, 1969c)

The amendments were submitted to Congress but were not adopted.

The problems continued to mount as interpretations of the law were not in occupational therapists' favor. Cromwell (AOTA, 1969) reported to the members of the Delegate Assembly that recent interpretations made by the Social Security Administration placed occupational therapy at a disadvantage of being the lone service in home health agencies. The interpretation continues to be an issue.

Association Response to External Events: Lobbying

The passage of the Medicare and Medicaid legislation brought to the attention of the Association that external events could have significant effect on the practice of occupational therapy. Because occupational therapists were not active in lobbying members of Congress at the time Medicare and Medicaid were passed, occupational therapy had no recognized status as a service provider in the new legislation. To correct the lack of lobbying presence at hearings for congressional bills, President Brunyate recommended a lobbyist be hired. In 1967, Russell J. N. Dean, Director of the Washington Consulting Service, was hired to represent the Association before Congress.

Other Legislation

Other legislation important to occupational therapy was the passage of the Community Mental Health and Mental Retardation Act in 1963 (Public Law 88-164), which provided money to establish community-based services for persons with psychiatric disorders and intellectual disabilities in place of institutionalization. This Act ultimately led to a reduction in size or closing of many state mental health facilities and the loss of jobs in mental health practice. Community-based facilities were funded on a sliding scale in which the federal government would pay most of the initial costs and the state was to pick up funding by the end of 7 years. Many states did not pick up funding, and the facility services were scaled back or closed, further reducing jobs for occupational therapy practitioners in mental health. In 1965, the Heart Disease, Cancer, and Stroke Amendments to the Regional Medical Programs (P.O. 89-239) was passed. The Act was designed to increase the study and research on the three conditions, all of which indirectly benefited occupational therapy practice. However, the focus on stroke was probably the greatest benefit. In 1966, the Allied Health Professions Act (Public Law 89-749) was passed, which provided funds to universities to start or strengthen allied health professional education. Many occupational therapy educational programs took advantage of the funding to initiate or expand the curriculum in occupational therapy.

TECHNOLOGY

During the 1960s, splinting materials improved with the introduction of more flexible plastics. Royalite (PolyOne) and Bakelite (Union Carbide) were the early versions. These plastics were less brittle and more flexible than the early acrylic and nitrocellulose plastics. However, the plastics did require heating to temperatures of 300° F to 350° F to become malleable. Such high temperatures limited forming the splint directly on the client because the skin would be burned (Koepke, Feallock, & Feller, 1963). Later, Prenyl (Larson Medical Products) and Orthoplast (Patterson Medical) became available (Kester, 1966; Willis, 1969). These plastics were the early low-temperature splinting materials that could be molded at temperatures around 150° F allowing the splint to be formed directly on the client.

RESEARCH

Research methods and studies began to change in the 1960s. Most research studies prior to the 1960s were survey questionnaires, program descriptions, or craft analyses. Beginning in the 1960s, articles in AJOT began to discuss methods of research and the attitude and skill sets necessary to conduct experimental research. For example, Reilly (1960, p. 206) stated there are three factors needed to nurture a climate for occupational therapy research : (1) at the clinical level, our minds should become dominated by the attitudes and methods of science; (2) at the school level, our curricula should contain knowledge both substantive and appropriate to the problems that are the responsibility of our profession to solve; and (3) at the administrative level, our national association should be so organized that our collective resources could be directed with more validity to the improvement of the occupational therapy service, which is to fill the health needs of patients for activity. She suggested that the research should focus on the assumptions that "man has a vital need for activity, and that activity enhances convalescence" (Reilly, 1960, p. 208). However, she also noted that occupational therapy practice lacked a theoretical base to organize its assumptions. She also stated that research requires a specific thinking process that occupational therapists would have to learn. To facilitate the learning process, Paolino (1962) discussed in detail how to take observational notes on a clinical session in occupational therapy. Llorens et al. (1964) reported the systematic evaluation of children using standardized tests of perceptual motor skills. Ayres (1966) reported the interrelationships among perceptual motor functions. Fox (1966) reported the computer simulation of neurophysiological processes. Although limited in scope, a research tradition was starting to grow within the profession.

ASSOCIATION

During the 1960s, the Association was concerned with maintaining and strengthening the objectives on which the organization was founded: educational and practice standards, credentialing (registration) of practitioners, and support of research. The policy statement in Table 6-3 presents the concerns expressed by the Board of Management. The primary concern was registration of qualified practitioners, followed by standards for educating therapists. Standards for occupational therapy programs and professional competence followed. Increasing the body of knowledge in general, and specifically to physicians, was viewed as important. Finally, the Association saw it

Table 6-4
PRESIDENTIAL INFLUENCES

Wilma West, 1961-1964

Major accomplishment: Bylaws that reorganized the Association.

    As a profession we should return to the principles of our founders who valued the therapeutic effect of occupations on health. Secondly, we need to return to the principle that education leads to practice, not vice versa. (AOTA, 1992)

Ruth Brunyate Wiemer, 1964-1967

Major accomplishment: Reorganized Association, moved to new quarters, and acquired more staff to provide better membership services.

    I think the association's greatest achievement was our move from a single agency to a business league and foundation... because it has enabled us to speak out on health issues and to facilitate our inclusion in significant legislation. At the same time it has helped us focus on research and therefore enhance our ability to clarify our philosophical base, our science, and our art. (AOTA, 1992)

Florence Cromwell, 1967-1973

Major accomplishment: Moving the Association headquarters from New York City to Washington, DC, increasing the profession's visibility and participation in federal legislation matters.

    The major accomplishment of AOTA and its members in 75 years is our return to the philosophy of our founders—believing in the curative effects of occupation—and a growing willingness to champion that principle in health maintenance and illness prevention. (AOTA, 1992)

Adapted from:

1969 election brochure

AOTA (1992). AOTA's hall of leaders. *OT Week, 6*(21), 40-43.

American Occupational Therapy Association (1967). Presidents of the American Occupational Therapy Association (1917-1967). *American Journal of Occupational Therapy, 21*(5), 290-298.

American Occupational Therapy Association (1967). Presidents of the American Occupational Therapy Association (1917-1967). *American Journal of Occupational Therapy, 21*(5), 290-298.

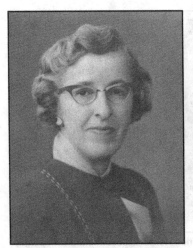

Figure 6-6. Wilma L. West, OTR, FAOTA. (Printed with permission from the Archive of the American Occupational Therapy Association, Inc.)

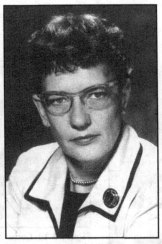

Figure 6-7. Ruth W. Brunyate (Wiemer), MEd, OTR, FAOTA, President of AOTA, 1964-1967. (Printed with permission from the Archive of the American Occupational Therapy Association, Inc.)

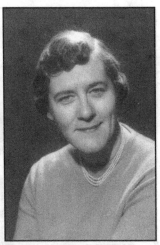

Figure 6-8. Florence S. Cromwell, MA, OTR, FAOTA, President of AOTA, 1967-1973. (Printed with permission from the Archive of the American Occupational Therapy Association, Inc.)

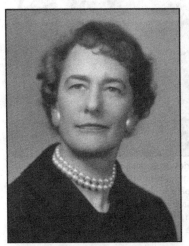

Figure 6-9. Marjorie B. Fish, OTR, Executive Director of AOTA, 1952-1964. (Printed with permission from the Archive of the American Occupational Therapy Association, Inc.)

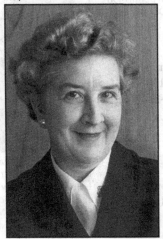

Figure 6-10. Frances Helmig, OTR, Executive Director of AOTA, 1964-1968. (Printed with permission from the Archive of the American Occupational Therapy Association, Inc.)

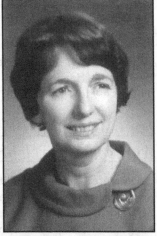

Figure 6-11. Harriet J. Tiebel, OTR, Executive Director of AOTA, 1968-1971. (Printed with permission from the Archive of the American Occupational Therapy Association, Inc.)

as a mission to consider the importance of environmental conditions in which practitioners and clients lived and worked, while continuing to focus on the direct treatment interaction between the practitioner and client. The Association was still concerned about any attempt by another health care organization to take over occupational therapy practice or practitioners.

There were three Presidents of the Association during the 1960s: Wilma L. West (1961-1964), Ruth Brunyate (1964-1967), and Florence S. Cromwell (1967-1970 [first term]) (Table 6-4; Figures 6-6 to 6-8; see Table 6-2). There were also three Executive Directors during the 1960s: Marjorie

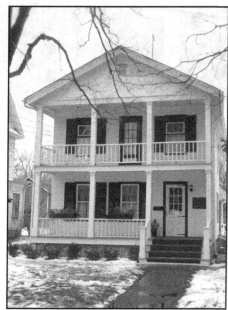

Figure 6-12. Consolation House, 16 Broad Street, Clifton Springs, New York. (Printed with permission from the Archive of the American Occupational Therapy Association, Inc.)

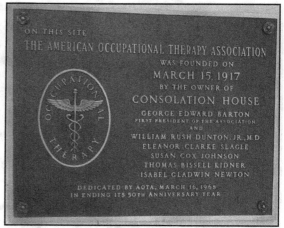

Figure 6-13. Consolation House plaque. (Printed with permission from the Archive of the American Occupational Therapy Association, Inc.)

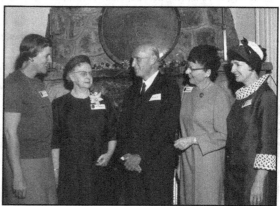

Figure 6-14. Dignitaries attending the 50th anniversary luncheon. From left to right: President Florence S. Cromwell; Mrs. Isabel Barton, widow of George Edward Barton; Dr. Sidney Licht, special guest; immediate Past President Ruth W. Brunyate; and Executive Director Mrs. Harriet Tiebel. (Printed with permission from the Archive of the American Occupational Therapy Association, Inc.)

Fish (1952-1964), Frances Helmig (1964-1968), and Harriet Tiebel (1968-1971) (Figures 6-9 to 6-11; see Table 6-2).

Founders' Day, 1967—50th Anniversary Celebration

On March 15, 1967, in Clifton Springs, New York, there was a chill in the air. The last evidence of a late winter snow was being washed away by a warm drizzle. By 10 a.m., people began assembling in front of the large white house at 16 Broad Street (Figure 6-12). George Barton had bought the house in 1912 and named it Consolation House, and there he offered services to those with disabling conditions. "The weather and quiet setting must have lent a surreal air to the gathering, a sense that the ghosts of people long gone were present once more. It was, as many would say later, a time for remembering" (AOTA at 70, 1987). However, to a passerby, the only evidence that something of significance might be happening was a "red velvet cloth covering a three-foot square on the wall of the front porch" (Neuhaus, 1968, p. 337; Figure 6-13). Guests were greeted at the door by Mr. and Mrs. Wright, the present owners of Consolation House (Neuhaus, 1968). It was Founders' Day, commemorating the first half-century of the Association. Those assembled included Isabel Goodwin Barton, George Barton's widow and the last survivor of the foundering members; Florence S. Cromwell, current AOTA President; Sidney Licht, MD, a long-time supporter of occupational therapy; Harriet Tiebel, AOTA Executive Director; Ruth Brunyate (later Wiemer), immediate past President; and about 45 other people (Figure 6-14). The purpose was to place a plaque on the right side of the door. At 11 o'clock, Mrs. Isabel Barton, President Florence Cromwell, and Margaret Zinsley, a student from the State

University of New York at Buffalo representing the future of the profession, stepped onto the porch to remove the velvet cloth over the plaque that would commemorate the place where the founders had met on March 15, 1917 (Figure 6-15). A reception followed at the Clifton Springs Hospital, originally a tuberculosis sanitarium where George Barton received treatment for his tuberculosis (Figure 6-16).

Bylaws of 1964

New bylaws were adopted at the 1964 annual meeting (AOTA, 1964, 1965a). These bylaws changed the organization and structure of the Association. New functions and powers listed in Article II of the bylaws were to improve and

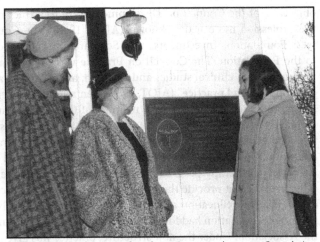

Figure 6-15. Dedication of 50th anniversary plaque at Consolation House. From Left to right: Florence S. Cromwell, AOTA President; Mrs. Isabel Barton, wife of founder George Edward Barton; and Margaret Zinsley, occupational therapy student at SUNY Buffalo. They represented the past, present, and future of occupational therapy. (Printed with permission from the Archive of the American Occupational Therapy Association, Inc.)

advance the practice of occupational therapy, improve and advance the education and qualification of occupational therapists, establish standards of performance, foster the research and study of occupational therapy, and engage in other activities to further the dissemination of knowledge of the practice of occupational therapy (AOTA, 1965a, p. 37). Emphasis was placed on the practice of occupational therapy as the first and foremost function of the Association. The Constitution in 1955 had a stated objective "to promote the use of occupational therapy" but did not specifically state the concept of improving and advancing the practice of occupational therapy. Also, a new function was added "to establish standards of performance" in occupational therapy practitioners in a variety of rules and functions in occupational therapy facilities. The emphasis on standards of education and training and on research remained the same. Other changes were that the House of Delegates became the Delegate Assembly, which became a legislative body to formulate policy, not just a recommending body as the House of Delegates had been. The Board of Management was renamed the Executive Board.

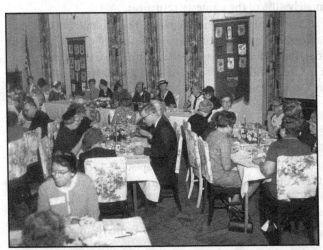

Figure 6-16. 50th anniversary luncheon celebration held at the Clifton Springs Sanitarium (now Hospital) in Clifton Springs, New York. (Printed with permission from the Archive of the American Occupational Therapy Association, Inc.)

The committee structure was streamlined from 36 separate committees listed on an organization chart in 1960 into four Councils: Development, Finance, Practice, and Standards (AOTA, 1960a, 1965a). The Council on Development included the AHA/AOTA Joint Committee, AJOT, History, International, Legislation, Recognitions, Recruitment, and Publicity. In a nutshell, the objectives of the Council on Development were to attract members, retain members, and make the profession more widely known (AJOT, 1968). The Council on Finance had three committees: Foundation, Investments, and Scholarship. Later the scholarships would be transferred to the Foundation. The Council on Practice was to "be concerned with treatment theories and methodologies, clinical studies and research, and planning and projection for future professional development and practice" (AJOT, 1968). Ten regions were created across the country, with a person representing each region as a member of the Council on Practice. The Council on Standards included the subcommittees on the standards for the profession, continuing education, basic professional education, occupational therapy assistants, registration and certification, and graduate education. The Council on Standards was to be concerned with the development of criteria for occupational therapy programs, including personnel, policies, administration, salaries, and all other aspects that provide the framework for clinical practice (AJOT, 1968). Of importance is the de-emphasis on education and the elevation of practice and practice-related issues. The previous Council on Education had four subcommittees and was a central reporting format for activities in the Association. Under the new structure, practice was given a prominent role.

The last House of Delegates meeting was held in Denver, Colorado, on October 25, 1964, with 39 member associations attending. The first Delegate Assembly was held in Miami Beach, Florida, on October 30, 1965, with 39 representatives of affiliated associations and four officers present (AOTA, 1967b, p. 9). The House of Delegates had been an advisory group to the Board of Management. The new Delegate Assembly had policy-making responsibilities, which resulted in the development of a number of documents (Table 6-5).

Amnesty and Reinstatement

In 1967, Resolution 121 was adopted for the purpose of encouraging therapists who had not been practicing for a while or had let their registration lapse to rejoin the profession to increase the number of practicing therapists. The resolution read as follows: "There will be a one-time only opportunity for all occupational therapists having at any time, met the qualifications for and been registered, to be granted during one membership years, eligibility for registered membership" (AOTA, 1968a, p. 112). The year was set for 1970 to allow preparation time. The total number of therapists who took advantage of the amnesty program was 378 (Neuhaus, 1971). States with the largest number of therapists reinstated were California, Wisconsin, New York, Massachusetts, and Pennsylvania, accounting for approximately 40% of the amnesty returnees.

To assist in the retry process, courses and textbooks were prepared. For example, a Refresher Course was given by the Southern California Occupational Therapy Association for 6 weeks to 13 nonpracticing therapists (AJOT, 1968). Publications prepared to assist in the amnesty program included the Professional Reactivation in Occupational Therapy (AOTA, 1969d) and the Reference Handbook on Continuing Education of Occupational Therapists (AOTA, 1970).

Registration and Membership

In 1964, there were 39 state associations represented in the House of Delegates. The total number of registered occupational therapists was 6,602; 4,527 occupational therapists and 768 occupational therapy assistants were members of AOTA. States with the highest number of registered occupational therapists were California (1,029), New York (723), Michigan (388), Illinois (378), Wisconsin (332), and Pennsylvania (300). States with the largest number of occupational therapy assistants were California (688), New York (487), Michigan (273), Illinois (272), and Pennsylvania (214).

Association Grants

Many activities of the Association were started and funded by grant money. In 1967, the Association received 4.2 million in grants and contracts. It was grant money that originally funded

Table 6-5
ASSOCIATION DOCUMENTS

YEAR	DOCUMENT	SOURCE
1960	Student's Report on Student Affiliation Center	Cited in *American Journal of Occupational Therapy, 16*(1), 40
1963	A Statement of Basic Philosophy, Principle & Policy	*American Journal of Occupational Therapy, 17*(4), 159 and *American Journal of Occupational Therapy, 18*(2), 88
1964	Guidelines for Developing a Training Program for the Occupational Therapy Assistant	Cited in *American Journal of Occupational Therapy, 18*(1), 45
1964	Report of Performance in Student Affiliations	*Manual for Supervision of Student Affiliations*, 1966
1965	Guidebook for an Accredited Educational Program for the Occupational Therapist	New York: American Occupational Therapy Association
1967	Eligibility for Writing the Examination for Registration	Delegate Assembly minutes
1967	Guide for Development and Use of Personnel Policies	*American Journal of Occupational Therapy, 21*(6), 406-408
1968	Classification Standards for Occupational Therapy Personal • Minimal Occupational Therapy Classification Standards for Staff Level Personnel: Staff Occupational Therapist I, II, & III and One Therapist Department • Minimal Occupational Therapy Classification Standards for Supervisory Administrative Level: Supervising Occupational Therapist I, II, and III • Minimal Occupational Therapy Classification Standards for Occupational Therapy Assistant I, II, & III • Minimal Occupational Therapy Classification Standards for Occupational Therapy Aide	
1968	Objectives of Occupational Therapy Education	AOTA, 1968b
1968	Standards for Occupational Therapy Service Programs	*American Journal of Occupational Therapy, 23*(1), 81-82
1969	Statement of Occupational Therapy Referral	AOTA, 1969b

ASSOCIATION DOCUMENTS		
1960	*Occupational Therapy Reference Manual for Physicians*	AOTA, 1960e
1962	*Manual for Supervision of Student Affiliations* (revised 1966)	Published by Wm. C. Brown, Dubuque, IA
1963	*Proceedings of Workshop on Graduate Education in Occupational Therapy*	New York: AOTA (VRA Training Grant OVR 62-80)
1963	*Students Affiliations*	Published by Wm C. Brown, Dubuque, IA
1966	*Occupational Therapy Teachers Institute: Concept of the Effective Teacher*	Wayne State University (VRA 66-66)
1966	*Bulletin on Practice*	Published by the Council on Practice (discontinued 1971)
1966	*Information Enclosure*	Published by the Council on Development (discontinued 1969)
1967	*The Application of Educational Objectives in Curriculum Construction*	University of Illinois (VRA 367-T-67)
1967	*Summer Experience in Occupational Therapy: Manual for Organizing a Program*	New York: AOTA (Ed. B. Neuhaus)
1969	*Methods and Media for Academic and Clinical Teaching, University of Utah*	New York: AOTA (VRA 367-T-69)

the education and continuing education programs. In fact, there were several years during the 1970s and 1980s when AOTA had more in grants than it did in its internal budget. Many of the functions of the Association were started with grants and later incorporated into annual budgets. Grant money was a double-edged sword. The money allowed the Association to start many programs that would not have been possible within the existing budget of the Association. However, when the grant money terminated, a decision had to be made to find money in the Association's budget or terminate the activity. Membership dues had to be increased and other sources of income found so that many of the services begun under various grants could be continued (AOTA at 70, 1987).

Changing Focus of the Association

The Association increasing transformed from a unifying force designed to serve the member needs for setting educational standards, certifying qualified practitioners, and providing placement services (job finding) to an advocate and leader in the health care community. Under the new bylaws (1964), the structure of the Association had changed. AOTA essentially became a business league composed of professionals serving common interests. The Association became a dynamic lobbyist on behalf of health-related legislation in which the profession had an active interest, such as legislation and regulatory guidelines supportive of occupational therapy and people with disabilities. The Association also was reorganized to allow the newly formed Foundation to respond to the need to meet an expanding mission to promote and sponsor scientific, literary, and educational programs to support the profession. In short, AOTA recognized it had a dual mission: to meet day-to-day membership needs and to plan for the long-range growth of the profession as a whole (AOTA at 70, 1987).

Recruitment and Manpower

A VRA grant (367-T-66) continued the work on recruitment (AOTA, 1966a). Four objectives are listed: (1) groundwork for two new and two repeat summer work experiences in occupational therapy programs for high school and college students, (2) continued liaison with the state and regional recruitment committees through telephone conferences, (3) contact with state health career councils, and (4) development of a new photograph library for loan or purchase by state associations. The summer work experience was report by Neuhaus (1965, 1969) as a success but was time consuming. In spite of the Association's efforts, manpower continued to be a major problem. An example is the study by Poole and Kassalow (1968), which reports that of those replying to the survey, 51% were not employed. Of the 177 respondents not working, only 104 indicated any interest in returning to the field sometime in the future. The current position held by a majority of respondents was housewife. In the 1960s, many women did not work after they were married and had children.

Consultants in Physical Disabilities and Neuropsychiatry

In 1957, the Association received a grant from the Office of Vocation Rehabilitation in the Health, Education, and Welfare Department to establish a position for a Field Consultant for a 5-year period in both physical disabilities and neuropsychiatry (AOTA, 1957). During the first 3 years, the grant money sponsored Irene Hollis, OTR, as a consultant in physical disabilities through 1960. The last 2 years were to fund a consultant in psychiatry. Mary Alice Coombs, OTR, served from 1960 until her death in 1964, and June Mazer served when the grant was renewed from 1964 to 1968 (AOTA, 1968a).

Graduate Traineeships

In 1960, the Association announced that a grant from the Office of Vocational Rehabilitation (later renamed the Vocational Rehabilitation Administration) had been received to make traineeships available to occupational therapists who were interested in advanced study on the master's or doctoral level. The area of study could be in occupational therapy or a related field that would "enable therapists to acquire the advanced knowledge and skills needed for teaching, clinical supervision, research, or other leadership positions in the field" (AOTA, 1960d). VRA grant 237-T-65

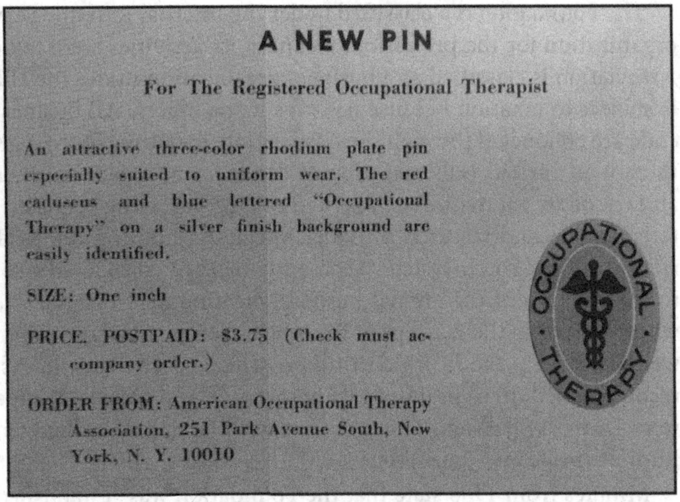

Figure 6-17. New occupational therapy pin, 1968. (Printed with permission from the Archive of the American Occupational Therapy Association, Inc.)

continued the funding for graduate traineeships (AOTA, 1966a). The traineeships were administered through the AOTA Committee on Graduate Study and continued to be available until 1972. Among the first-year recipients was Jerry Ann Johnson, future AOTA President, for master's degree study (AOTA, 1960c).

AOTA Membership in Other Organizations

In 1967, the Delegate Assembly passed Resolution 173, which gave authority to the Executive Board to select which external organizations and associations AOTA would join as members or which meetings and conferences they would attend (AOTA, 1968a). The task of selection was viewed as impractical for the Delegate Assembly to attempt. Thereafter, the Executive Board made the decision not to affiliate with or attend meetings of activity-based groups, such as those for recreation or music. Instead the focus was on organizations dealing with health, disability, or rehabilitation (Figure 6-17).

FOUNDATION

At the annual conference in Denver in October 1964, the Association authorized the formation of a foundation for the purpose of education and research (AOTA, 1964). At the midyear meeting in Des Moines, Iowa, the Foundation Committee submitted a report and incorporation papers to the Executive Board. The Executive Board was to serve as the incorporators, and the Foundation was incorporated in the state of Delaware on April 14, 1965 (AOTA, 1965c). The purpose of the Foundation was stated as follows:

The corporation is organized exclusively for charitable, scientific, literary and educational purposes, including for such purposes the making of distributions to organizations that qualify as exempt organization under Section 401(c) (3) of the Internal Revenue Code of 1954. The particular business and objects of the corporation shall be to advance the science of occupational therapy and increase the public knowledge and understanding thereof by the encouragement of the study of occupational therapy (1) through the provision of scholarships, (2) by engaging in studies, surveys and research, and (3) by all proper means." (Annual report to the membership, 1965, p. 14)

The Foundation is a classified under the Internal Revenue Service (IRS) tax code as a charitable organization for the profession, meaning its activities were tax exempt under the IRS code. The Association is classified as a business organization under the IRS tax code for the profession and is subject to taxation because it serves its members. All business activities as defined in the IRS code are conducted through the Association, including lobbying Congress to include occupational therapy in various bills and provide funds for occupational therapy services. The Foundation is able to conduct activities such as fund raising, receiving bequests, and administering grants related to education and research activities, including housing the AOTA/AOTF library and computerized database search system. Such activities are considered tax exempt. The history is reported in the minutes of the annual business meeting on November 1, 1965. A lawyer raised the issue when reviewing the concept of the single-fee structure. He said the objectives of the Association were changed in the 1955 Constitution, which could make the Association liable for back taxes; he recommended division into a business league and charitable organization. The original Directors were Dean Tyndall and Florence Cromwell (1965), Alice Jantzen and Ethel Huebner (1966), and Ruth Brunyate and Janet Stone (1967).

Minutes from 1968 state that the Foundation was "established in order to advance the science of occupational therapy and increase the public knowledge and understanding of occupational therapy in the service of mankind" (AOTA, 1968a). The Association established the Foundation to encourage the professional growth of occupational therapy by providing financial support for research education and professional publications. By housing such activities in the Foundation, the Association was able to establish itself as a business league. This designation "means that the Association can devote more of its resources to activities of direct benefit to its membership in such areas as legislation, personnel policies, etc." (p. 121). In 1969, the Delegate Assembly adopted Resolution 229, which states that 2% of Association dues would go to the Foundation to establish a financial base for the Foundation (AOTA, 1969b).

The American Occupational Therapy Foundation was designed to serve the profession rather than individual members and therefore sponsor educational and research programs designed to expand the contributions of occupational therapy to society and secure the profession's future position in the non-health care community. The Foundation could award scholarships and produced publications designed to promote greater awareness of the benefits of occupational therapy (AOTA at 70, 1987).

REFLECTION

The 1960s were a time of rapid change in the profession and the Association. Disorders that had formed a large portion of the client population seen by occupational therapy practitioners decreased substantially, such as tuberculosis and acute poliomyelitis, but other disorders such as neurological disorders, especially stroke and an emphasis on acute care facilities, increased. Education of therapists changed to focus more on dysfunction occurring as a consequence of a disease rather than on the disease itself. Clinical affiliations (field work) were changed to align with the concept of dysfunction and were shortened. Legislation related to health care, such as Medicare and the Community Mental Health Act, would change the focus of the Association from an internal direction to an external outlook. Lobbying on behalf of member interests would create a new outlook on what the Association needed to do to help members provide occupational therapy services and increase employment. The federal tax code created a need to divide the focus between membership services and professional development. The Foundation was created as a charitable organization on behalf of the professional research and education, whereas the Association concentrated on enhancing membership services.

REFERENCES

Ackley, N. (1962). The challenge of the sixties. *American Journal of Occupational Therapy, 15*(6), 273-281.

Albee, G.W. (1969). Emerging concepts of mental illness and models of treatment: The psychological point of view. *American Journal of Psychiatry, 125*(7), 42-48.

American Medical Association, Council on Medical Education and Hospitals. (1949). Essentials of an acceptable school of occupational therapy. *Journal of the American Medical Association, 141*(16), 1167.

American Occupational Therapy Association. (1955). *Proceedings of the Occupational Therapy Institute: A reassessment of professional education and practice in occupational therapy as related to rehabilitation.* New York, NY: Author.

American Occupational Therapy Association. (1957). OVR grant for field consultant in psychiatry. *Newsletter, 19*(11), 2.

American Occupational Therapy Association. (1958a). Curriculum study gets under way. *Newsletter, 18*(8), 1.

American Occupational Therapy Association. (1958b). Curriculum study staff. *Newsletter, 18*(7), 2.

American Occupational Therapy Association. (1958c). Summary of Medical Advisory Council meeting. New York, NY: Author.

American Occupational Therapy Association. (1960a). AOTA organization chart. New York, NY: Author.

American Occupational Therapy Association. (1960b). *Occupational therapy reference manual for physicians.* Dubuque, IA: Wm. C. Brown Book Co.

American Occupational Therapy Association. (1960c). OVR traineeship awards. *Newsletter, 20*(7), 2.

American Occupational Therapy Association. (1960d). OVR traineeships available. *Newsletter, 20*(3), 1.

American Occupational Therapy Association (1960e). *The occupational therapy reference manual for physicians.* Dubuque, IA: Wm. C. Brown

American Occupational Therapy Association. (1961). *Facts...about occupational therapy.* New York, NY: Author.

American Occupational Therapy Association. (1963). A statement of basic philosophy, principle and policy. *American Journal of Occupational Therapy, 17*(4), 159.

American Occupational Therapy Association. (1964). Report of the 1964 annual conference in Denver. *Newsletter, 24*(11), 1.

American Occupational Therapy Association. (1965a). Bylaws of American Occupational Therapy Association. *American Journal of Occupational Therapy, 19*(1), 37-41.

American Occupational Therapy Association. (1965b). *Guidebook for an accredited curriculum in occupational therapy.* New York, NY: Author.

American Occupational Therapy Association. (1965c). *AOTA Annual report to the membership.* New York, NYC: Author.

American Occupational Therapy Association. (1966a). AOTA-VRA grants. *Newsletter, 26*(1), 1.

American Occupational Therapy Association. (1966b). Delegate Assembly minutes. *American Journal of Occupational Therapy, 20*(1), 49-53

American Occupational Therapy Association. (1966c). Notes on Medicare for the occupational therapist. New York, NY: Author.

American Occupational Therapy Association. (1967a). Highlights of the curriculum study conference, Part II. *American Journal of Occupational Therapy, 21*(3), 179-181.

American Occupational Therapy Association. (1967b). *50th Anniversary: Then - and now!: 1917-1967.* New York, NY: Author.

American Occupational Therapy Association. (1968a). Minutes of the annual business meeting. *American Journal of Occupational Therapy, 22*(2), 109-123.

American Occupational Therapy Association. (1968b). Objectives of occupational therapy education- edited 1968. *American Journal of Occupational Therapy, 22*(6), 540-542.

American Occupational Therapy Association. (1969a). AOTA Executive Board. Official definition. *Newsletter, 22*(2), 1.

American Occupational Therapy Association. (1969b). Delegate Assembly minutes. *American Journal of Occupational Therapy, 23*(6), 520-531.

American Occupational Therapy Association (1969c). Delegate Assembly minutes. *American Journal of Occupational Therapy, 23*(2), 162-185.

American Occupational Therapy Association (1969d). *Professional reactivation in occupational therapy.* Dubuque, IA: Kendall/Hunt Publishing

American Occupational Therapy Association. (1969e). Statement on occupational therapy referral. *American Journal of Occupational Therapy, 23*(6), 530-531.

American Occupational Therapy Association (1970). *Reference handbook on continuing education of occupational therapists.* Dubuque, IA: Kendall/Hunt Publishing

American Occupational Therapy Association. (1986). 1980 Statement of occupational therapy referral. In: *Reference manual of the official documents of the American Occupational Therapy Association* (p. IX.1). Rockville, MD: Author.

American Occupational Therapy Association. (1992). AOTA's hall of leaders. *OT Week, 6*(21), 40-43.

American Occupational Therapy Association at 70. (1987). *Occupational Therapy News, 41*(11), 7.

Anderson, A. G. (1959, October). *Report of the "basic approach" committee.* New York, NY: American Occupational Therapy Association.

Appleby, L., Morton, J. E., Lawson, R. E., Loudon, R. G., & Brown, J. (1960). Toward a therapeutic community in a tuberculosis hospital. *American Journal of Occupational Therapy, 14*(1), 117-120.

Ayres, A. J. (1963a). The development of perceptual-motor abilities: A theoretical basis for treatment of dysfunction. *American Journal of Occupational Therapy, 17*(6), 221-225.

Ayres, A. J. (1963b). Occupational therapy directed toward neuromuscular integration. In H. S. Willard & C. S. Spackman (Eds.), *Occupational therapy* (pp. 358-466). Philadelphia, PA: Lippincott.

Ayres, A.J. (1966). Interrelations among perceptual-motor abilities in a group of normal children. *American Journal of Occupational Therapy, 20*(6), 288-292.

Ayres, A. J. (1968). Sensory integrative processes and neurophysiological learning disabilities. In J. Hellmuth (Ed.), *Learning disabilities* (Vol. 3, pp. 41-68). Seattle, WA: Special Child Publications.

Barnes & Noble (1996). *Webster's new universal unabridged dictionary.* New York: Barnes & Noble Books.

Barton, W.E. (1955). Medical supervision in occupational therapy. *American Journal of Occupational Therapy, 9*(2, Pt. 1), 53-56, 79

Brunyate, R. (n.d.). *Review of the status of occupational therapy.* New York: American Occupational Therapy Association.

Conte, W.R. (1960). The occupational therapists as a therapist. *American Journal of Occupational Therapy, 14*(1) 1-3, 12.

Diasio, K. (1967). Psychiatric occupational therapy: Search for a conceptual framework in light of psychoanalytic ego psychology and learning theory. *American Journal of Occupational Therapy, 22*(5), 400-407.

Fidler, G.S. (1963). Nationally speaking: The prescription in occupational therapy. *American Journal of Occupational Therapy, 17*(3), 122-124.

Fidler, G. S. (1966). Learning as a growth process: A conceptual framework for professional education. *American Journal of Occupational Therapy, 22*(1), 1-8.

Fidler, G.S., & Fidler, J.W. (1963). *Occupational therapy: A communication process in psychiatry.* New York: Macmillan.

Fox, F. H. (1966). Computer simulation of neurophysiological processes: Implications for research in occupational therapy. *American Journal of Occupational Therapy, 20*(6), 274-279.

Franciscus, M.L. & Abbott, M. (1968). *Opportunities in occupational therapy.* New York, NY: Vocational Guidance Manuals.

Grinker, R. R. (1969). Emerging concepts of mental illness and models of treatment: The medical point of view. *American Journal of Psychiatry, 125*(7), 37-41.

Halford, M. A. (1957). I had polio. *American Journal of Occupational Therapy, 11*(3), 129-130, 166.

Howe, M., & Dippy, K. (1968). The role of occupational therapy in community mental health. *American Journal of Occupational Therapy, 22*(6), 521-524.

Kester, D. L. (1966). New product makes splinting easier. *American Journal of Occupational Therapy, 20,* 43-44,

Kilburn, V. (1966). Highlights of the curriculum study conference: Part 1. *American Journal of Occupational Therapy, 21*(2), 102-105.

Koepke, G. H., Feallock, B., & Feller, I. (1963). Splinting the severely burned hand. *American Journal of Occupational Therapy, 17,* 147-150.

Llorens, L. A., Rubn, E. Z., Braun, J., Beck, G., Mottley, N., & Beall, D. (1964). A preliminary report on training in cognitive-perceptual-motor functions. *American Journal of Occupational Therapy, 18*(5), 202-208.

Mase, D. J. (1968). The growth and development of the allied health schools. *Journal of the American Medical Association, 206*(7), 1548-1550.

Matthews, M. E. (1959, April). *Basic approach in occupational therapy: Final report.* New York, NY: American Occupational Therapy Association.

Mazer, J. & Goodrich, W. (1958). The prescription: An anachronistic procedure in psychiatric occupational therapy. *American Journal of Occupational Therapy, 12*(4, Pt. 1), 165-170

Mosey, A. J. (1967). Recapitulation of ontogenesis: A theory for practice of occupational therapy. *American Journal of Occupational Therapy, 22*(5), 426-432.

Neuhaus, B. E. (1965). Recruiting occupational therapy students through a vacation work program. *Journal of Rehabilitation, 31,* 26-27.

Neuhaus, B. E. (1968). Founders' day at Clifton Springs. *American Journal of Occupational Therapy, 22*(4), 337-339.

Neuhaus, B. E. (1969). Summer experience: A positive approach to the manpower dilemma. *American Journal of Occupational Therapy, 23*(1), 65-68.

Neuhaus, B. E. (1971). Implementation of Resolution #121. *American Journal of Occupational Therapy, 25*(7), 378-380.

Owen, C. M. (1968). An analysis of the philosophy of occupational therapy. *American Journal of Occupational Therapy, 22*(6), 502-505.

Nichols, V.L. (1960). Keynote address: The therapist and the profession. In: *Proceedings of the 1960 annual conference* (pp. 1-4). New York: American Occupational Therapy Association.

Paolino, A. F. (1962). Prospects for research in occupational therapy. *American Journal of Occupational Therapy, 16*(4), 167-170.

Peters, C. O. (2011). Powerful occupational therapists: A community of professionals, 1950-1980. *Occupational Therapy in Mental Health, 27,* 199-410.

Poole, M. A., & Kassalow, S. (1968). Manpower survey report: Wisconsin Occupational Therapy Association. *American Journal of Occupational Therapy, 22*(4), 304-306.

Reed, K. L., & Sanderson, S. R. (1980). Defining occupational therapy. In *Concepts of occupational therapy* (pp. 1-8). Baltimore, MD: Williams & Wilkins.

Reilly, M. (1960). Research potentiality of occupational therapy. *American Journal of Occupational Therapy, 14*(4), 206-209.

Reilly, M. (1962). Occupational therapy can be one of great ideas of 20th century medicine. *American Journal of Occupational Therapy, 16*(1), 1-9.

Reilly, M. (1966). A psychiatric occupational therapy program as a teaching model. *American Journal of Occupational Therapy, 20*(2), 61-67.

Sloane, R.B. (1969). The converging paths of behavior therapy and psychotherapy. *International Journal of Psychiatry, 7*(7), 493-501.

Smith, A. R., & Tempone, V. J. (1967). Psychiatric occupational therapy within a learning theory context. *American Journal of Occupational Therapy, 22*(5), 415-420.

Spackman, C.S. (1952). Occupational therapy for patients with physical disabilities. Par 1. In H.S. Willard & C.S. Spackman (Eds.), Principles of occupational therapy (pp. 169-255). Philadelphia: Lippincott

Spackman, C. S. (1963). Co-ordination of occupational therapy with other allied medical and related services. In H. S. Willard & C. S. Spackman (Eds.), *Occupational Therapy* (3rd ed., pp. 1-14). Philadelphia, PA: Lippincott.

Spackman, C.S. (1963b). Occupational therapy as a supportive measure in the general hospital. In H.S. Willard & C.S. Spackman (Eds.), *Occupational Therapy* (3rd ed., pp. 115-138). Philadelphia: Lippincott.

Spackman, C.S. (1971). Occupational therapy—Its relation to allied medical services. In H.S. Willard & C.S. Spackman (Eds.), *Occupational therapy* (4th ed., pp. 1-11). Philadelphia: Lippincott.

VanderBos, G.R. (Ed.). (2007). *APA Dictionary of psychology.* Washington, D.C.: American Psychological Association.

Wegg, L. S. (1960). The essentials of work evaluation. *American Journal of Occupational Therapy, 14*(2), 65-70.

West, W. L. (1968). Professional responsibility in times of change. *American Journal of Occupational Therapy, 22*(1), 9-15.

Willis, B. (1969). The use of Orthoplast Isoprene splints in the treatment of the acutely burned child: Preliminary report. *American Journal of Occupational Therapy, 23,* 57-61.

Yasumura, M., & Baldwin, J. S. (1953). Occupational therapy for rheumatic and cardiac children. *American Journal of Occupational Therapy, 7*(2, Part 1), 62-67, 80.

Yerxa, E. J. (1967). Authentic occupational therapy. *American Journal of Occupational Therapy, 21*(1), 1-8.

Zimmerman, M. E. (1960). Devices: Development and direction. In *Proceedings of the 1950 annual conference of the American Occupational Therapy Association* (pp. 17-24). New York, NY: American Occupational Therapy Association.

Zimmerman, M. E. (1963). Occupational therapy in the A.D.L. program. In H. S. Willard & C. S. Spackman (Eds.), *Occupational therapy* (pp. 329-357). Philadelphia, PA: Lippincott.

BIBLIOGRAPHY

American Occupational Therapy Association. (1958). *The objectives and functions of occupational therapy.* Dubuque, IA: Wm. C. Brown.

American Occupational Therapy Association. (1969). Delegate Assembly minutes. *American Journal of Occupational Therapy, 23*(2), 162-185.

American Occupational Therapy Association. (1969). 1969 annual election. New York, NY: Author.

Anderson, A. G. (1960). *A discussion of the pilot study on basic approach. Proceedings of the 1960 annual conference.* New York, NY: American Occupational Therapy Association.

Medical Education, Section V. (1969). Educational programs in areas allied with medicine. *Journal of the American Medical Association, 210*(8), 1524-1529.

Robinson, R. A. (1958). A general approach in occupational therapy. In *Proceedings of the 1956 Regional Occupational Therapy Institutes: Denver, Los Angeles, Madison, Richmond and Annual Institute, Minneapolis* (p. 4). Dubuque, IA: Wm. C. Brown.

7

Back to Philosophical Base
1970s to 1980s

Key Points

- The national office moved from New York City to Rockville, Maryland, in 1972.
- The Philosophical Base Project was implemented to identify assumptions and principles of occupational therapy.
- The Association adopted a positive stance toward state licensure, and states began passing legislation to license occupational therapy personnel.
- A lobbyist was hired by the Association to advocate for congressional legislation favorable to occupational therapy.
- Code of Ethics statements were separated from bylaws to create a standalone document in 1977.
- The Uniform Terminology document adopted in 1979 became a forerunner of the Occupational Therapy Practice Framework.
- The number of therapists increased significantly during the 1970s.
- The number of educational programs increased significantly for both therapists and assistants.
- The Roster of Fellows and Roster of Honor were created in 1970s. Other award programs followed.
- The Association became a major publisher of occupational therapy literature.

Highlighted Personalities

- Lela Augustine Llorens, theorist
- Anne Cronin Mosey, theorist
- Florence S. Cromwell, AOTA President, 1970-1973 (second term)
- Jerry Ann Johnson, AOTA President, 1973-1976
- Mae Dorothy Hightower Vandamm, AOTA President, 1976-1982
- Leo Fanning, AOTA Executive Director

- James Garibaldi, AOTA Executive Director
- Phillip Shannon, Chair of Philosophical Base Project
- Alice C. Jantzen, AOTF President
- Elizabeth J. Yerxa, AOTF President
- Myra L. McDaniel, AOTF President
- Nancy V. Snyder, AOTF President
- Wilma L. West, AOTF President

Andersen, L. T., & Reed, K. L.
The History of Occupational Therapy: The First Century (pp. 195-228).
© 2017 Taylor & Francis Group.

Key Places

- Rockville, Maryland—New headquarters office on Executive Boulevard in the Wilco Building, 1972

Political Events/Issues

- Florida and New York passed legislation to license occupational therapists in 1975.
- Between 1976 and 1979, nine more states passed state licensure laws.
- The Rehabilitation Act of 1973 (Public Law 93-112) was passed, which included Section 504 on architectural design and provision of independent living.
- Education for All Handicapped Children Act passed in 1975

Economic Events/Issues

- Passage of the Education for All Handicapped Children expanded job opportunities for occupational therapy personnel in schools.
- The Health Maintenance Organization was created to limit health care costs in 1973.
- Various agencies of the federal government continued to provide grant money to the Association for several projects.

Educational Issues

- Essentials of an Accredited Education Program for the Occupational Therapist were revised in 1972.
- Standards and Guidelines of an Occupational Therapy Affiliation Program were adopted in 1973.
- Document of Advanced Professional Education in Occupational Therapy was adopted in 1972.
- The number of educational programs continued to increase.

Key Times/Events

- Meeting of Slagle lecturers to discuss philosophical base

Sociocultural Events/Issues

- Task Force reports were published on social issues, target populations, and mental health.
- Terminology adopted by the National Commission on Accreditation changed the concept of registration to certification: Registration Exam became Certification Exam.
- The Coalition of Independent Health Professions was created in 1970.

Technological Events/Issues

- Early computer-assisted programs began appearing in the literature.

Practice Issues

- The number of practicing therapists increased 135% between 1972 and 1982.
- The issue of qualifications to maintain competency of practice was discussed throughout the 1970s.
- The first Uniform Terminology document was adopted in 1979.
- The Code of Ethics document was adopted in 1977.
- The Role Delineation Study was completed.

Foundation Issues

- The Foundation began awarding scholarships.
- The Foundation published its first public information brochure.
- A paid funding coordinator was hired to relieve volunteers of some responsibilities of running the Foundation.

Association Issues

- The Association's national office was moved to Rockville, Maryland, to be closer to Capitol Hill and the seat of the U.S. government.
- The Delegate Assembly passed Resolution 400 supporting the adoption of state licensure legislation for occupational therapy personnel in 1974.
- The Delegate Assembly became the Representative Assembly in 1977.
- The Council on Standards developed plans to maintain eligibility for certification (re-certification program).
- The Model Practice Act to guide state associations in writing licensure legislation was adopted in 1975.
- The Association created the Legislative Affairs Division in 1972 to address issues related to occupational therapy practice in congressional legislation. (The name has changed several times since.)
- Career mobility criteria were developed for assistants to sit for the therapist certification examination.
- A study of entry-level functions of therapists, assistants, and aides was completed.
- A terminology report was accepted changing the term registration to certification in 1973.
- Proficiency Testing and Career Laddering programs were developed but were ultimately rejected by the Representative Assembly in the 1980s.
- The bylaws formally recognized affiliate associations as entities; prior status was primarily concerned with determining delegate eligibility—1972
- The bylaws created the Committee of State Association Presidents in 1976.
- The bylaws created Special Interest Sections in 1976.

INTRODUCTION

The United States celebrated 200 years of independence—the Bicentennial—in 1976. The Vietnam War finally came to an end in 1975 after 15 years of warfare. The Camp David Accords were signed in 1978 by Egyptian President Anwar al Sadat and Israeli Prime Minister Menachem begin to reach a settlement between Israel and Egypt, with President Jimmy Carter presiding over the event. Iran took 63 Americans hostage in November 1979; they were not released until January 1981.

A major decision for occupational therapy practitioners in the 1970s was accepting licensure after 2 decades of active opposition by the national Association. State licensure decreased the therapists' dependency on the continuing certification but increased the demand on the state associations to initiate and then monitor the licensure process. Many state associations were small and struggling. Licensure, however, provided a potential unifying effect because all practitioners were affected by the licensure law in their state or jurisdiction.

In 1977, the Representative Assembly created the Special Interest Sections (SIS) to support the advancement of special practice areas. Five specialty areas were initially approved: developmental disabilities, gerontology, mental health, physical disabilities, and sensory integration. Others would be added later.

The occupational therapy workforce grew 230% between 1966 and 1978, according to data collected for the manpower study conducted in 1984 (American Occupational Therapy Association [AOTA], 1985).

For the profession there would be a continued process of growth and change. Part of the process was related to the general recognition by society of the potential contributions of the different members of the health care team, but a major part was the result of efforts within the profession itself. Increased emphasis on improving standards, competency, and education for the members of the profession and greater effectiveness in the overall administration of the Association contributed to the growth and viability of the profession and the Association.

Publications would increase the literature base of the profession. Mosey (1970) published a book describing three theories or frames of reference for occupational therapy practitioners to apply in the practice of mental health. Ayres (1972) published a book describing the theory of practice called sensory integration to address problems described as sensory integration dysfunction. The fourth edition of the textbook by Helen Willard and Clare Spackman was published in 1971, the last edition by the original authors and editors. The fifth edition published in 1978 was edited by new authors, Helen Hopkins and Helen Smith. A textbook devoted to the practice of occupational therapy for physical dysfunction edited by Catherine Trombly and Anna Scott was published in 1977.

As one effort to address the shortage of therapists, the Delegate Assembly designated 1970 as an amnesty or reinstatement year for therapists who had let their registration (now certification) lapse. Formerly registered therapists could re-register without having to take the registration (now certification) examination again. According to the final report, 378 therapists took advantage of the offer (Neuhaus, 1971). In the same year, the presidents of the state associations developed a propose and function document to create a meeting format at the annual conference to discuss issues of mutual concern, share information and ideas, and make recommendations for actions to the Delegate Assembly and Executive Board. The following year, 1971, the Delegate Assembly passed Resolution 300 on continuing certification and registration because there was growing concern about the maintenance of qualifications to practice beyond the point of initial credentialing. Harriet Tiebel resigned as Executive Director in 1971, and Leo Fanning, the first non-therapist to lead the Association, started his tenure the following year. To better access Congress, the Association move its headquarters to Rockville, Maryland, in 1972, ending 46 years of having a New York City address for the official office. Also in 1972, a formal definition of occupational therapy was adopted and published (AOTA, 1972c). The next year, 1973, the Delegate Assembly approved a resolution encouraging states to seek licensure laws to describe the practice of occupational therapy and credentials of qualified practitioners for the benefit and protection of consumers. The same year, the first group of therapists was named to the Roster of Fellows and began using the initials FAOTA behind their names. The Occupational Therapy Newspaper began publication in 1973, and the old News Letter or Newsletter, published from 1938 to 1973, was discontinued.

By 1979, 13 states and the District of Columbia would pass licensure laws. The Delegate Assembly would become the Representative Assembly and, in 1977 for the first time, all 50 states plus the District of Columbia and Puerto Rico would have a Representative seated in the Representative Assembly, making for a truly nationwide representation of occupational therapists and assistants. The Representative Assembly adopted for the profession the first official Code of Ethics as a separate document from the bylaws in 1977. A major challenge was to keep up with the rapid expansion of educational program at all three levels: assistant, master's, and post-professional. Cordelia Myers retired as editor of American Journal of Occupational Therapy in 1975, and Elaine Viseltear became editor. Recruitment changed from a lack of applicants to an overabundance of applications in the early 1970s (Fanning, 1972). A major problem in education became a lack of qualified faculty.

EDUCATION

Educational Programs

Educational opportunity in occupational therapy was expanding. In 1970, there were 36 accredited educational programs for occupational therapists, and by 1979 there were 53. There were 43 occupational therapy assistant programs in 1979. Thirty states had an occupational therapy program, and 24 states had an occupational therapy assistant program. However, 28 states had neither an occupational therapy nor an occupational therapy assistant program within the state borders. Lack of educational programs in each state continued to be a barrier in developing occupational therapy service programs throughout large parts of the country, especially the Western states. There were no occupational therapy educational programs at either the professional or technical level in 10 Western states, including Iowa, Nebraska, South Dakota, Utah, Montana, Idaho, Nevada, Arizona, New Mexico, and Wyoming.

Revision of the Essentials

The Essentials of an Acceptable Education Program for the Occupational Therapist was revised for the fourth time in 1973. Essentials for the occupational therapy assistant were developed with the American Medical Association (AMA) in 1976.

The Ad Hoc Committee on Education created by the Executive Board in 1977 identified six issues and made 16 recommendations. The six issues related to (1) faculty characteristics and responsibilities, (2) faculty shortage, (3) multiple entry routes leading to certification as an OTR, (4) lack of research, (5) external influences and forces, and (6) AOTA member readiness to decide on semiprofessional or professional status. The recommendations were:

- The AOTA Commission on Education (COE) and the Division of Education (in the National Office) should immediately identify external resources needed to better prepare faculty members and curriculum directors for their functions and responsibilities in university environments.
- The Essentials should reflect the necessity and importance of (a) faculty research involvement in patient practice or related areas, and (b) faculty engagement in research and scholarly endeavors.
- The Essentials must delineate more clearly the functions, responsibilities, and value orientations for faculty in university settings.
- Faculty members should identify the qualifications and criteria utilized by their colleges and universities to award tenure, grant promotions, and recognize faculty and program competence.
- Clinical and educational representatives to COE and their colleagues should explore the costs, efficacy, and liability of retaining current field work patterns.
- It is recommended that fieldwork experience be a requirement for certification rather than for graduation and that it become a responsibility of AOTA rather than of the individual occupational therapy programs. (Note: This recommendation was never implemented.)
- Members of AOTA should develop, adopt, and implement a coherent educational system leading from entry into the profession through various stages or steps to the highest desirable levels, with one step leading logically to another.
- A 2-year moratorium should be placed upon the establishment and/or recognition of new programs for occupational therapy assistants or occupational therapists at the associate of arts and baccalaureate degree levels.
- Additional data about occupational therapists should be obtained, including the attrition rates of OTRs and COTAs and reasons for attrition (raising families with intent to return to practice later versus leaving the profession).

- Review and reconsider the functions and educational preparation of COTAs, including the possibility of a return to specialty training for COTAs. Preparation of the OTR for entry into the profession should continue to focus on generalist professional education, with a liberal arts base. Advanced professional education should lead to specialization and research.

- Evaluate the various options for entry into the profession, including the proficiency examination, especially in relation to the data base being collected about occupational therapists.

- Postpone decision of whether or not to adopt a proficiency examination as a mode of entrance until such time as the data requested in this report are available and the members of the Association can make basic decisions about entry into the profession.

- Faculty members, particularly in graduate programs, should emphasize the need for faculty and graduate research related to direct and indirect services as opposed to opinion polls, attitude surveys, and studies.

- It is recommended that members of AOTA adopt the concept of moving toward full professional status.

- It is recommended that the master's degree be considered as the point of professional entry into occupational therapy.

- The Commissions of Education and Practice should promote utilization of therapists within a realistic reliable and viable framework and should be charged to develop a master plan for levels of function and performance of occupational therapy. (Johnson, 1978)

Revision of the Certification Examination

In 1975, the content, format, and type of questions used on the certification (registration) examination for occupational therapists was substantially modified for the first time since the examination process was developed in 1947 (AOTA, 1975d). The old content consisted of three sections of approximately equal weight: Basic Knowledge, Clinical Conditions, and Occupational Therapy Principles and Practice. The new content was divided into four sections with several subsections. The four major sections and percentage of questions were: Occupational Therapy Services–Evaluation (30%), Occupational Therapy Services–Planning (30%), Occupational Therapy Services–Implementation (30%), and Program Support Services/Professional Development (10%). Evaluation included occupational performance, performance components (developmental, measurable, or gradable functions), and life space. Planning included goal setting, selection of objectives, and methodology for attainment of identified performance in selected occupation and performance component tasks. Implementation included development, maintenance, and restoration of function in identified occupations and performance components. Program support included management, communication, and professional development. The change was designed to better reflect the process of occupational therapy practice as opposed to a collection and accumulation of facts, data, and information.

The format of questions changed from a focus on knowledge and memorization to a focus on application and problem solving. In other words, knowledge was considered necessary but not sufficient to practice occupational therapy. The practitioner must be able to apply the knowledge to a problem (dysfunction, disorder, condition) presented by the client, develop an intervention plan, and implement the intervention plan to address the client's problem. In the example below, the first question (old format) can be answered by reading the information in a standard textbook, which anyone with appropriate reading skills could do. No application or problem-solving skills are needed. The second question (new format) requires an understanding of the problem (dysfunction) experienced by a person with the disorder of carpal tunnel syndrome and what intervention plan and intervention strategy or strategies an occupational therapy practitioner could use to address or correct the problem. Focusing questions on application as opposed to knowledge alone was an attempt to make the examination more closely align with the real world of occupational therapy practice. The sample questions are as follows:

Old format:
What nerve is affected by carpal tunnel syndrome?
   A. Radial
   B. Ulnar
   C. Median*
   D. Musculocutaneous

New format:
Treatment after carpal tunnel syndrome repair should concentrate on strengthening:
   A. Gross grasp
   B. Precision finger skills*
   C. Wrist extension
   D. Wrist flexion

Although the changes in content, format, and type of question were developed for the occupational therapist examination, the changes were incorporated in the development of the examination for occupational therapy assistants. Prior to June 1977, there was no uniform requirement for assistants to pass a written examination. In 1975, the Delegate Assembly passed Resolution 471-76, which established the new certification requirement that assistants, as well as occupational therapists, take a certification examination to practice occupational therapy (AOTA, 1976a).

PRACTICE

Practice by the Numbers

According to the 1977 AOTA membership survey, the most common diagnoses seen by occupational therapists were stroke/hemiplegia (26.7%), cerebral palsy and psychosis (12.4%), and intellectual disability (10.2%). For occupational therapy assistants, the most common diagnoses seen were cerebrovascular accident/hemiplegia (23.7%), arteriosclerosis (12.9%), mental retardation (11.6%), and psychosis (9.5%). Note the changing terminology in Table 7-1. Cerebrovascular accident (CVA) is more commonly called stroke, mental retardation is now called intellectual disability, and arteriosclerosis was a general term for dementia. Although practitioners saw a range of ages in clients, occupational therapists saw more children, and assistants saw more elderly clients. Combining categories results in the following: 76.8% physical disabilities and 23.2% mental health problems seen by occupational therapists and 72.8% physical disabilities and 27.2% mental health problems seen by assistants (AOTA, 1978a). Additional factors and figures about practitioners from 1971 are presented in Table 7-1 and from 1977 are presented in Table 7-2.

State and Jurisdiction Licensure

In 1969, the Delegate Assembly adopted a position of neutrality (AOTA, 1969a, p. 528). The action was taken in response to a licensure bill passed in Puerto Rico. A formal statement was issued in a position paper entitled "Licensing and Standards of Competency in Occupational Therapy"

Table 7-1 THE PROFESSION BY THE NUMBERS (1971)		
	OCCUPATIONAL THERAPISTS	OCCUPATIONAL THERAPY ASSISTANTS
Female	96%	89%
Average years of experience	7.64	7.04
Major clinical interests	• Physical dysfunction, 39% • Psychosocial dysfunction, 26.5% • Perceptual-motor, 11% • Chronic illness, 5% • Community mental health, 5%	• Psychosocial dysfunction, 31% • Physical dysfunction, 19% • Mental retardation, 14% • Community mental health, 8% • Medical/surgical, 7% • Addiction/alcoholism, 5%
Primary age of clients	• Adults, 42% • Mixed ages, 27% • Pediatrics, 20% • Aged, 7% • Adolescents, 4%	• Mixed ages, 34% • Adults, 29% • Aged, 27% • Pediatrics, 6% • Adolescents, 4%
Employment status	• Working full-time, 50% • Not presently employed, 33% • Employed part-time, 14% • Student, 2% • Self-employed, 1%	• Working full-time, 72% • Not presently employed, 12% • Employed part-time, 8% • Other, 6% • Student, 2%
Employer type	• State facility, 22% • Voluntary or proprietary, 22% • City or county facility, 21% • Federal facility, 11% • Educational facility, 9% • Self-employed, 4% • Other, 11%	• Private, 37% • State facility, 33% • City or county facility, 16% • Federal facility, 6% • Other, 8%
Salary	81% of salaries between $7,000 and $12,500	69% of salaries between $4,800 and $8,000
Major function	• Clinical practice, 58% • Administration, 18% • Education, 9% • Consultation, 8% • Research, 1% • Other, 6%	• Provide treatment, 46% • Conduct activity program, 44% • Administration, 5% • Preparation, 2% • Maintenance, 1% • Other, 2%

Adapted from American Occupational Therapy Association. (1971). Reports to the Delegate Assembly: the Executive Director. *American Journal of Occupational Therapy, 25*(7), 377-378.

(AOTA, 1969a). In 1971, a follow-up statement was written to further clarify the Association's position, entitled "Statement on Licensure of Occupational Therapists" (AOTA, 1971b).

Three years later, the position would be changes to support licensure as the states of New York and Florida both passed licensure bills (AOTA, 1975c). The rationale in support was written as the public need for occupational therapy services of uniformly high quality, contemporary problems of obtaining reimbursement for occupational therapy services, and the need to protect the public from unqualified practitioners (Johnson, 1975a).

To mitigate some of the concerns West had described in her statement of opposition to licensure, a Model Practice Act was adopted, including a model definition of occupational therapy, to guide therapists and legislators in preparing licensure bill (AOTA, 1969b). The Model Practice Act was revised many times over the years and was never officially published after the initial version but rather acted as a guide to respond to issues related to defining occupational therapy and others terms commonly used in licensure laws, stating qualifications for practitioners, and suggesting the

Table 7-2
THE PROFESSION BY THE NUMBERS (1977)

	OCCUPATIONAL THERAPISTS	OCCUPATIONAL THERAPY ASSISTANTS
Female	95%	88%
Degree	Baccalaureate degree, 89%	Associate degree, 67%
Median age	31.5 years	25.5 years
Median salary	$14,500	$10,500
Employed	75%	
Provide direct service to clients	68%	86%
Practice in a hospital setting	30%	
Primary area of practice	• Physical disabilities, 65% • Mental health, 35%	
Employed by government agency (city, county, state, or federal)	48%	41%
Employed by private, nonprofit organization	36%	35%

Adapted from: American Occupational Therapy Association. (1978-1979). *Annual report*. Rockville, MD: Author.

national certification examination be adopted as a major entry criterion. As a result, reciprocity among occupational therapy practitioners has been more uniform, and the cost of preparing licensure bills has been manageable by the states and jurisdictions seeking licensure.

By 1979, 13 states and two jurisdictions (Puerto Rico and the District of Columbia) were licensed. Table 7-3 presents a summary by decade of the progress toward state and jurisdiction licensure. Table 7-4 presents a brief summary of the actions by the Association regarding licensure.

Definitions of Occupational Therapy Practice

Adequate definitions to describe the essence of occupational therapy, while at the same time describing the breadth and depth of the profession, continue to be a challenge. Several definitions published during the 1970s are presented in Table 7-5. The definition used in the Occupational Therapy Handbook, a recruitment brochure, describes occupational therapy as a "health profession" that uses "selected activity" while working with a variety of health and other professions to promote health, to evaluate behavior, and to treat and prevent disability (AOTA, 1970a). Mentioning team members is not usual in the definition of occupational therapy. The 1970 definition also uses the word "participation," which would be used frequently in definitions published after the year 2000. However, the context would be changed from participation in activity to participation in daily life. In 1971, the definition of occupational

Table 7-3
PROGRESS IN ACHIEVING LICENSURE LAWS IN STATES AND JURISDICTIONS

YEARS	NO. OF STATES	NO. OF JURISDICTIONS
1968-1979	13	2
1980-1989	22	
1990-1999	6	1
2000-2009	7	
2010-2015	2	
Total	50	3 (Guam, Puerto Rico, DC)

	Table 7-4
	SUMMARY OF LICENSURE ACTIONS BY DATE
1951	West statement as Executive Director opposing licensure *AJOT, 5*(2), 60-63
1969	Motion and Position paper (negative position continued) AOTA, (1969a). Minutes of the Delegate Assembly, Resolution 230-69. *AJOT, 23*(6), p. 528 & AOTA. (1969b). Position Paper. Licensing and standards of competency in occupational therapy. *AJOT, 23*(6), 529-530 (adopted by the Delegate Assembly June, 1969)
1974	Resolutions 376-74 neutral on licensure and 400-74 supporting licensure AOTA (1974). Minutes of the Delegate Assembly, Resolution 376 Licensure and other Credentialing Mechanisms (neutral stand on licensure). *AJOT, 28*(9), 564. Johnson, J.A. (1975). Nationally speaking. *AJOT, 29*(2), 73. AOTA (1975). Minutes of the Delegate Assembly, Resolution 400-74 Licensure. (adoption of licensure). *AJOT, 29*(3), 154-155 Resolution 230-69 was rescinded

therapy appearing in the issue of the Journal of the American Medical Association (JAMA) on medical education incorporated the term *purposeful activity*. Purposeful activity as a phrase began appearing in the occupational therapy literature in 1922 when Edith Bowman, a psychologist, explained that "the fundamental principle of occupational therapy is a psychological principle: the substitution of a coordinated, purposeful activity, mental or physical, for scattered activities or the idleness which comes with weakened body or mind" (Bowman, 1922, p. 172). The phrase *purposeful activity* would appear frequently in definitions in the 1980s.

In 1972, the Legislation Committee developed an official statement on occupational therapy, which was presented to the Committee on Ways and Means in the U.S. House of Representatives as it considered national health insurance legislation. The legislation failed, but the work by the Association to define occupational therapy to Congress was important in presenting occupational therapy practice to external groups. Also in 1972, the Council on Standards developed a definition that would be expanded and published in the 1973 Essentials of an Accredited Education Program for the Occupational Therapist. In 1974, the Task Force on Social Issues created a definition specifically for the discussion of social issues, which stressed the scientific aspect of occupation as a health determinant. In 1975, the first definition of occupational therapy was published to be used as a model for state licensure laws. The focus on "work assessment" would be changed in later definitions to a focus on activities of daily living, as noted in the 1977 revision. Note that the 1976 definition appearing in a publication not under the control of the Association still focuses on occupational therapy as a "medically directed treatment" (U.S. House of Representatives, 1976). No mention is made of the use of occupational therapy in educational environment because the Education for All Handicapped Act had only been passed the previous year.

Practice Models

In 1977, Kielhofner and Burke attempted to explain the two major theoretical viewpoints that had influenced the development of occupational therapy practice in mental health over the years, which they labeled *humanistic moral treatment school* and *scientific school* (Kielhofner & Burke, 1977).

Under the humanistic tradition, the knowledge base for occupational therapy intervention was governed by the process of studying and examining man's behavior while acting in the environment. Thus, the view of man involved an environmental focus on the total organization of behavior. Problems occurred as a result of wrong habits of living and reactions to stress. Intervention

	Table 7-5
	DEFINITIONS OF OCCUPATIONAL THERAPY IN THE 1970S
1970	Occupational therapy is a health profession which contributes to the physical and emotional independence and well-being of an individual through the use of selected activity. The occupational therapist evaluates each individual to determine the current level of functioning. As a member of the treatment team, he works in collaboration with the physicians, the physical and speech therapists, nurses, psychologists, social workers, vocational counselors and other specialists to plan a therapeutic activity program with the following objectives: • To promote and maintain health • To evaluate behavior • To treat physical and emotional disability • To prevent further disability Through participation in supervised activity, singly, or in groups, the individual is health to solve some of his own programs (AOTA, 1970b).
1971	Occupational therapy is concerned with the use of purposeful activity in the promotion and maintenance of health, the prevention of disability, the evaluation of behavior, and as treatment of persons with physical or psychosocial dysfunction. This is accomplished by using a wide spectrum of treatment procedures based on activities of a creative, social, self-care, educational, and vocational nature (American Medical Association, 1971).
1972	Occupational therapy is the art and science of directing man's participation in selected tasks to restore, reinforce and enhance performance, facilitate learning of the skills and functions essential for adaption and productivity, diminish or correct pathology and to promote and maintain health (AOTA, 1972d).
1972	Occupational therapists serve today at all levels of health care: in planning, in screening, in programs preventing health deterioration or injury, in diagnostic, evaluative, treatment, rehabilitation, and health advocacy services. They function in hospitals, extended-care facilities, clinics, public and special schools, rehabilitation centers, and home health agencies. A wide variety of patients are referred to occupational therapists including those who are blind, infants born with physical deformities or brain dysfunction, persons whose life style has been permanently altered by serious illness, such as cancer or stroke, those who are emotionally ill, those who are permanent or temporarily incapacitated by accidents, persons who are mentally retarded, and many others." Occupational therapists work with physicians, nurses, speech and audiology, physical therapy, nutrition, psychology and social work (AOTA, 1972c).
1973	Occupational therapy is the art and science of directing man's participation in selected tasks to restore, reinforce and enhance performance, facilitate learning of those skills and or correct pathology, and to promote and maintain health. Reference to occupation in the title is in the context of man's goal-directed use of time, energy, interest, and attention. Its fundamental concern is the development and maintenance of the capacity throughout the life span, to perform with satisfaction to self and others those tasks and roles essential to productive living and to the mastery of self and the environment (AOTA, 1973c).
1974	Occupational therapy is the science of using occupation as a health determinant. Integration of the individual's psychobiological systems is promoted through selected purposeful use of occupation. Occupational therapy enhances an individual's ability to perform with satisfaction those tasks and roles essential to productive, acceptable living (AOTA, 1974b).

(continued)

methodology focused on activity in normal, temporal, physical, and social settings. The goal was to maintain and restore healthy habits of living.

In contrast, the scientific school of theory suggested that the knowledge base for intervention should be governed by rules of rational inquiry called the scientific method. The view of man focused on brain and body rather than the environment. Problems were described in terms of diseases, such as neurological lesions. Intervention entitled drugs, surgery, and custodial care. The goal was to alter brain tissues and cells through the use of one or more of the intervention protocols.

Table 7-5 (continued)
DEFINITIONS OF OCCUPATIONAL THERAPY IN THE 1970S

1975	Occupational therapy means the application of knowledge of the effects of occupation upon human beings to facilitate the integration of biological, social and psychological systems to help them attain or maintain maximum functioning in their daily life tasks. It includes, but is not limited to such techniques as work assessment, assessment of play and leisure performance, the manipulation of objects, the development of self-care and capacity for independence through the dynamics of occupational involvement such techniques being applied in the treatment of individual patients or clients, in groups, or through social systems (AOTA, 1975g).
1976	Occupational therapy: medically directed treatment of physically and/or mentally disabled individuals by means of constructive activities designed and adapted by a professionally qualified occupational therapist to promote the restoration of useful function (U.S. House of Representatives, 1976).
1977	Occupational therapy is the application of occupation, any activity in which one engages, for evaluation, diagnosis and treatment of problems interfering with functional performance in persons impaired by physical illness or injury, emotional disorders, congenital or developmental disability, or the aging process tin order to achieve optimum functioning and for prevention and health maintenance. Specific occupational therapy services include but are not limited to, activities of daily living (ADL), the design, fabrication and application of splints; sensorimotor activities; the use of specifically designed crafts; guidance in the selection and use of adaptive equipment; exercises to enhance functional performance; prevocational evaluation and training; and consultation concerning the adaptation of physical environments for the handicapped. These services are provided to individuals or groups through medical, health, educational and social systems (AOTA, 1977d).

Occupational therapy practitioners were often caught between the theoretical viewpoints. Were environmental factors or brain functions more responsible for mental illness? Could activity such as occupational performance complete with drugs and surgery in improving mental health? Kielhofner and Burke suggested that the crisis for occupational therapy practitioners to solve revolved around the concepts of holism versus reductionism—that is, does a person function as an internal whole in adapting to both internal and external environments, or does a person function as a collection of internal tissue parts without regard for external environment influences? Kielhofner and Burke favored the former viewpoint based on holism and humanism as a basis for future occupational therapy theory development. Both were students of Mary Reilly, which likely influenced their choice of theory construction.

Another strong influence on theory and practice were the expanding ideas about the importance of human developmental theories on occupational therapy practice. Llorens (1970) highlighted the potential use of developmental theories throughout the lifespan for organizing the process of evaluating, planning and intervening to influence behavior expectations and adaptive skills (Figure 7-1). She expanded

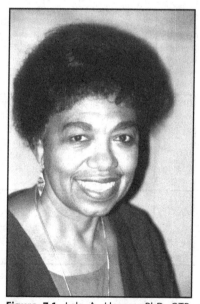

Figure 7-1. Lela A. Llorens, PhD, OTR. (Printed with permission from the Archive of the American Occupational Therapy Association, Inc.)

her ideas in a follow-up article in 1977 in which she outlined 10 premises on which developmental theory was based (Llorens, 1977). Clark (1979a, 1979b) expanded the use of human development theory in her articles describing a practice model she entitled human development through occupation. Clark suggested that human development and adaptation was facilitated by the capacity of

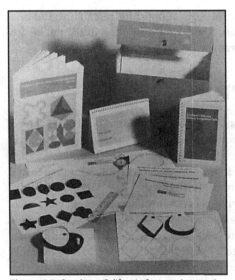

Figure 7-2. Southern California Sensory Integration Tests by A. Jean Ayres, published in 1972. (Printed with permission from the Archive of the American Occupational Therapy Association, Inc.)

a person to purposefully affect his or her own world of self, culture, and environment. The long-range goal of occupational therapy was to enhance the individual's occupational role performance appropriate to the person's developmental stage.

The model of sensory integration was increasing in popularity. In 1972, Ayres published the Southern California Sensory Integration Tests (SCSIT), a compendium of tests she had originally published as separate instruments (Ayres, 1972). The SCSIT was the first test battery published by an occupational therapist (Figure 7-2).

Mosey (1970) attempted to organize three of the major models of practice used by occupational therapists in mental health (Figure 7-3). The models as she named them were object relation analysis, a psychoanalytic approach; action-consequence, a learning theory; and recapitulation of ontogenesis, a developmental theory.

Mental Health Practice

In May 1974, the Executive Board created a Task Force on Mental Health that was charged with identifying current issues of concern in the practice of occupational therapy in mental health and to recommend solutions to the identified problems. The Task Force members quickly identified that the major problem confronting mental health practitioners, and the profession as a whole, was "a failure to delineate the foundation of our practice" (AOTA, 1976b, p. 6). In addition, there was no clear delineation nor documentation in the occupational therapy literature for the theoretical assumptions suggested by Reilly (1962) that man, through the use of his hands, could influence the state of his health or that occupation was essential to human health and function. Although all of the published models of practice promised improvement, none had standardized clinical techniques that could be used to establish the validity of the profession.

A core problem identified by the Task Force members was undergraduate preparation, which provided practitioners with skills to practice but not the skills to advance the profession's knowledge base. To address the problem in mental health, the Task Force members suggested a 5-year program be implemented to refine the knowledge base and strengthen the technology by selecting a target population, such as schizophrenia, to be a focus of study. Recommendations were also made that the preparation of therapists move to master's level entry, that the national office create a position for a Research Coordinator, that specialty practitioners be educated beyond entry level, and that continuing education opportunities be focused on mental health. Although the Task Force suggested dates for implementing that recommendations, the Association was unable to meet any of them by the date specified in the report. Instead, the Task Force report added to the growing body of evidence that work was needed in several areas to

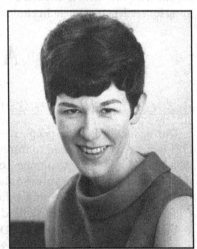

Figure 7-3. Anne C. Mosey, PhD, OTR. (Printed with permission from the Archive of the American Occupational Therapy Association, Inc.)

advance the profession. Master's level entry would occur in 1999. Support for research would be a target area in the Foundation, but not in the Association. Specialized education in mental health would be recognized in the specialty certification program.

LEGISLATION

According to the September 1979 Data Line, the passage of the Education of all Handicapped Act (Public Law 94-142) in 1975 opened hundreds of positions throughout the country for practitioners to work in school settings. Occupational therapy was classified as a related service. Another piece of legislation with job opportunities for practitioners was the Rehabilitation, Comprehensive Services, and Developmental Disabilities Amendments of 1978 (Public Law 95-602). Title III related to Comprehensive Services for Independent Living provides for payment of services such as occupational therapy for those clients who can increase their level of independence, although they many have no vocation potential. One change in the regulations is a change in definition of a developmental disability from a short list of diagnoses to a functional definition, thereby expanding the covered population and thus the demand for occupational therapy services (AOTA, 1979b). Table 7-6 summarizes the legislation affecting occupational therapy during the 1970s.

TECHNOLOGY

Articles on the use of computers in occupational therapy began appearing in the 1970s. One of the first articles to discuss the use of computers in occupational therapy practice appeared in 1975 (English, 1975). English summarized examples of use such as recording functional status, use of computers by individuals with disabilities to learn work tasks such as data entry, and adaptation of computers to modify input and feedback to the user. The article predates the wider use of personal computers with Microsoft and Apple software. The use of FORTRAN (formula translation) or COBOL (common business-oriented language) was discussed instead. The use of computers for data entry by individuals with disabilities had been previously discussed by Smith (1973). Use of voice as a modified input system is discussed by Glenn, Miller, and Broman (1976). Use of computer programming for student placement in clinical settings is discussed by Hawkins and Hawkins (1978).

ASSOCIATION

Association Reorganization

During the 1970s, three people served as President of the Association: Florence Cromwell, 1970-1973 (second term); Jerry A. Johnson, 1973-1978 (Figure 7-4); and Mae D. Hightower-Vandamm, 1978-1982 (Figure 7-5). A summary of their accomplishments appears in Table 7-7. Table 7-8 provides brief biographies. Figure 7-6 shows the members of the Executive Board during Cromwell's second term, and Figure 7-7 shows the six of the past Presidents of the Association: Ruth Brunyate Wiemer, Wilma West, Helen Willard, Jerry Johnson, Ruth Robinson, and Florence Cromwell.

Two people served as Executive Director of AOTA during the 1970s: Leo Fanning, 1972-1975 (Figure 7-8); and James Garibaldi, 1975-1987 (Figure 7-9). Fanning and Garibaldi were not occupational therapists. A significant change for the Association was moving the its headquarters from New York City to Washington, DC, in 1972 (AOTA, 1972a). The new office building in shown in Figure 7-10.

Table 7-6
LEGISLATION ADOPTED IN THE 1970S THAT HAD EFFECTS ON OCCUPATIONAL THERAPY

1970	Developmental Disabilities Act (P.L. 91-517). Focus was on meeting needs of persons with developmental disabilities by addressing gaps in service.
1970	Elementary and Secondary Education Act Amendments (P.L. 91-230). Created Title VI called Education of the Handicapped, which consolidated special education programs.
1972	Social Security Act Amendments (P.L. 92-223). Intermediate care facilities could be created for people with mental retardations.
1972	Social Security Act Amendment (P.L. 92-603). Established supplemental security income to people on standardized assistance programs.
1973	Rehabilitation Act Amendment (P.L. 93-112). Two parts are important. First, the Architectural and Transportation Barriers Compliance Board was established to enforce standards on publicly funded buildings and transpiration. The Act prohibits discrimination against people with disabilities in any program that receives federal funding. Employers could not discriminate and governments must provide equal opportunity and access to programs. The standards in Section 504 established the groundwork for the standards included in the Americans with Disabilities Act. Second, services were to focus on independent living, aligning with the deinstitutionalization that occurred, and shifting control from the provider to the consumer. Also, the term vocational was dropped from the title of the Act.
1973	Health Maintenance Organization Act (P.L. 93-222). Established foundation for managed care in the insurance industry with a focus on controls for costs and coverage.
1974	Elementary and Secondary Education Act Amendments to Title VI (P.L. 93-380). Introduced the concepts of due process, least restrictive environment, child find, nondiscriminatory testing/evaluation, child identification, and full service goals.
1975	Developmental Disabilities Assistance and Bill of Rights Act (P.L. 94-103). Institutes with university-affiliated facilities can provide full service to people with developmental disabilities. These facilities also offered continuing education for professionals working in the industry. Created state systems for protection and advocacy. Outlined rights of those who have developmental disabilities.
1975	Education for All Handicapped Children (P.L. 94-142). The Act increased the opportunity for occupational therapists to work with children with disabilities in schools, to help them participate in school setting based upon their Individualized Education Program. Part D added training for special education, related services, and early intervention providers.
1978	Rehabilitation Comprehensive Services and Developmental Disability Act (P.L. 95-602). National Institute of Handicapped Researched was established for purpose of grants and research projects. Redefined developmental disabilities to emphasize severity of impairment functions, NOT the diagnosis.

Adapted from:

Lohman, H. (2014). Payment for services in the United States. In B. A. Boyt Schell, G. Gillen, & M. E. Scaffa (Eds), *Willard & Spackman's occupational therapy* (12th ed., pp. 1051-1067). Philadelphia, PA: Wolters Kluwer.

Reed, K. L. (1992). History of federal legislation for persons with disabilities. *American Journal of Occupational Therapy, 46*(5), 397-408.

Van Slyke, N. (2001). Legislation and policy issues. In M. Scaffa (Ed.), *Occupational therapy in community-based practice settings* (pp. 85-94). Philadelphia, PA: F. A. Davis.

Mission and Goal Statement

In 1975, the Delegate Assembly adopted a mission and goal statement for the Association (Resolution 437-75), which is "to serve as an advocate for occupational therapy to enhance the health of the public in the medical, community, and education environments through research, education, action, and service" (AOTA, 1975f; Johnson, 1975b, p. 261). Goals of the Association are:

- To provide opportunities for the expression of member concerns, to anticipate emerging issues, to facilitate decision making, and to expedite the translation of those decisions into action

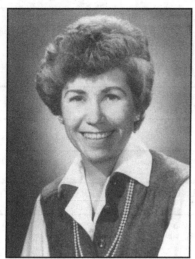

Figure 7-4. Jerry A. Johnson, EdD, MBA, OTR, FAOTA, President of AOTA, 1973-1978. (Printed with permission from the Archive of the American Occupational Therapy Association, Inc.)

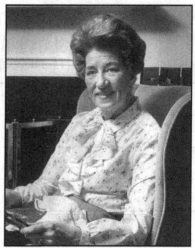

Figure 7-5. Mae Hightower-Vandamm, OTR, FAOTA, President of AOTA, 1978-1982. (Printed with permission from the Archive of the American Occupational Therapy Association, Inc.)

Table 7-7
PRESIDENTS AND MAJOR ACCOMPLISHMENTS
Florence Cromwell, 1970-1973 (second term)
Cromwell continued to address the external organizations that interacted with the Association to develop health care policy and set health care standards.
Jerry A. Johnson, 1973-1978
"During her tenure, she identified issues related to entry level into the profession, ambivalence regarding licensure, and a need for AOTA to be responsive to the needs and interests of all members. Her major goal was to move entry to the profession to the master's level because she felt the change would contribute most to professional growth." Dr. Johnson attended a meeting with President Ford as the AOTA representative of the Coalition of Independent Health Professions (AOTA, 1976c, 1992b).
Mae D. Hightower-Vandamm, 1978-1982
"Under her leadership, the vision for more membership rights and participation became reality. During her tenure, the office building that houses both AOTA and the Foundation was purchased. Quote: "We're recognized now as a vital profession to the treatment of almost every disability... I think we're headed toward graduate level certification.""
Adapted from AOTA, 1992; 1992b.

- To support the development of research and knowledge bases for the practice of occupational therapy, and to promote the dissemination and sharing of such information
- To facilitate and support an educational system for occupational therapy which responds to current needs, and anticipates, plans for, and accommodates to change
- To promote occupational therapy as a viable health profession
- To facilitate the formation of partnerships with consumers to promote optimal health conditions for the public (Johnson, 1975b, p. 161)

Overall, the goals were consistent with the roles of the Association as outlined by Cromwell (1972): (1) to establish standards of education for its practitioners, for their practice, and for

Table 7-8
PRESIDENTIAL BIOGRAPHIES

JERRY ANN JOHNSON

September 21, 1931–November 23, 2012

Born in Lubbock, Texas. She attended Levelland High School in Lubbock and received her undergraduate degree in occupational therapy from Texas Woman's University when the university was called Texas State College for Women in Denton, Texas. She earned a Master's of Business Administration from Harvard Business School and then a doctorate in education from Boston University. She received the Distinguished Alumni award from Texas Woman's University in 1984. She was president from 1973 to 1978, gave the Eleanor Clarke Slagle lecture in 1972, was a charter member of the Roster of Fellows in 1973, received the Award of Merit in 1979, and was named a Fellow in 1973. She was chair of the Department of Occupational Therapy at Boston University, Director of the program in occupational therapy at Washington University in St. Louis, and taught at Thomas Jefferson University in Philadelphia. She was a veteran of the U.S. Navy and served in the U.S. Naval Reserve. She received the National Defense Serve Medal. She wrote several chapters and articles published in the occupational therapy literature. Wellness was one of her favorite topics.

MAE DOROTHY HIGHTOWER-VANDAMM

November 11, 1926–November 20, 2014

Born in Dublin, Georgia. She received a bachelor's degree from Wesleyan College and a master's degree from Columbia University. She served as Association president from 1978 to 1982, served on the Finance and Budget Committee, was named to the Roster of Fellows in 1976, and received the Award of Merit in 1983. She wrote about independent living for the disabled. She served as Executive Director of the Delaware Curative Workshop for more than 30 years. A building at the Workshop is named in her honor. She was a champion of the cause of disabled children, and the Mae Hightower-Vandamm Pediatric Fund was formed in recognition of her commitment. She was elected to the Hall of Fame of Delaware Women, served as a docent at the Delaware Art Museum, and was a Supporter of the Brandywine Conservancy and Winterthur. She served on the board of the First State Miniature Club and was a member of the National Association of Miniature Enthusiasts. She was recognized for her award-winning needlework, serving on the Board of Directors of the Main Line Chapter of the American Needlepoint Guild.

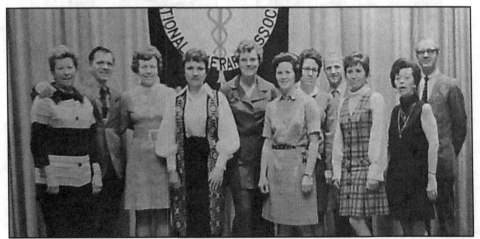

Figure 7-6. Executive Board. From left to right: Myra McDaniel, Fred Odner, Marion Crampton, Joane Wyrick, Florence Cromwell, Nedra Gillette, Nancy Snyder, Robert Bing, Jerry Johnson, Gail Fidler, and Clyde Butz. (Printed with permission from the Archive of the American Occupational Therapy Association, Inc.)

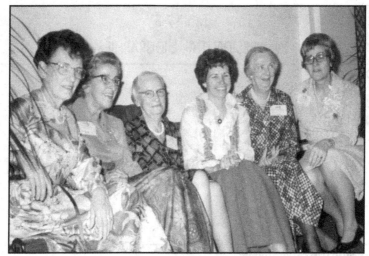

Figure 7-7. Past Presidents of AOTA at an AOTA conference. From left to right: Ruth Brunyate Wiemer, Wilma L. West, Helen S. Willard, Jerry A. Johnson, Ruth A. Robinson, and Florence S. Cromwell. (Printed with permission from the Archive of the American Occupational Therapy Association, Inc.)

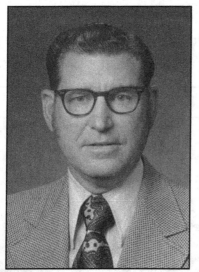

Figure 7-8. Leo C. Fanning, Executive Director of AOTA. (Printed with permission from the Archive of the American Occupational Therapy Association, Inc.)

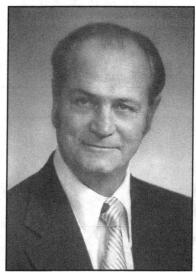

Figure 7-9. James Garibaldi, Executive Director of AOTA. (Printed with permission from the Archive of the American Occupational Therapy Association, Inc.)

their recognition to practice; (2) to provide ongoing support for excellence of practice; and (3) to design, prepare for, and implement change strategies to keep the profession timely (p. 3A). Major themes continued to be education, practice, research, and standards. The newly stated themes were (1) addressing membership concerns, (2) viewing occupational therapy as a health profession, and (3) fostering consumer partnerships to promote health. These goals were translated in priorities for each year. An example is shown in Table 7-9.

Recognition of Student Members and State Association Presidents

The bylaw changes in 1976 (AOTA, 1977c) formalized the organization of two important constituencies in the Association for the first time. Student members of the Association became members of the Student Committee under the Representative Assembly.

> The Student Committee shall conduct the business of the occupational therapy and occupational therapy assistant student groups as it related to student issues and concerns .... The committee shall be chaired by a student member of the Association ... and shall be a member of the Assembly with vote (AOTA Bylaws, Article 10, Section 1H).

Thus, student members had a recognized role within the Association. The second constituency was the State Association Presidents who were formally organized as the Committee of State Association Presidents (CSAP) under the Executive Board (AOTA Bylaws, Article 10, Section 2C). All presidents of state associations were considered members. "The committee shall facilitate sharing of plans and ideas, serve as a forum for the discussion of relevant current issues and serve as a centralized source of information and materials which may be utilized by State Association presidents" (Section 2C). Although informal sharing of ideas and materials had occurred between states over the years, CSAP provided a formal mechanism for sharing and also provided another link between members and the officers of the Association. Ideas coming through the Delegate Assembly had to be presented as formal motions called Resolutions, whereas ideas coming through CSAP could be presented as

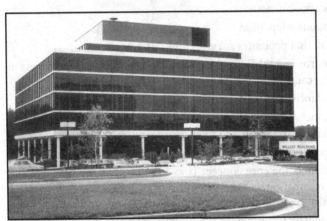

Figure 7-10. National Office, Executive Boulevard, Rockville, Maryland, 1972-1980. (Printed with permission from the Archive of the American Occupational Therapy Association, Inc.)

Table 7-9
PRIORITIES IN 1971-1972

- More intensive public education relating occupational therapists' service and roles to health and to the evolving system of health care
- Increased engagement in external affairs—where health planning and health systems are being discussed
- Extensive information sharing with members to broaden their perspectives about their own and the profession's roles in the evolving health system
- Long-range planning for manpower needs—kinds, levels, how to education, how to certify, how to utilize urgently needed information to blend with community and national programs
- Encouragement of continued professionalization through more and intensified research in both education and practice
- Better feedback systems throughout the Association and profession to reinforce self-confidence in these turbulent times and to spark more innovative models of practice
- Continued attention to standards at all levels of function; update, improve, and disseminate them; and give evidence of our interest in peer review and public audit
- Capitalization on our image change made possible by the community health model, our extra-hospital engagement, our humanistic practitioner roles now becoming increasingly evident

Cromwell, F. S. (1972). Nationally speaking. *American Journal of Occupational Therapy, 26*(2), 3A-6A.

items for discussion without presentation as a formal motion. Both sources increased the information available to the Association to act and react to issues of concern to therapists and assistants.

Philosophy of the Profession Project

In 1979, the Representative Assembly adopted Resolution 531-79, entitled the Philosophical Base of Occupational Therapy, and Resolution 531-79, entitled Occupation as the Common Core of Occupational Therapy (AOTA, 1979a, p. 785). The philosophical statement includes eight points in the form of assumptions about the basic philosophy of the profession:

- Man is an active being whose development in influenced by the use of purposeful activity.
- Human beings are able to influence their physical and mental health and their social and physical environment through purposeful activity.
- Human life is a process of continuous adaptation.
- Adaptation is a change in function that promotes survival and self-actualization.
- Biological, psychological, and environmental factors may interrupt the adaptation process at any time throughout the life cycle, causing dysfunction.
- Purposeful activity facilities an adaptive process.
- Purposeful activity (occupation), including its interpersonal and environmental components, may be used to prevent and mediate dysfunction and to elicit maximum adaptation.
- Activity as used by the occupational therapist includes both an intrinsic and therapeutic purpose.

The second resolution on occupation as the core concept is as important as the first. For the first time, the Association stated that occupation was the core concept of occupational therapy. At the same time, the lack of clarity remains because the resolution used the term purposeful activity rather than occupation. The failure to clarify terminology and underlying assumptions is an ongoing issue within the profession itself, as well as within the professional association.

Discussion of philosophy began in 1977, with the formation of the Ad Hoc Committee for Identifying the Philosophy of Occupational Therapy, chaired by Philip Shannon under the direction of the Commission on Practice (AOTA, 1977a). The need had been identified in the Task Force on Social Issues report (AOTA, 1972b). The purposes of the Committee were to define the parameters of occupational therapy, develop an interface between practice and education and generate theory from which multiple models might emerge, and provide direction for the association in legislative issues (AOTA, 1979c).

The final report was given to the Representative Assembly in 1983 (AOTA, 1983). Although the Executive Board recommended publication of the final report in the journal, it was never published. Part of the problem occurred when the 10 former Slagle lecturers met in July 1982 to identify philosophy (Figure 7-11). Mary Reilly objected to the transcripts of the session being published

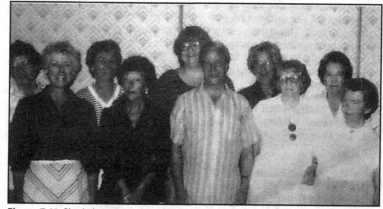

Figure 7-11. Slagle lecturers who participated in the Philosophical Base Project. From left to right: (back row) Ruth Wiemer, Jerry Johnson, Carolyn Baum, Wilma West, and Mary Reilly; (front row) Betty Yerxa, Gail Fidler, Bob Bing, Muriel Zimmerman, and Lorna Jean King. (Printed with permission from the Archive of the American Occupational Therapy Association, Inc.)

and made the Association promise not to publish the content for 25 years. Another problem was the relatively negative tone of the report, suggesting the literature of occupational therapy did not yield a very useful result.

A few general statements can be made about the outcome of the project. Philosophy was defined as the "reason for existence, the broad thrust of a profession in relationship to society and the individual" (AOTA, 1982b, p. 3). Statements from the literature were organized into five categories: the relation of occupational therapy to man; the relationship of occupational therapy to society; the role of occupational therapy; assumptions, hypotheses, proposition-supporting programs, techniques, and methodologies; and Association policies. The review of literature was limited to three publications: *Archives of Occupational Therapy* (1922-1924, 18 issues), *Occupational Therapy & Rehabilitation* (1925-1951, 162 issues) and the *American Journal of Occupational Therapy* (1947-1978, 220 issues). Articles published in other journals such as the *Maryland Psychiatric Quarterly*, *Trained Nurse and Hospital Review*, and *Modern Hospital* were not reviewed, thus excluding many early articles written by the founders when the formative ideas about occupational therapy were first published.

Task Force Reports

The 1970s were the era of the Task Force Reports. There were three: Social Issues (AOTA, 1972b), Target Populations #1 (AOTA, 1974a) and #2 (AOTA, 1974c), and Mental Health (AOTA, 1976b). The Task Force on Social Issues was charged to identify and document social, legislative, humanitarian, professional, political, education, and financial forces, trends, and other issues that may have an impact on health care in the coming decades; to identify changes in the health care system; and to identify present, emerging, and potential roles of occupational therapy and propose recommendations for study and change to the Executive Board of the Association. The number one issue was legislation, and the recommendation was that the Association, at all levels of the organization, become more active in the decision-making and policy-making aspects of legislation affecting health care delivery. The second issue was that occupational therapy practitioners needed to become more active "in the development of accepted theoretical frames of reference, theories, standardized evaluation and treatment procedures, research, special studies and publication" (AOTA, 1972b, p. 355). The third issue was to increase involvement in identifying conditions that contributed to illness and disability, especially those in the environment. Occupational therapy practitioners could help develop new theories and intervention strategies relating disability to environmental influences. The fourth issue was to assist practitioners to identify employment opportunities in new areas and models of practice and to attain the skills to perform the new roles. Fifth, education and practice needed to be based on theory rather than being technique oriented, and Association documents on education and practice standards should state and support the theoretical base. Sixth, manpower needed to be increased, but also the level of performance needed to change from a technical level to a professional level. Occupational therapists needed to know how to function in leadership roles and delegate responsibilities. Seventh, communication about the Association needed to improve, and more information about occupational therapy practice needed to be made available. Eighth, the gap between the Association and individual members might be decreased if more activities occurred at a regional rather than national level. As with other reports, many good ideas were generated to solve identified problems, but acceptance and integration of the ideas into Association activities was slow.

In 1973, the Delegate Assembly adopted Resolution 367-73 to identify client populations needing the expertise that occupational therapy was uniquely qualified to address to acknowledge publicly the rank order of their priority, to influence Association legislation activities, and to establish program development activities compatible with the established priorities (AOTA, 1974a). The Task Force began by asking the following questions: What is an occupational therapist and what does an occupational therapy do? The answers were organized into a set of assumptions that were illustrated in a diagram called the Occupational Therapy Process. Although the charge was to identify client populations that occupational therapy was uniquely prepared to address, the Task Force members recommended that the Association direct its energies instead to accomplishing the following specific objectives:

- To undertake activities which will enable occupational therapy to become a uniquely definable, independent health profession
- To further examine, refine, and validate theories related to the practice of occupational therapy to strengthening the educational programs by ensuring the curricula and field placement centers utilize such frames of reference as the foundation for educational planning
- To continue to identify and understand human health needs and those factors which influence such needs, particularly as these impinge upon occupational performance
- To meet with competence and responsibility, the consumer health needs which are uniquely responsive to occupational therapy services (American Journal of Occupational Therapy [AJOT], 1974b)

Once again, the Association and the profession were directed to establish and delineate the theoretical base and framework underpinning the practice of occupational therapy. The task force could not identify the clients that occupational therapy was uniquely qualified to serve because the profession had not sufficiently stated and supported through research and publication what it was uniquely qualified to do. Because there was no list of client populations to be served, there was no way to prioritize which clients should be served, to publicly announce the list, and to focus the Association resources to that list.

Special Interest Sections

In 1975, the Council on Practice formed a task force to make recommendations regarding the development of SIS as an organizational part of AOTA. Based on the information provided by the Council on Practice, the Representative Assembly approved the establishment of the SIS in October 1976. In January 1977, AOTA President Jerry Johnson appointed an Ad Hoc Committee on Special Interest Sections to develop a workable structure for the SIS. Based on the Committee's work, a draft of the structure was development, including issues such as membership selection, funding, and basic philosophy (AOTA, 1992a).

The Representative Assembly approved the development of five SIS initially: Developmental Disabilities, Gerontology, Mental Health, Physical Disabilities, and Sensory Integration. President Johnson appointed Chairs for the SIS in their initial year of operation. Thereafter, the Chairs were to be elected by the SIS members. Membership in the SIS is a voluntary benefit that provides continuing education through presentations at the annual conference and a newsletter.

The Developmental Disabilities SIS provides information on habilitation and prevention issues by promoting knowledge and skills in services for people who have developmental disabilities. Practitioners in school-based settings could join the subsection on school systems.

The Gerontology SIS provides members with current information and resources on practice, research, and legislation of interest to therapists working with elderly patients. Information and activities include those related to education and training, practice models, intervention approaches, reimbursement, service delivery systems, and external organizations concerned with aging.

The Mental Health SIS includes the entire range of mental health practice services in multiple settings for clients with mental illness and developmental disabilities. Topics covered include practice models, clinical education, legislative issues, payment systems, research, and recruitment and retention issues.

The Physical Disabilities SIS provides a forum for sharing information and ideas about physical disabilities practice. The SIS promotes practice interests through its active members and steering committee.

The Sensory Integration SIS represents the interests of therapists using Ayres' sensory integration approach to evaluate and intervene across multiple age groups and diagnoses. The SIS offers resources on practice trends, networking, and continuing education.

Registration and Membership

The total number of occupational therapists with membership in AOTA in 1970 was 9,688, and the total number of occupational therapy assistants was 1,545. States with the largest occupational therapist memberships were California (1,505), New York (977), Michigan (592), Illinois (495), Wisconsin (476), and Pennsylvania (409). States with the largest number of occupational therapy assistants were New York (297), Wisconsin (201), Minnesota (76), and Texas (56). Membership in the Association continued to be concentrated in the Northeast, North Central, and California in the far West.

Product Output Reporting System and Uniform Terminology Project

In October 1977, Congress passed Public Law 95-142, the Medicare and Medicaid Anti-Fraud and Abuse Amendments. As part of the Amendments, the Secretary of the Department of Health and Human Services was required to establish regulations for uniform reporting systems for all hospital departments. Specifically, the stipulations were that "in reporting under such a system, hospitals shall employ such chart of accounts, definitions, principles, and statistics as the Secretary may prescribe" (Public Law 95-142). At the time the law was passed, no national system for reporting productivity of hospital based occupational therapy services existed. Although the above statement refers to hospitals, all services reimbursed by Medicare or Medicaid, including hospitals, skilled nursing and intermediate care facilities, and home health agencies, were to have uniform reporting systems (AOTA, 1986a).

As with any federal directives, it took a while for them to be put into action. At the July 1978 Board meeting, President Mae Hightower stated that she had received reports from Francis Acquaviva, National Office Operations Research; letters from the Washington State Occupational Therapy Association; and a phone call from John Farace, Chair of the Commission on Practice, all concerned with actions being taken by the Health Care Financing Administration (HCFA) to prepare the proposed Uniform Hospital Reporting Manual (AOTA, 1978b). Acquaviva had been informed by Kathy McFarland from Washington State that the HCFA intended to use the Washington State Relative Value System in the proposed Uniform Hospital Reporting Manual to be used by all Medicare-certified providers. McFarland wanted the Association to be aware of proposed HCFA action because the results would affect occupational therapy departments across the country. Because the comment period regarding the proposed actions was short, comments were solicited from each of the major Association commissions and committees, and Acquaviva wrote a reply to HCFA stating membership concerns and requesting funding for a proposal to complete a project aimed at validating, replicating, and/or developing uniform terminology and a uniform reporting system for occupational therapy services. Major concerns were that (1) a system developed in one state (Washington) was proposed to be implemented across the country with no input or validation from any other state, (2) relative values were being assigned to various items of terminology rather than numbers of treatment units, (3) the administrative costs of a new system on occupational therapy departments that probably already had a reporting system would be high, and (4) the new definition of occupational therapy for licensure adopted by the Association had not been used.

In August 1978, the Executive Board charged the Commission on Practice to form a task force to review the existing occupational therapy terminology and relative value reporting systems and develop a proposal for a national occupational therapy product output report system (AOTA,

1983). The task force was chaired by Sylvia Harlock, a member of the Commission on Practice and the Washington State Occupational Therapy Association. The purpose of the task force was to create a national system that could become part of the U.S. Health Care Finance Administration Manual (AOTA, 1978-1979). The Occupational Therapy Product Output Reporting System, including the Uniform Terminology System for Reporting Occupational Therapy Services, was adopted by the Representative Assembly in April 1979 (AOTA, 1979a, p. 805). The document called the Uniform Occupational Therapy Evaluation Checklist, adapted from the Uniform Terminology System, was approved by the Representative Assembly in March 1981. The documents printed in the Occupational Therapy Newspaper (AOTA, 1981) and in the Reference Manual of Official Documents of the American Occupational Therapy Association in 1983 and 1986 (Hopkins & Smith, 1983) but were never officially published in AJOT. The Uniform Terminology documents were never published by the HCFA because the Uniform Hospital Reporting Manual, for which the documents had been written, never materialized due to congressional concerns about antitrust issues related to potential price fixing (AOTA, 1989). Although the initial rationale for a reimbursement reporting system did not occur, the projects was not a total loss because the Uniform Terminology document helped create a base of consistent terminology that was used in many documents to follow. The Uniform Terminology document itself was revised in 1989 and 1994 (AOTA, 1989, 1994).

The uniform terminology system was organized into seven categories of service: occupational therapy assessment, occupational therapy treatment, patient/client-related conferences, travel, patient treatment related, service management, and education and research. The first four categories were considered to be direct service care to patients or clients, whereas the remaining three were viewed as indirect patient care. Treatment was subdivided into six components, including independent living/daily living skills, sensorimotor, cognitive, psychosocial, therapeutic adaptation, and prevention. A total of 84 terms were defined or described (AOTA, 1981, 1983, 1986a).

Proficiency Testing and Career Laddering for Persons Not Educated as Occupational Therapists

In 1971, the Association became involved in the federal program called Proficiency Testing or Competency-Based Qualification. The Association received a government contract (AOTA, 1972b). The purpose was to develop an examination that a person could take to qualify as an occupational therapist without having to complete the required educational program. Phase I was completed in 1973. Field testing began 2 years later (AOTA, 1975e). A year later, the Association accepted another Department of Health, Education, and Welfare contract for the final development of the competency-based criterion-referenced examination (AOTA, 1977b). However, the membership was not pleased with the results of either project. In 1978, the Representative Assembly voted that "any grants or contracts applied for and awarded would not obligate the Association to use or accept resulting products, methods or objectives inconsistent with existing policies and procedures" (AOTA, 1978b). Finally, in 1979, the Representative Assembly voted that proficiency testing was not an acceptable method of entry into the profession (AOTA, 1979a).

As West (1992) points out, accepting and completing the work of grants on proficiency and competency testing "may not have been in the best interests of the profession" (p. 1068). In a 1985 "The Issue Is" article, Hinojosa states that competency-based education does not meet the "needs of a profession regarding accountability and mastery of methodological techniques" and does address a profession's philosophical base, theoretical concerns, ethical issues, and affective functions (p. 541). Credit is due to members of the Association to recognize and correct errors in judgment (AOTA, 1975a).

Awards

The Representative Assembly established the Roster of Fellows in 1970 with resolution 263-70 and began in 1973 to honor those who had made a significant contribution to the Association and the profession. From 1973 to 1979, 183 people were named Fellows and permitted to use FAOTA (Fellow of the American Occupational Therapy Association) after their names. Other new Association awards include the following:

- 1973—Certificate of Appreciation
- 1976—COTA Award of Excellence
- 1978—Roster of Honor for Occupational Therapy Assistants
- 1978—Cordelia Myers Writer's Award

Continuing Certification (Resolution 300-71 and Recertification)

The continuing certification process started in 1965 with a motion made by Mildred Sleeper adopted at the first Delegate Assembly, which stated that the Assembly was to "authorize the appropriate Councils of the association to establish realistic standards for an effective means of maintaining eligibility for the annual renewal of registration and membership" (AOTA, 1966, p. 50). A second motion (Resolution 155) that was defeated in 1967 contained a proposal stating that the minimum requirements for registration were to be completed every 3 years. The responsibility for submitting proof of fulfillment of the requirements would remain with the individual member. A Committee on Continuing Registration and Certification was to be established to implement the policy of recertification (AOTA, 1968, p. 520). The issue of continuing certification was renewed in 1971 with the passage of Resolution 300-71. The aim of the Resolution was "to improve, promote and insure, insofar as is possible, the provision of quality care to consumers of occupational therapy services by competent, qualified occupational therapy personnel" (Johnson, 1972).

In 1975, the report stated that the Continuing Certification Program staff had been working with six task forces to develop general standards of practice in the areas of developmental disabilities, mental health, and physical disabilities and specific standards in the areas of stroke, arthritis and home health (AOTA, 1975a). A pilot study for a recertification program was to begin in 1976. Other portions of the program included the development of a self-assessment instructional package for therapists practicing in mental health. The program was funded through a 2-year Department of Health, Education, and Welfare contract (NO1-AH-44116).

Resolution 540-79 was adopted in April 1979 and stated that the recertification process was a high priority. The process when fully implemented was to be "mandatory, attainable, accessible, and cost effective all members and administratively manageable" (AOTA, 1979a, pp. 793-794). Alternative means were to be allowed to demonstrate continuing competency such as courses for credit, research, publication, professional participation, honors, exam(s), field work, continuing education, self-study, and conducting workshops. Self-assessment materials were to be made available to members as soon as possible. As part of the continuing study by the Recertification Task Force created in 1980, they studied aspects related to feasibility and suitability of recertification methods, including mandatory continuing education, written examination, on-the-job performance evaluation, and peer review/chart audit. A summary of the studies was printed in the Occupational Therapy Newspaper from May through August 1981 (Recertification Study Reports, 1981). Two plans were presented: Plan A was Voluntary Recognition and Plan B was labeled Research & Development to further study the ramifications of recertification.

In 1982, Resolution 582-82 brought an end to the study of continuing certification and recertification, stating that (1) it was expensive to develop an acceptable and reliable recertification or voluntary recognition program, (2) the recertification program may not be necessary in the field of occupational therapy because there was little evidence that therapists or assistants were not maintaining their competency to practice, and (3) there were other growth-enhancing programs and services that could be developed for the benefit of therapists and assistants. Therefore, the resolution dictated that "no further AOTA studies on recertification methods be done until there is an evidence need for such studies" (AOTA, 1982a, p. 813). Although not stated in the resolution, another important factor was the increase in the number of states with licensure laws that would set the requirements for renewing a license within that state. Such requirements would have greater impact on the practice of occupational therapy than any program developed or implemented by the Association. Other factors mentioned in final report in 1981 were the mixed reactions regarding the acceptance by the membership, lack of validity of many of the suggested assess-ment measurements, and uncertainty regarding public acceptance (Recertification Study Reports, 1981). Ultimately, the National Board for Certification in Occupational Therapy would develop a voluntary recertification program, and state associations were able to use the accumulated data in developing the requirements for recertification within each state.

Career Mobility Program

In 1971, the Delegate Assembly adopted Resolution 311-71, which directed the Council on Standards to develop procedures whereby certified occupational therapy assistants could qualify to sit for the registration examination and thus become registered occupational therapists with-out having to return to a formal academic setting (AOTA, 1971a, p. 374). The Career Mobility Program was developed in response to the resolution and was administered by the Career Mobility Review Committee, a subcommittee of the Certification Committee. In addition, AOTA adopted a Statement on Career Mobility in 1973 (AOTA, 1973b).

According to the Annual Report (AOTA, 1978-1979) from 1971 to 1978, 43 certified occu-pational therapy assistants successfully met the work experience, field work, and examination requirements to become registered occupational therapists through the Career Mobility Program. Sixty certified occupational therapy assistants had applied and were participating in the program.

The Career Mobility Program was not without controversy. One concern was the criteria used to determine successful completion of fieldwork experience. To correct some perceived weak-nesses, additional resolutions were adopted in 1975 (Resolution 451-75). The criteria were changed to require the following:

- Current certification by AOTA as an occupational therapy assistant
- Accumulation of not less than 4 years of occupational therapy practice as a certified occupa-tional therapy assistantA
- Evidence of having fulfilled current fieldwork experience requirement stipulated in the Essentials of an Accepted Educational Program for the Occupational Therapist, which may have been fulfilled within the 4 years of occupational therapy practice (AOTA, 1975b, p. 559)

Role Delineation Study

The Role Delineation Study began in 1976. Its purpose was to serve as the basis for a criterion-referenced entry examination for occupational therapy assistants under a grant contract with the Department of Health, Education, and Welfare (Shapiro & Brown, 1981). As part of the contract, both levels (therapists and assistants) of practice were described. In addition, Mae Hightower-Vandamm, Association President, charged the investigators to delineate the differences and simi-larities between the two levels of practice. The Professional Examination Service conducted the study using several separate methodological steps: worker logs, observation/interview, supervisors' structured checklists, role defined by experts, and role verification. The study results were summa-rized into 108 tasks statements encompassing the role of occupational therapy practitioner prac-ticing in entry-level positions where both therapists and assistants were working together. Fifty tasks were considered to be a part of the evaluation function of occupational therapy practitioners,

12 tasks were considered a planning function, and 46 were labeled as intervention and program termination functions. Of the 108 tasks, 80 were reported as being done by both therapists and assistants. Both levels were responsible for evaluation, planning, and intervention. However, assistants performed the tasks under supervision of a therapist and were not responsible for determining that the task needed to be done or how it was to be performed. Therapists were seen as involved more often in intervention programs aimed at correcting, improving, or maintaining the components of performance, whereas assistants were seen as involved more in programs aimed at improving or maintaining function in occupational performance. Occupational performance was defined as planning and participation in everyday activities such as self-care, work, academic, homemaking, leisure, and play (AOTA, 1981, p. 310). Performance components were defined as "learned and/or inherent elements of behavior that permit the planning and participation in everyday activities" (AOTA, 1981, p. 311). The difference between the two levels was further articulated in the degree of responsibility, amount of supervision required, and objective or goal of the intervention program. Because the purpose of the study was to develop examinations based on entry-level skills only, the study could not be used to generalize beyond the intent to prepare an examination process. However, the same or similar methodology was used in a study of roles and functions in the education of school-based practice (Gilfoyle & Hays, 1979) and student achievement in occupational therapy courses (Borg & Bruce, 1981).

Delegate Assembly

In 1975, there were 44 associations represented at the Delegate Assembly meeting. The following year, 1976, all 50 states had established state associations as part of the renamed Representative Assembly. Those with two associations within one state boundary (California, Pennsylvania, and New York) combined to form one association, and those representing two states (Dakota representing both North and South Dakota, and Alabama-Mississippi) were separated into individual state associations (AOTA, 1976a). Finally, all states had functioning occupational therapy state associations within the state boundary.

The Delegate Assembly become a functioning policy body and began adopting standards, policy statements, and position papers on a number of topics related to issues of concern to occupational therapy and practice. Table 7-10 summarizes the documents by year of adoption, title, and location of published document, if known.

Register Publication and Registration Examination

Registers were published in 1970, 1972, and 1974-1975. The last Register was published in 1980. Thus, the publication of the names of qualified practitioners, which had begun in 1932, ended. The expense in terms of time and money was no longer considered cost effective. As states became licensed, initial certification became less important as a statement of qualification because licensure had to be renewed on a regular basis to practice in the state. In addition, state licensing boards maintained a list of all licensed therapists and assistants in that state, further reducing the need for a national list.

The registration examination process was transferred to an outside firm in 1972, marking the first time the examination process was handled outside the Association (Cromwell, 1972, p. 4A). The transfer was necessary because the process of getting examination questions together for each examination; getting the examination forms printed; getting packets of examinations ready for each school; making sure the packets arrived on time; getting packets returned and scored; and notifying schools, individuals, and state licensure boards of the results was beginning to be a time-consuming project for the Association staff as the number of schools and applicants increased. Outsourcing the process to a company that specialized in test construction, administration,

Table 7-10

DOCUMENTS PUBLISHED BY THE ASSOCIATION DURING THE 1970S

1970	• Educating the Occupational Therapy Assistant: A Guide (AOTA, 1973a Appendix 6, Ch 3) • Guidelines for Continuing Education Experiences (AOTA, 1973a, Appendix 8, Ch 3 • Standards and Guidelines of an Occupational Therapy Affiliation Program (AJOT, 25(6), 313-315; AOTA 1973b, Appendix 3, Ch 3
1971	• Statement on Licensure of Occupational Therapists, February 19, 1971 Source? Check this • The Role of Occupational Therapy in Health Maintenance. Index of AOTA Official Documents, 1978
1972	• Advanced Professional Education in Occupational Therapy (AOTA, 1973a Appendix 2 Ch 2. • Consumer Involvement. AJOT, 1973, 27(1), 48 • Essentials of an Accredited Educational Program for the Occupational Therapists. Index of AOTA Official Documents, 1978 • Occupational Therapy: Its Definition and Functions. Index of AOTA Official Documents, 1978. Reference Manual of the Official Documents of the American Occupational Therapy Association, 1980) • Quality of Care in Occupational Therapy (Lyla Spelbring) Index of AOTA Official Documents, 1978
1973	• Clarification of Terminology (AOTA, 1973a Ch 1) based on Terminology Report to Executive Board • Consumer Involvement. AJOT, 1973, 27(1), 48 • Entry Level Functions of the Registered Occupational Therapy, Certificated Occupational Therapy Assistant and Occupational Therapy Aide. Index of AOTA Official Documents, 1978 • Occupational Therapy Newsletter started • Philosophy of Basic Professional Education in Occupational Therapy. (AOTA, 1973a Appendix 1 Cj 2 • Standards for Occupational Therapists Providing Direct Service (AOTA, 1973a) Appendix 18 Ch 3) • Statement on Advanced Professional Education. AJOT, 1973, 27(3), 158. • Statement on Career Mobility, (AOTA, 1973a, Appendix 7, Ch 3) AJOT, 1073, 27(3), 157. • Statement on Medical Malpractice, AJOT, 1973, 27(1), 49-50. • Statement on Proficiency and Equivalency Measures. AJOT,1973, 27(6), 411. • Statement on SASHEP commission Report, AJOT, 1973. 27(3), 156-159.
1974	• Guidelines for an Occupational Therapist Providing Services as a Supervisor Index of AOTA Official Documents, 1978.
1975	• Essentials of an Approved Educational Program for the Occupational Therapy Assistant. Index of AOTA Official Documents, 1978. (AJOT, 1975, 29(8), 485-496). • Guidelines and Format for AOTA Position Papers. AJOT, 1975, 29(1), 53 • Guidelines for AOTA Recognitions. AJOT, 1975, 29(10), 632-635 • Model Occupational Therapy Practice Act. AJOT, 1975, 29(1), 48-52. • Philosophy and Concerns Regarding Education of the Handicapped. Index of AOTA Official Documents, 1978 • Policy Governing Lapse Certification of Occupational Therapists and Occupational Therapy Assistants (unpublished)
1976	• AOTA Certification Requirements (Index of AOTA Official Documents; 1980 Reference manual) • Essentials of an Approved Education Program for the Occupational Therapy Assistant, AJOT, 1976,30(4), 245-263. • Proposed Standards of Occupational Therapist working in home health: Job description. Index of AOTA Official Documents, 1978.

(continued)

Table 7-10 (continued) DOCUMENTS PUBLISHED BY THE ASSOCIATION DURING THE 1970S	
1977	• Guide for Graduate Education in Occupational Therapy Leading to the Master's Degree (1986 Reference Manual) • Guide to the Preparation of Fieldwork Objectives for Occupational Therapy Students & Fieldwork Performance Report Form • Principles of Occupational Therapy Ethics. Reference Manual of the Official Documents of the American Occupational Therapy Association, 1980. (Revised 1979) • Proposed policy statement – National Health Insurance, AJOT, 31(2), 110
1978	• The Role of the Occupational Therapist in the Promotion of Health and Prevention of Disabilities • Standards of Practice: Physical disabilities, Developmental Disabilities, Mental Health, Home Health
1979	• Enforcement Procedures for Principles of Occupational Therapy Ethics • Occupational Therapy for Sensory Integrative Dysfunction • The Role of Occupational Therapy in Home Health Care • The Role of Occupational Therapy in the Vocational Rehabilitation Process

scoring, and notification made good sense. Occupational therapy practitioners were still involved in writing the actual questions but experts in testing helped to edit the questions and organize the content of the examination forms.

AMERICAN OCCUPATIONAL THERAPY POLITICAL ACTION COMMITTEE

The American Occupational Therapy Political Action Committee (AOTPAC) was formed in the spring of 1978 and announced in the May issue of the Occupational Therapy Newspaper. The announcement stated the AOTPAC was the members' "opportunity to bring the profession of occupational therapy and its concerns to the attention of elected officials" (AOTA, 1978c, p. 1). All Association members were encouraged to donate to the AOTPAC because its purpose was to be "the political action arm of AOTA" (AOTA, 1978d, p. 2). The primary focus was on influencing passage of federal legislation that promoted the used of occupational therapy services. Changes to Medicare to increase occupational therapy services was one of the primary objectives (AOTA, 1978b) (Figure 7-12).

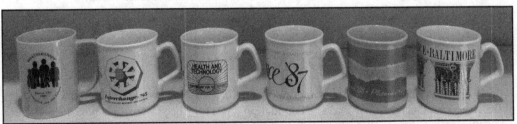

Figure 7-12. AOTPAC coffee mugs. AOTPAC sold coffee mugs at annual AOTA conferences for a number of years to raise money for the PAC. (Copyright © Dr. Lori T. Andersen. Reprinted with permission.)

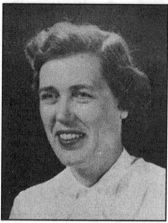

Figure 7-13. Alice C. Jantzen, PhD, OTR, first President of AOTF, 1965-1966. (Printed with permission from the Archive of the American Occupational Therapy Association, Inc.)

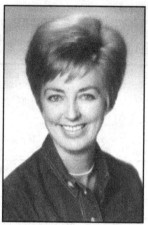

Figure 7-14. Elizabeth J. Yerxa, EdD, OTR, second President of AOTF, 1966-1968. (Printed with permission from the Archive of the American Occupational Therapy Association, Inc.)

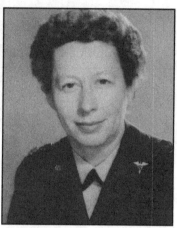

Figure 7-15. Myra L. McDaniel, Lt. Col., AMSC, OTR, third President of AOTF.

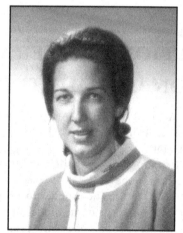

Figure 7-16. Nancy V. Snyder, OTR, fourth and seventh President of AOTF, 1969-1972 and 1986-1988. (Printed with permission from the Archive of the American Occupational Therapy Association, Inc.)

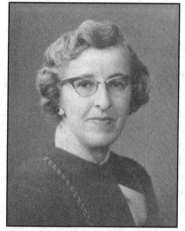

Figure 7-17. Wilma L. West, OTR, fifth President of AOTF, 1972-1982. (Printed with permission from the Archive of the American Occupational Therapy Association, Inc.)

FOUNDATION

In 1975, the Foundation had been functioning for 10 years. Five people had served as President of the American Occupational Therapy Foundation (AOTF): Alice C. Jantzen, 1965-1966 (Figure 7-13); Elizabeth J. Yerza, 1966-1968 (Figure 7-14); Myra L. McDaniel, 1968-1969 (Figure 7-15); Nancy V. Snyder, 1969-1972 (Figure 7-16); and Wilma L. West, 1972-1982 (Figure 7-17). The fund balance had grown from $2,068 in 1955 to $156,488 in 1975. Scholarship awards started in 1969. The first scholarship award, the OT Affiliate and Student Club Award, was given in June 1959. The second was the Pauline Gundersen Scholarship for study in the field of psychiatry. In October 1959, the Carolyn W. Kohn Scholarship Fund was announced. By 1975, 10 scholarship funds had been established (AOTF, 1975). In 1970, the Foundation moved beyond its first two commitments—education and research—and began to address the objective of increasing public knowledge and understanding of the profession. The first publication was a pamphlet titled "The Child With Minimal Brain Dysfunction" published in July 1974. By 1974, the work of the Foundation became more than the volunteer officers and directors could handle. A full-time Funding Coordinator was hired. Funding was shared with the Association.

REFLECTION

The 1970s were a time of rapid change for the profession and the Association. The headquarters moved from New York City to Rockville, Maryland to facilitate interaction with Congress and influence health care legislation favorable to occupational therapy education and practice. The Association approved the concept of state licensure to better define the practice of occupational therapy and describe the qualifications of practitioners to participate in state health care laws and regulations. The number of educational programs and practitioners rose rapidly during the 1970s as recruitment efforts began to have results and reimbursement through insurance increased revenues for rehabilitation workers such as occupational therapy practitioners as a result of federal legislation, especially Medicare, Medicaid and the Education for All Handicapped Act. Other events included the philosophy of the profession project and the recognition of practitioners through the establishment of the Roster of Fellows for therapists and the Roster of Honor for assistants.

REFERENCES

American Medical Association Medical education. (1971). Occupational therapist. *Journal of the American Medical Association, 208*(9), 1270.

American Occupational Therapy Association. (1966). Delegate Assembly minutes. *American Journal of Occupational Therapy, 20*(1), 49-53.

American Occupational Therapy Association (1968). A new pin for the registered occupational therapist. *American Journal of Occupational Therapy, 22*(6), 520.

American Occupational Therapy Association. (1969a). Licensing and standards of competency in occupational therapy. *American Journal of Occupational Therapy, 23*(6), 529-530.

American Occupational Therapy Association. (1969b). *Model occupational therapy practice act.* Rockville, MD: Author.

American Occupational Therapy Association. (1970a). *Occupational therapy handbook.* New York, NY: Author.

American Occupational Therapy Association. (1970b). *Occupational therapy handbook* (p. 2). New York, NY: Author.

American Occupational Therapy Association. (1971a). Delegate Assembly minutes. *American Journal of Occupational Therapy, 25*(7), 371-382.

American Occupational Therapy Association. (1971b). *Statement on licensure of occupational therapists.* Rockville, MD: Author.

American Occupational Therapy Association. (1972a). From program development—contract awarded. *Newsletter, 24*(8), 2.

American Occupational Therapy Association. (1972b). Report of the task force on social issues. *American Journal of Occupational Therapy, 26*(7), 332-359.

American Occupational Therapy Association (1972c). *Report on legislation.* New York: American Occupational Therapy Association.

American Occupational Therapy Association: Council on Standards (1972d). Occupational therapy: Its definition and functions. *American Journal of Occupational Therapy, 26*(4), 204-205.

American Occupational Therapy Association. (1973a). *Reference manual for occupational therapy educators.* Rockville, MD: Author.

American Occupational Therapy Association. (1973b). Statement on career mobility. *American Journal of Occupational Therapy, 27*(3), 157-158.

American Occupational Therapy Association. (1973c). Essentials of an Accredited Education Program for the Occupational Therapist. *American Journal of Occupational Therapy, 27*(2), 117-120.

American Occupational Therapy Association. (1974a). Association task force on target populations—report 1. *American Journal of Occupational Therapy, 28*(3), 158-163.

American Occupational Therapy Association. (1974b). Association task force on target populations—report 1. *American Journal of Occupational Therapy, 28*(3), 160.

American Occupational Therapy Association. (1974b). Association task force on target populations—report 2. *American Journal of Occupational Therapy, 28*(4), 231-236.

American Occupational Therapy Association. (1975a). *Annual report 1975.* Rockville, MD: Author.

American Occupational Therapy Association. (1975b). Delegate Assembly minutes. *American Journal of Occupational Therapy, 29*(9), 552-564.

American Occupational Therapy Association. (1975c). Delegate Assembly: Resolution 400-74 Licensure. *American Journal of Occupational Therapy, 29*(3), 154-155.

American Occupational Therapy Association. (1975d). Exam changes for OTRs. *Occupational Therapy Newsletter, 29*(10), 3.

American Occupational Therapy Association. (1975e). Field testing of proficiency examinations for entry level OTs is completed by PES, final report available. *Occupational Therapy Newspaper, 29*(4), 10.

American Occupational Therapy Association. (1975f). Delegate assembly minutes. *American Journal of Occupational Therapy, 29*(3), 153-159.

American Occupational Therapy Association. (1975g). Model Occupational Therapy Practice Act. *American Journal of Occupational Therapy, 29*(1), 48-49.

American Occupational Therapy Association. (1976a). Letters to the editor. *American Journal of Occupational Therapy, 30*(2), 110-112.

American Occupational Therapy Association. (1976b). Report of the mental health task force. *Occupational Therapy Newspaper, 30*(9), 6-7.

American Occupational Therapy Association. (1976c). President Ford addresses CIHP Members. *Occupational Therapy Newsletter, 30*(5), 5.

American Occupational Therapy Association. (1977a). In search of a philosophy. *Occupational Therapy Newspaper, 31*(10), 11.

American Occupational Therapy Association. (1977b). Proficiency testing update. *Occupational Therapy Newspaper, 31*(2), 6.

American Occupational Therapy Association. (1977c). Bylaws. *American Journal of Occupational Therapy, 31*(2), 111-118.

American Occupational Therapy Association. (1977d). Representative Assembly Minutes. *American Journal of Occupational Therapy, 31*(9), 585-606.

American Occupational Therapy Association. (1978a). 1977 membership data survey. Bethesda, MD: Author.

American Occupational Therapy Association. (1978b). Minutes of conference call (of the Executive Board) dated July 18, 1978. Bethesda, MD: AOTA/AOTF Library.

American Occupational Therapy Association. (1978c). Political action mailing. *Occupational Therapy Newspaper, 32*(5), 1.

American Occupational Therapy Association. (1978d). Political action—a tool for OT. *Occupational Therapy Newspaper, 32*(7), 2.

American Occupational Therapy Association. (1978-1979). *Annual report.* Rockville, MD: Author.

American Occupational Therapy Association. (1979a). 1979 Representative Assembly, 59th Annual Conference. *American Journal of Occupational Therapy, 33*(12), 780-813.

American Occupational Therapy Association. (1979b). Data Line: Manpower needs for OT personnel. *Occupational Therapy Newsletter, 33*(9), 3.

American Occupational Therapy Association. (1979c). Project to identify the philosophy of occupational therapy. *Occupational Therapy Newsletter, 33*(9), 1-6.

American Occupational Therapy Association. (1981). Uniform terminology for reporting occupational therapy services and uniform occupational therapy evaluation checklist. *Occupational Therapy Newspaper, 39*(11), 9-12.

American Occupational Therapy Association. (1982a). 1982 Representative Assembly—62nd annual conference. *American Journal of Occupational Therapy, 36*(12), 809-820.

American Occupational Therapy Association. (1982b). *Introduction to AOTA project to identify the philosophy of occupational therapy* (p. 3). Rockville, MD: Author.

American Occupational Therapy Association. (1983). Development of proposed occupational therapy product output reporting system. In *Reference manual of the official documents of the American Occupational Therapy Association* (pp. 29-36). Rockville, MD: Author.

American Occupational Therapy Association. (1985). *Occupational therapy manpower: A plan for progress.* Rockville, MD: Author.

American Occupational Therapy Association. (1986a). Development of proposed occupational therapy product output reporting system. In *Reference manual of the official documents of the American Occupational Therapy Association* (pp. VIII.19-21). Rockville, MD: Author.

American Occupational Therapy Association. (1986b). Occupational therapy product output reporting system and uniform terminology for reporting occupational therapy services. In *Reference manual of the official documents of the American Occupational Therapy Association* (pp. VIII.11-18). Rockville, MD: Author.

American Occupational Therapy Association. (1989). Uniform terminology for occupational therapy, 2nd edition. *American Journal of Occupational Therapy, 43*(2), 808-815.

American Occupational Therapy Association. (1992a). An historical look at special interest sections. *OT Week, 16*, 6-7.

American Occupational Therapy Association. (1992b). AOTA's Hall of leaders. *OT Week, 6*(21), 40-43

American Occupational Therapy Association. (1994). Uniform terminology for occupational therapy, 3rd edition. *American Journal of Occupational Therapy, 48*(11), 1055-1059.

American Occupational Therapy Foundation. (1975). The first decade: 1965-1975. *American Journal of Occupational Therapy, 39*(10), 636-640.

Ayres, A.J. (1972). *Southern California Sensory Integration Tests.* Los Angeles, CA: Western Psychological Services.

Ayres, A.J. (1972). *Sensory integration and learning disorders.* Los Angeles, CA: Western Psychological Services

Borg, B., & Bruce, M. A. (1981). Criterion-reference measurement in the college classroom. *American Journal of Occupational Therapy, 35*(5), 321-327.

Bowman, E. (1922). Psychology of occupational therapy. *Archives of Occupational Therapy, 1*(3), 171-178.

Clark, P. N. (1979a) Human development through occupation: Theoretical frameworks in contemporary occupational therapy practice—part 1. *American Journal of Occupational Therapy, 33*(8), 505-514.

Clark, P. N. (1979b). Human development through occupation: A philosophy and conceptual model for practice—part 2. *American Journal of Occupational Therapy, 33*(9), 577-585.

Cromwell, F. S. (1972). Nationally speaking. *American Journal of Occupational Therapy, 26*(2), 3A-6A.

English, C. B. (1975). Computers and occupational therapy. *American Journal of Occupational Therapy, 39*(1), 423-447.

Fanning, L. C. (1972). Executive director report – Mid year, p. 17. New York, NY: American Occupational Therapy Association

Gilfoyle, E. M. N., & Hays, C. A. (1979). Occupational therapy roles and functions in the education of school-based handicapped students. *American Journal of Occupational Therapy, 33*(9), 565-576.

Glenn, J. W., Miller, K. H., & Broman, M. T. (1976). Voice terminal may offer opportunities for employment to the disabled. *American Journal of Occupational Therapy, 30*(5), 308-312.

Hawkins, J. M., & Hawkins, B. (1978). Clinical placements by computer program. *American Journal of Occupational Therapy, 32*(6), 390-394.

Hinojosa, J. (1985). The issue is: Implications for occupational therapy of a competency-based orientation. *American Journal of Occupation Therapy, 39*(8), 539-541.

Hopkins, H. & Smith, H.D. (Eds.). (1978). *Occupational therapy,* 3rd ed. Philadelphia, PA: Lippincott.

Hopkins, H., & Smith, H.D. (Eds.). (1983). Appendix D: Uniform terminology for reporting occupational therapy services; Appendix E: Occupational therapy product output reporting system; Appendix F: Uniform occupational therapy evaluation checklist. In *Willard and Spackman's occupational therapy* (6th ed., pp. 899-914). Philadelphia, PA: J. B. Lippincott.

Johnson, J. A. (1972). Summary of interim planning committee activities for Resolution #300-71, June 1971–February 1972: Addendum to Executive Director report—Midyear conference. New York, NY: AOTA.

Johnson, J. A. (1975a). Nationally speaking: Licensure. *American Journal of Occupational Therapy, 29*(2), 73.

Johnson, J. A. (1975b). Nationally speaking: Mission and goal statements. *American Journal of Occupational Therapy, 29*(5), 261.

Johnson, J. A. (1978). Nationally speaking: Issues in education. *American Journal of Occupational Therapy, 32*(6), 355-358.

Kielhofner, G., & Burke, J. P. (1977). Occupational therapy after 60 years: An account of changing identify and knowledge. *American Journal of Occupational Therapy, 31*(1), 675-689.

Lee, H. S., Robinson, R. A., Whitcomb, B., & Lovett, H. M. (1968). The period of stabilization, July 1953 to January 1961. In R. S. Anderson, H. S. Lee, & M. L. McDaniel (Eds.), *Army Medical Specialist Corps* (pp. 391-430). Washington, DC: Office of the Surgeon General, Department of the Army.

Llorens, L. A. (1970). Facilitating growth and development: the promise of occupational therapy. *American Journal of Occupational Therapy, 24*(2), 93-101.

Llorens, L. A. (1977). A developmental theory revised. *American Journal of Occupational Therapy, 31*(10), 656-657.

Mosey, A. C. (1970). *Three frames of reference for mental health.* Thorofare, NJ: Charles B. Slack.

Neuhaus, B. E. (1971). Implementation of Resolution #221. *American Journal of Occupational Therapy, 23*(1), 65-68.

Recertification Study Reports (1981). *Occupational Therapy Newspaper, 35*(5), 1, 13; *35*(6), 7; *35*(7), 3, *35*(8), 3; *35*(9), 5.

Reilly, M. (1962). The Eleanor Clarke Slagle: Occupational therapy can be one of the great ideas of 20th century medicine. *American Journal of Occupational Therapy, 26*(1), 1-9.

Shapiro, D., & Brown, D. (1981). The delineation of the role of entry-level occupational therapy personnel. *American Journal of Occupational Therapy, 35*(5), 306-311.

Smith, E. I. (1973). The employment and functioning of the homebound disabled in information technology. *American Journal of Occupational Therapy, 27*(5), 232-238.

Trombly, C.A. & Scott, A.D. (1977). *Occupational therapy for physical dysfunction.* Baltimore, MD: Williams & Wilkins.

U.S. House of Representatives. Committee on Interstate and Foreign Commerce. (1976). *A discursive diction of healthcare* (p. 112). Washington, D.C.: Superintendent of Documents.

West, W. L. (1992). Ten milestone issues in AOTA history. *American Journal of Occupational Therapy, 46*(12), 1066-1074.

Willard, H.S. & Spackman, C.S. (Eds.). (1971). *Occupational therapy,* 4th ed. Philadelphia, PA: Lippincott.

BIBLIOGRAPHY

American Occupational Therapy Association. (1973). Continuing certification program to involve practice interests, membership. *Occupational Therapy Newspaper, 27*(2), 1.

American Occupational Therapy Association. (1976). *Annual report.* Rockville, MD: Author.

American Occupational Therapy Association. (1976). Delegate Assembly minutes. *American Journal of Occupational Therapy, 30*(3), 168-180.

American Occupational Therapy Association. (1976). OTAs to take certification exam. *Occupational Therapy Newspaper, 30*(6), 1.

American Occupational Therapy Association. (1986). Uniform occupational therapy evaluation checklist. In *Reference manual of the official documents of the American Occupational Therapy Association* (pp. VIII.22-23). Rockville, MD: Author.

8

Search for a Unifying Theory
1980s to 1990s

Key Points

- The Association purchased a building to house national office activities and staff for the first time.
- Association membership increased significantly.
- The American Occupational Therapy Certification Board (AOTBC) was created in 1986. (Forerunner of the National Board for Certification in Occupational Therapy.)
- *Uniform Terminology II* was published in 1989.
- There was an increased use of computers and physical agent modalities in occupational therapy service delivery.
- The library was organized and materials catalogued to create an archive and library of occupational therapy letters, documents, journals, books, and artifacts—1980.
- The Academy of Research was established by the Foundation in 1983.
- The number of journals focused on occupational therapy rapidly increased beginning in 1980.

Highlighted Personalities

- Gary Wayne Kielhofner, theorist
- Elizabeth June Yerxa, theorist
- Claudia Kay Allen, theorist
- Carolyn Manville Baum, AOTA President, 1982-1983

- Robert Kendall Bing, AOTA President, 1983-1986
- Elnora M. Gilfoyle, AOTA President, 1986-1989
- Jeannette Bair, AOTA Executive Director
- Martha Moersch, AOTF President

Key Places

- The Association bought a headquarters building in Rockville, Maryland.

Andersen, L. T., & Reed, K. L.
The History of Occupational Therapy: The First Century (pp. 229-260).
© 2017 Taylor & Francis Group.

Political Events/Issues

- Concern about anti-trust issues led to the certification process being separated from Association membership.
- The Omnibus Reconciliation Act of 1980 included payment for occupational therapy services in comprehensive outpatient rehabilitation facilities and home health.
- Occupational therapy was a qualifying service for home health under Medicare starting in 1981.
- Occupational therapy was covered in hospice care under Medicare in 1982.

Economic Events/Issues

- Reimbursement for occupational therapy services
- Diagnostic Related Groups (DRGs) implemented

Association Issues

- Manpower Study, 1983-1985
- Policy on use of physical agent modalities adopted by Representative Assembly
- Occupational Therapy Directions for the Future Project completed
- Professional and Technical Role Analysis (PATRA) project completed
- Task Force on OT/PT Issues reported findings
- Uniform Occupational Therapy Evaluation Checklist published in 1981
- Second edition of Uniform Terminology document adopted, 1989

Foundation Issues

- Archival materials, monographs (books), and serials (journals) were formally organized and catalogued into a library within the Foundation, 1980
- Computerized online database of library materials created
- Academy of Research established in 1983
- Developing working relationship with the Association

Key Times/Events

- Certification and membership fees separated in 1986: Membership dues could be paid without paying for continuing certification as state licensure became primary means of establishing continuing competence to practice.

Sociocultural Events/Issues

- Home computer age expanded rapidly with the introduction of the IBM model 8088.
- With an increase in geriatrics, there was recognition that the population was aging.

Technological Events/Issues

- Computers become a major medium in occupational therapy practice.
- Electronic media enhance self-care devices for client service.

Educational Issues

- *Essentials and Guidelines of an Accredited Education Program for the Occupational Therapist*—revised in 1983
- *Essentials and Guidelines of an Approved Educational Program or the Occupational Therapy Assistant*—revised in 1983

Practice Issues

- Approximately 40% of hospitals and 30% of nursing homes offered occupational therapy services.
- Hospitals, school settings, and nursing homes were major employers.
- De-emphasis on the use of crafts in favor of modalities with more direct measurement potential, especially in physical disabilities practice
- Theories based on principles of occupational therapy were created.

"Occupational Therapy—A Vital Link to Productive Living"
–New slogan adopted by AOTA, 1986

INTRODUCTION

President Ronald Reagan served two terms, from 1980 to 1988. During the 1980s, the Cold War between the Soviet Union and the United States thawed out on the military front, ending with the fall of the Berlin Wall in 1989. At the same time, interest heated up on the space shuttle technology front. A new era of technology emerged with the creation of the first personal computer by IBM in 1981. The development of the Internet began to change communication systems in ways not previously imagined possible. Technological advances led to improvements in health care, but the costs of health care would greatly increase. New approaches to reimbursement from per diem rates to per service costs would force occupational therapy practitioners to demonstrate evidence that showed their services to be of value in promoting health and wellness as well as decreasing the impact of disability. The challenge to explain increased as occupational therapy practitioners both expanded their service roles and began to specialize in different areas of practice. The efforts made to establish a unifying scope of practice led to a paradigm shift away from the mechanistic, biomedical view toward a more holistic and client-centered approach to practice and serve delivery. New ideas such as the Model of Human Occupation (Kielhofner), clinical reasoning (Rogers), and occupation science (Yerxa) expanded the concepts about how occupational therapy should be explained and what processes were needed to implement occupational therapy services. State licensure continued to be an issue and further challenged occupational therapy practitioners to identify what constituted occupational therapy service and what identified a competent occupational therapy practitioner. The impact of Public Law 94-142 (Education for All Handicapped; now Individuals with Disabilities Act) increased the role of occupational therapy in the school system as the concept of self-care became important for children to function successfully in the school environment.

CHANGING TRENDS

Bair (1982) suggested there were 10 topics related to changes in practice affecting occupational therapy in the 1980s:

- Age of the population: The population continues to age, growing from 10% in 1975 to an expected 20% by 2030. The number of long-term care facilities will grow as a result. Treatment focusing on home care will increase. For older individuals, the issues of self-reliance and mobility are major considerations.
- Consumer awareness: Increased public education and awareness will result in people being more aware of self-responsibility for personal health. Wellness and prevention concepts are increasing accepted for both philosophical and economic reasons.
- Technology: Improved technology will help more people to survive catastrophic illness. However, the cost may restrict access to new technology for some clients.
- Business influence: Business leaders favor a more competitive health care market as a means of reducing or controlling costs. Businesses are providing more health maintenance programs to employees. Strategic planning, marketing, productivity, and accountability are becoming important aspects of the health care industry.

- Environmental and economic disasters and dislocation: Concern that environmental disasters and economic disasters could impact health care delivery, especially as people move to the sun belt.
- Shift in personal values and lifestyles: There has been a gradual shift in Americans' values away from materialistic attainment toward more community-directed and spiritual goals. More people are interested in holistic medicine, nutrition, exercise, and health promotion.
- Hospitals: More hospitals are becoming part of corporate groups to face complex regulatory demands and cost constraints. In 1958, 200 hospitals were grouped in a formal system, but by 1981, there were 34 investor-owned systems managing 900 hospitals and 300 not-for-profit facilities. The number of acute beds is expected to decrease while the number of emergency centers, wellness and fitness, and home health care programs is expected to increase.
- Long-term care: The number of long-term care facilities is expected to grow rapidly as the elderly become a more powerful political and lobby group. There will more focus on the total needs of the elderly.
- Psychiatric mental health facilities: The growth is in drug addiction and alcoholism programs.
- Hospice: From 1974 to 1981, the number of hospice programs grew from 1 to more than 800. Most programs are free—standing even if they are hospital affiliated.

The challenges included keeping pace with the changes in health care delivery. Occupational therapy personnel became more actively involved in cardiac rehabilitation, stress reduction, working with the elderly, pain management programs, and promoting early infant development. Other challenges included the development and use of technological advances in rehabilitation such as bioelectric limbs, computers, and computer-based communication systems.

In an article focusing on the growth of the profession during the 1980s, Gilfoyle (1987) outlined the challenges facing the profession. The challenges have been reordered to group them together into those that must be addressed within (I [internal]) the profession and those that require interaction with external groups (E). There should be an increased focus on:

- Demonstrating accountability for occupational therapy services, including effectiveness and efficacy (I)
- Developing a scientific foundation regarding use of human occupation throughout the lifespan (I)
- Establishing new priorities to meet members' needs to respond to a consumer-driven health care environment supporting health promotion, disease prevention, and productive living (I)
- Decreasing dependence on the medical system for delivery of services as have been in the past: focus on becoming a health-related and human service profession (I)
- Continuing to focus on standards of practice, Code of Ethics, and the credentialing process (I)
- Improving public's awareness and understanding of occupational therapy services by reaching out to various publics with whom we work (E)
- Engaging in interprofessional collaboration with other health and human service organizations (E)
- Focusing on consumer collaboration to advocate for the rights of special populations (E)

EDUCATION

Number and Location of Educational Programs

The number of educational programs increased from 57 professional programs (including Puerto Rico) and 52 assistant-level programs in 1980 to 68 professional programs and 68 assistant programs (AOTA, 1980-1981, 1989a). Thirty-three states plus the District of Columbia and Puerto Rico had at least one professional level program operating within the state (AOTA, 1989a). Thirty states had an assistant-level program operating within the state. Western states composed the largest group of states with no occupational therapy education program within the state at either the professional or assistant level. Western states with no professional-level program included Alaska, Idaho, Montana, Wyoming, South Dakota, Nevada, Utah, Arizona, New Mexico, and Iowa. Eastern states included Kentucky, Mississippi, South Carolina, West Virginia, Vermont, Delaware, and Rhode Island. Figures 8-1 and 8-2 show the location of the professional- and technical-level programs.

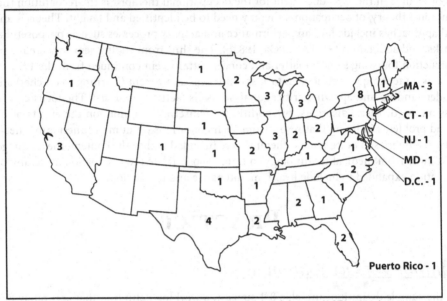

Figure 8-1. Location of professional education in occupational therapy (AOTA, 1989a).

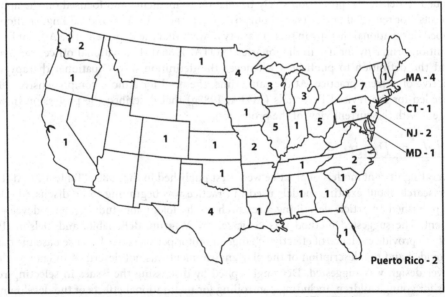

Figure 8-2. Location of occupational therapy assistant programs (AOTA, 1989a).

Essentials Revision

In 1983, the Essentials and Guidelines of an Accredited Education Program for the Occupational Therapists were revised for the fifth time the original document was developed in 1935 (AOTA, 1983a). Previous revisions since the original document was developed in 1935 were in 1943, 1949, 1965, and 1973. The Essentials and Guidelines of an Approved Educational Program for the Occupational Therapy Assistant were also revised for the fifth time since the original document was approved in 1958 (AOTA, 1983b). Previous revisions were in 1962, 1967, 1970, and 1975. A major change in the 1983 document for the occupational therapist is the recognition that theories, not just theory, of occupational therapy need to be identified and taught. Theories and theoretical approaches include human performance and activity processes such as purposeful activity, life tasks, and adaptation (AOTA, 1983a, 1983b). The shift from stating semester credits or hours of instruction to listing subject matter and concept attainment continued from the 1973 revision. The focus on techniques was less on task-specific skill attainment (learning to crochet) and more on understanding and applying critical analysis skills (activity analysis). The focus continued to be less on the diseases, disorders, or conditions themselves and more on the effects of dysfunction and problems in living that result from such conditions on human functioning, health, and society. As theories in occupational therapy were included within the content, the language began to shift away from medical terminology to terminology related to occupational therapy practice. Intervention expanded to include health maintenance and prevention.

PRACTICE

Definitions of Occupational Therapy

As the sample definitions in Table 8-1 suggest, a working definition that accurately described the current state of occupational therapy was inconsistent at best. Whereas the Association struggled to redefine the profession as focusing on health using a variety of media and methods, others continued to define the profession solely in relation to medicine and focused on the application of "objects" for remedial or diversional purposes (Kamenetz, 1983). Standard English dictionaries described occupational therapy in such a variety of ways that the Representative Assembly adopted a definition primarily for use in dictionaries (AOTA, 1986a). The national office was instructed to send the definition to publishers whenever the definition of occupational therapy was not descriptive of current practice. At the same time, the need for a more comprehensive definition was needed for the revised Essentials (AOTA, 1983g) that described the profession in wording consistent with the current view of the profession.

Models of Practice

Several significant models of practice were first published in the 1980s (Table 8-2). At the same time, research about existing models used in practice was beginning to be discussed. DeGangi (1983) published an article describing a research methodology for studying neurodevelopmental treatment. The suggested method was criticized by Magrun, deBenabib, and Nelson (1983) as unlikely to provide evidence of effective change in motor performance because baseline data were not provided and the description of the play environment was not described in enough detail. A crossover design was suggested. DeGangi replied by discussing the issues in selecting research designs for young children, including controlling for maturational effects of the developing child and selecting observations of motor performance that can be reliably observed for measurement (DeGangi, 1983).

Table 8-1 DEFINITIONS OF OCCUPATIONAL THERAPY IN THE 1980s	
1981	Occupational therapy is the use of purposeful activity with individuals who are limited by physical injury or illness, psychosocial dysfunction, developmental or learning disabilities, poverty and cultural differences or the aging process in order to maximize independence, prevent disability and maintain health, etc. (AJOT, 35(12) Resolution 572-81.)
1983	A system of medically prescribed activities, typically involving the use of objects to increase coordination, range of motion, power, and function, or for diagnostic, psychiatric, or other therapeutic purposes. (Kamenetz, H.L. (19783). Dictionary of rehabilitation medicine, p. 214. New York: Springer.)
1983	Occupational therapy is the art and science of directing man's participation in selected tasks to restore, reinforce and enhance performance, facilitate learning of those skills and functions essential for adaptation and productivity, diminish or correct pathology, and to promote and maintain health. Reference to occupation in the title is in the context of man's goal-directed use of time, energy, interest, and attention. Its fundamental concern is the development and maintenance of the capacity throughout the life span, to perform with satisfaction to self and others those task and roles essential to productive living and to the mastery of self and the environment. (Essentials and guidelines of an accredited educational program for the occupational therapist, AJOT, 1983, 37(12), 817-823.)
1984	Occupational therapy is a specialized health care service whose practitioners treat people who have physical, emotional and developmental disabilities. Occupational therapists and occupational therapy assistants help disabled people of all ages acquire or regain the skills they need to live independent, productive, and satisfying lives. (AJOT Calendar. The World of Occupational Therapy, 1984)
1986	Occupational therapy: Therapeutic use of self-care, work, and play activities to increase independent function, enhance development, and prevent disability. May include adaptation of task or environment to achieve maximum independence and to enhance quality of life. (AOTA Representative Assembly minutes, AJOT 40(12), 852)

Table 8-2 MODELS OF PRACTICE	
1980	Model of human occupation (Kielhofner et al.)
1981	Spatiotemporal adaptation (Gilfoyle & Grady)
1982	Ecological systems model (Howe & Briggs)
1985	Cognitive disability (Allen)
1988	Occupational form and occupational performance (Nelson)
1989	Occupational science (Yerxa et al.)

Blakeney, Strickland, and Wilkinson (1983) published an article on the use of sensory integrative techniques with adults diagnosed with schizophrenia. Rosenthal (1983) cautioned that other approaches may be as effective at improving adaptive responses such as improved posture and gait, decreased psychomotor retarding, and normalization of behavior in general. She stated that a diagnostic-prescriptive physical activity program could produce similar results and reminded the reader that sensory integration should not be used as a panacea.

Gary Kielhofner (Figure 8-3) and colleagues published a series of four articles presenting the Model of Human Occupation (MOHO) (Kielhofner, 1980a, 1980b; Kielhofner & Burke, 1980; Kielhofner, Burke, & Igi, 1980). Although Kielhofner was a

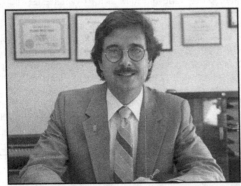

Figure 8-3. Gary Kielhofner, PhD, OTR. (Printed with permission from the Archive of the American Occupational Therapy Association, Inc.)

Table 8-3
PERSONALITIES

GARY WAYNE KIELHOFNER

February 15, 1949–September 2, 2010

Born in Oran, a small farming community in southeastern Missouri. He was the only boy with four sisters. He earned a degree in psychology from St. Louis University in 1974, a master's degree in occupational therapy from the University of Southern California in 1974, and a doctorate in public health from the University of California Los Angeles in 1980. He was a faculty member at Virginia Commonwealth University and Boston University before joining the faculty at the University of Illinois in Chicago in 1986 and becoming Head of the Department of Occupational Therapy, a job he held for 20 years. He was a Wade/Meyer Chair in Occupational Therapy. He learned about occupational therapy while working on a rehabilitation unit in a St. Louis hospital to fulfill the obligation for community service as a conscientious objector during the Vietnam War. In 1980, he and Janice Burke introduced a theoretical model called the Model of Human Occupation (MOHO), designed to fill a gap in understanding and address clients with psychosocial challenges in the rehabilitation process. The model provided a guide to assessment and a reasoning process to measure the impact of intervention. The model was originally published in four articles in AJOT and later in four book editions. The model became popular and was used widely across many countries. In addition to the model, he also published articles and books on research techniques and books on conceptual models used in occupational therapy. He was named to the Roster of Fellows in 1983 and to the Academy of Research in 1984.

(Braveman, B., Fisher, G., & Suerez-Balcazar, Y. (2010). "Achieving the ordinary things": A tribute to Gary Kielhofner. American Journal of Occupational Therapy, 64[6], 638-631.)

ELIZABETH JUNE YERXA

Born August 18, 1930

Born in Pasadena, California. She graduated from the University of Southern California with a bachelor's degree in occupational therapy in 1952. She earned a master's in 1967 and a doctorate in 1970 in education psychology from Boston University. She worked in the cerebral palsy unit of the Los Angeles Orthopedic Hospital and for the California Elks Association cerebral palsy mobile unit in Lancaster, California. She was employed as an instructor in occupational therapy at the University of Puget Sound in Tacoma, Washington. She worked for 15 years as an instructor, educational coordinator, and research coordinator in the Occupational Therapy Department of Rancho Los Amigos Hospital in Downey, California. She was professor and Chairperson, Department of Occupational Therapy, University of Southern California, from 1976 to 1988. She served as Chairman of the Committee on Student Affiliations; was a member of the Council on Education and the Developmental Advisory Committee; was a member-at-large of the Board of Management; and was Vice President of the Association. She presented the Eleanor Clarke Slagle lectureship in 1966 and was named to the Roster of Fellows in 1973 and the Academy of Research as a charter member in 1983. She was the second President of the AOTF in 1967.

(AJOT, 15(4), 174; 16(4), 210 and 22(2), 62. Photo AJOT, 1967, 21(5), 299)

CAROLYN MANVILLE BAUM

Born March 24, 1943

Born in Chicago, Illinois, and grew up in Winchester, Kansas. She graduated from Winchester High School in 1961. She received her bachelor's degree in occupational therapy from the University of Kansas in 1965, a master's degree in health management from Webster University in 1979, and a doctorate in social work from Washington University in St. Louis, Missouri, in 1993. She worked at the University of Kansas Medical Center and at the Research Medical Center in Kansas City until 1976, when she joined the faculty at Washington University School of Medicine as the Director of Occupational Therapy Clinical Services. In 1988, she was appointed Director of the Program in Occupational Therapy. She served as President twice: once in 1982-1983 to complete the term of office for Mae Hightower-Vandamm when the bylaws were changed from a 2-year term to a 3-year term, and then a full term from 2004-2007. She received the Eleanor Clarke Slagle lectureship in 1980 and was named to the Roster of Fellows in 1975. She received the Award of Merit in 1984. She is also a member of the AOTF Academy of Research. She has co-authored several textbooks with Charles Christiansen.

(continued)

Table 8-3 (continued)
PERSONALITIES

ROBERT KENDALL BING

March 2, 1929–May 15, 2003

Born in Cambridge, Nebraska. He graduated from Central High School in Cape Girardeau, Missouri, in 1947. He attended college at Southeast Missouri State University and received a degree in occupational therapy at the University of Illinois under Beatrice Wade. He served as President from 1983-1986 and was named to the Roster of Fellows in 1973. He earned his Master of Arts degree at the Institute for Child Study at the University of Maryland College Park in 1954 and his Doctor of Education degree from the University of Maryland in 1961. His doctoral dissertation was a study of the life of William Rush Dunton, Jr., with whom he lived for several years. He joined the U.S. Army Medical Service and worked at Fitzsimmons Army Medical Center in Denver. He taught on the faculty at Richmond Professional Institute, University of Florida, and University of Illinois at Chicago, where he was also Director of Activity Therapy at the Illinois State Psychiatric Institute. He was Dean of the first school of Allied Health Sciences in the Southwestern states at the University of Texas Medical Branch in Galveston from 1968 to 1980 and was later awarded the title of Professor and Dean Emeritus. He taught briefly at Elizabethtown College in Pennsylvania but remained active as Visiting Professor, Occupational Therapy, University of South Dakota for several years. He was awarded the Eleanor Clarke Slagle lectureship in 1981, received the Award of Merit in 1987, and was named a charter member of the Roster of Fellows in 1973. He was recognized for his knowledge in the history of health, social welfare, and occupational therapy. In 1999, he established the Bing Scholar scholarship program. He was a member of Phi Kappa Pi honorary fraternity.

ELNORA MAE CLAUSING GILFOYLE

Born May 19, 1934

Born in Tennessee. She graduated from the University of Iowa program in occupational therapy. She served as President and Secretary of the Association. She received the Eleanor Clarke Slagle lectureship in 1984 and was named a charter member of the Roster of Fellows in 1973. She received the Award of Merit in 1991. She worked at the University of Colorado Health Sciences Center and then taught at Colorado State University. She served as Dean of the College of Applied Human Sciences at Colorado State University and as Provost and Academic Vice President of Colorado State University. She was inducted into the Colorado Women's Hall of Fame in 1994. She was interested in leadership and creative partnerships and established the Institute for Women and Leadership at Colorado State University in 1995. With Ann P. Grady and Josephine C. Moore, she authored two editions of Children Adapt: A Theory of Sensorimotor Development. She also wrote Mentoring Leaders with Ann Grady and Cathy Nielson.

student of Mary Reilly at the University of Southern California, MOHO would not be viewed as a successor to her model of occupational behavior but as a new approach that Kielhofner hoped would act as a unifying theory for the profession. A short biographic sketch appears in Table 8-3.

Yerxa (Figure 8-4) and colleagues at the University of Southern California published a model called occupational science in 1989, which was designed to support the academic discipline in the university setting by organizing the academic subjects and their relationship to the education of practitioners in occupational therapy (Yerxa et al., 1989) (see Table 8-3).

Problems in Practice

The Education for All Handicapped Children Act of 1975 was implemented in 1978. Many opportunities for occupational therapy practitioners became available. However, some school officials stated that occupational therapy constituted "medical" treatment and therefore was not a responsibility of the school. Some therapists were instructed to bill the

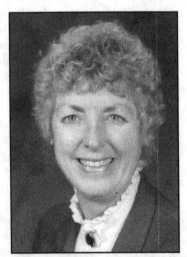

Figure 8-4. Elizabeth J. Yerxa, EdD, OTR. (Printed with permission from the Archive of the American Occupational Therapy Association, Inc.)

family's medical insurer (Hightower-Vandamm, 1980a, p. 308). Still other school officials wanted a prescription or referral from a physician for occupational therapy services, reinforcing the concept of occupational therapy as a medical intervention. As Hightower-Vandamm cautioned, practice in the school systems must support the education of the disabled child, and practitioners must demonstrate that occupational therapy can support educational objectives or the role of occupational therapy in the schools might decrease.

Teachers and educators also had mixed reactions to occupational therapy practitioners entering the schools (Hightower-Vandamm, 1980a, p. 309). Some teachers welcomed the added help in identifying and addressing learning and behavior problems in the classroom, whereas others did not think anyone but a teacher should be managing learning and behavior in the classroom. Teachers who thought occupational therapy practitioners were going to "take over" the classroom and its students and tell the teachers what to do were likely to resent any evaluation or intervention by occupational therapy practitioners. In some cases, occupational therapy practitioners were welcomed only if they acted as consultants or in-service instructors but did not actually see, talk to, or touch a child.

At the same time, physicians were beginning to doubt and question the value of occupational therapy for children with sensory integrative problems. Issues included the lack of recognition by physicians that a sensory integration problem existed because physicians were not trained to evaluate such dysfunction, lack of understanding of the potential relationship between sensory function and learning, and resistance or reluctance to refer or give up some control to occupational therapy practitioners because the physician did not believe in treatment effectiveness for sensory integrative dysfunction (Hightower-Vandamm, 1980a, p. 308).

Another problem area was vocational and work-related evaluation. Although occupational therapists had been active in evaluating potential for work and vocational training for many years, as Hightower-Vandamm (1980a, p. 309) pointed out, the area of practice was increasingly being lost to occupational therapy practitioners. Vocational evaluation was being performed by specialists with a master's degree in vocational evaluation. The tools developed by occupational therapists many years ago in psychiatric hospitals were now being used by persons trained in another discipline.

Another area of practice that developed during the 1980s was that of facilitating independent living because of the 1978 amendments to the Rehabilitation Act of 1973 that provided clients with services for independent living even if no vocational goal was defined (Hightower-Vandamm, 1980a, p. 309). Occupational therapy practitioners needed to understand that the goal of independent living was to move the person out of institutional settings such as state hospitals or nursing homes. The goal was NOT to enable them to live alone, by themselves, without anyone else in the household. For some clients, living alone may be the best solution, but for others, having a roommate or caregiver or both may be the best arrangement. The focus was on noninstitutional living, not living "all by myself."

Perhaps most significant was the change from large general hospitals to a variety of settings, often in the community. Tables 8-5A and 8-5B show the trend away from institutions and in-patient settings to community and outpatient settings.

Manpower

According to statistics reported by the American Hospital Association (AHA) in 1980, of the 6,965 registered hospitals in the United States, 31.1% (2,167) employed occupational therapists and 18.8% (1,307) employed occupational therapy assistants or aides (AHA, 1980). Unfortunately, the survey did not differentiate between assistants and aides. Among hospitals employing occupational therapists, 21.9% had vacant positions and 11.5% had vacant positions for assistants or aides. Among hospital-based therapists, 6,882 worked full-time and 10,367 worked part-time. Among assistants and aides, 4,024 worked full-time and 454 worked part-time (AOTA, 1982a).

From 1981 to 1987, the percentage of hospitals with occupational therapy services increased over the country from 41.8% to 49%. The New England states had the highest percentage at 74.7%, whereas the East South Central states had the lowest at 25.5%. Hawaii has the highest percent at 95.5%, whereas Mississippi had the lowest at 14.3% (AHA, 1988). In 1982, the states with the largest percentage increase in occupational therapists from 1972 to 1982 were Louisiana (445%), Wyoming (418%), South Carolina (382%), Oklahoma (343%), and Utah (300%). States with the largest number of occupational therapists were California (3,442), New York (2,318), Michigan (1,531), Massachusetts (1,310), and Texas (1,288). States with the largest number of certified occupational therapy assistants were New York (962), Minnesota (701), Wisconsin (554), California (394), and Massachusetts (346).

Manpower Study

According to Acquaviva and Presseller (1983), nearly 40% of hospitals and about 30% of nursing homes and home health agencies had occupational therapy services. These percentages are slightly higher than those reported in data prepared by the AHA. The number of therapists per population varied from 1 per 4,000 in New Hampshire to 1 per 59,000 in Mississippi. At the same time, the growth of the professional education slowed substantially. Only 1,900 to 2,000 students were graduating per year from 1975 to 1981. Faculty members stayed steady at about 520. The number of qualified applicants declined. Some educational programs were not filling all available positions.

Langwell, Wilson, and Deane (1981) reported that approximately 56% of counties in the United States had no registered occupational therapists working in those counties. The authors stated that, based on the analysis of the data available, occupational therapists worked primarily in facilities such as hospital departments, rehabilitation centers, nursing homes, or psychiatric inpatient facilities. Therefore, employment patterns depended on the location of such facilities. In addition, the distribution of occupational therapists was associated with per capita income of the population. Counties with higher per capita incomes were more likely to have several occupational therapists working in them and to have more facilities with occupational therapy departments. Client ability to pay for services was suggested as a major factor. Thus, job opportunities were more likely to be available in counties with higher per capita income and more health care facilities. Conversely, counties with lower per capita incomes tended to have fewer facilities for health care services, no or limited occupational therapy services, lack or limited payment for occupational therapy services, and few opportunities for employment in occupational therapy service programs.

Recommendations of the Manpower Study (Masagatani, 1985) were the following:

- Increase the numbers of occupational therapy personnel
- Encourage the expansion of the occupational therapy education system
- Expand Association activities aimed at recruiting more students for occupational therapy programs
- Increase the number of qualified occupational therapy faculty members
- Monitor the number and characteristics of the pool of field work centers
- Modify the credentialing politics to facilitate the movement of additional personnel into the U.S. workforce
- Modify the characteristics of occupational therapy personnel to most effectively meet the needs of the population and changing service delivery patterns
- Expand the Association's efforts in continuing education
- Encourage the occupational therapy educational system to prepare graduates to practice in new service delivery environments
- Review and document the current behavior of the health care system and its potential effect on the number and characteristics of occupational therapy personnel as part of the Association's annual planning process

- Increase research and promotional activities aimed at expanding the availability of occupational therapy services to meet the needs of persons presently unserved or underserved
- Produce valid information on the efficacy and cost of occupational therapy treatment that can be used in promoting the development or expansion of services
- Focus promotion efforts on the most rapidly growing components of health care delivery
- Take a more active role in enhancing the public and professional awareness of the issues involved in meeting the needs of minorities

Recommendations from the Manpower Study were summarized into the following three main statements with several subtopics:

- Increase the number of occupational therapy personnel to meet population needs and unmet demands through such means as increasing the number of educational programs, recruiting more students, increasing the number of qualified faculty, monitoring the characteristics of field work sites, and modifying credentialing mechanisms
- Modify the characteristics of occupational therapy personnel to most effectively meet population needs and changing service delivery patterns through such means as expanding continuing education offerings, engaging educational programs to prepare graduate to practice in new service delivery environments, and reviewing changes in the health care system for potential effect on occupational therapy
- Increase research and promotional activities aimed at expanding the availability of occupational therapy services to meet the needs of persons presently unserved or underserved through such means as producing valid information of the efficacy of occupational therapy treatment, focusing on the most rapidly growing components of the health care delivery system, and enhancing public and profession awareness of issued involved in meeting the needs of minorities (Masagatani, 1985)

Work Settings

A survey of new graduates in 1989 showed that entry-level occupational therapists were working primarily in hospital settings (64%), followed by school systems (12%), nursing homes (5%), and other (19%). Entry-level occupational therapy assistants were also employed primarily in hospitals (34%), followed by school systems (19%), nursing homes (18%), and other (29%). Other work settings included community mental health centers, outpatient clinics, residential care facilities, and sheltered workshops (Silvergleit, 1990).

The membership survey in 1986 provides a more comprehensive list but does not separate occupational therapists from assistants (Table 8-4). Hospitals and school systems are the major work sites by category, but nearly 38% of practitioners were working in settings not on the lists.

Table 8-4
1986 MEMBER DATA SURVEY: WORK SETTING

Setting	Percentage
General hospitals	22%
School systems	17%
Rehabilitation centers	10.5%
Psychiatric settings	6.9%
Rehabilitation units	4.2%
Pediatrics	1.7%
Other[a]	37.7%

[a]Includes sheltered workshops, home health care, skilled nursing facilities, senior centers, early intervention programs, and others.

De-emphasis on Crafts

The de-emphasis on crafts is documented beginning in 1951, when an editorial appeared in AJOT suggesting that practitioners should not discuss treatment media but treatment results. The suggestion was the following:

Pick two or three interesting work products and explain the results of the work in relation to the case treated. Did the patient get the desired muscle recovery through that one activity or was another necessary to supplement the treatment, what effect on the patient's personality was evidenced by the activity? In other words, the practitioner should express the work as a treatment medium in which you cooperated with the physician for a desired result. (Editorial, 1951, p. 39)

To rephrase, the outcome should be stressed more than the medium or technique used to obtain the desired results.

The concern about the role of crafts in occupational therapy practice increased during the 1980s. In a letter to the editor, Walker et al. (1982) stated that they "believe that the strong use of craft activities seriously weakens our professional credibility" (p. 48). Craft activities were not seen as real treatment media in medical settings. They further stated that "efficiency and cost effectiveness dictate a sharp reduction in use of crafts, with substitution of activities that lend themselves to reliable standardization" and that a return to a crafts emphasis would be impractical (p. 48). In other words, craft activities were not viewed as being subject to critical measurement using the same standards, such as of range of motion in degrees, muscle strength in pounds per square inch of pressure, or endurance in minutes or hours of exercise or work activity. They summarize their argument by stating that "it is enough of a dilemma for the practitioner to convince the patient, physician, and administration of the credibility of occupational therapy as a medically oriented discipline, rather than as a traditional diversional orientation, without feeling that the AOTA is divided on the scope of our practice" (p. 49). They wanted the Association to support the practice of therapy "as a well-defined treatment to improve patients' daily life skills," rather than encouraging what they believed to be a regressive step toward crafts therapy (p. 49). Clearly, craft activities were seen as lacking in the production of defined results that would be acceptable to medical consumers, practitioners, payers, and administrators. In the authors' view, crafts were diversional in nature without redeeming qualities in reducing identified pathological conditions or facilitating activities of daily living.

The reaction against crafts may have been in part the result of lack of education or lack of learning objectives presented in lecture, laboratory, or fieldwork education. In a letter to the editor, Clopton (1981) states that she was "expected to be an expert on the therapeutic aspects of crafts without knowing why they were therapeutic unless it was to divert the mind from facing one's problems" (p. 669). The therapeutic value of crafts had been published in articles in Occupational Therapy and Rehabilitation. The Committee on Installations and Advice (1928, 1929) published a series of reports on the analysis of 12 crafts, including instructions on analyzing craft activities. In his chapters on prescription, Dunton (1950, 1957) included a section on the use of crafts in function restoration and examples of analysis. However, other textbooks on occupational therapy published after 1929 did not include the information on analysis of crafts the Committee used or examples of analyses.

Clopton (1981) also stated that when she returned to get additional education after raising a family, the "new therapeutic techniques involving reflexes and development, as well as an expanded view of neurology and perception, would make a return to the use of crafts as an exclusion occupational therapy treatment medium prohibitive" (p. 669). The implication was that crafts were the only medium or modality used in occupational therapy practice, a fact that may have been true in some but not all practice settings.

In 1979, Eliason and Gohl-Giese did a survey of the use of media and modalities used in occupational therapy. There were 76 replies from therapists working in physical dysfunction and 45 from those working in psychiatry. The media or modalities used by at least 90% or more of respondents in psychiatric facilities were needlework, leatherwork, copper tooling, woodworking, tile work, macramé, ceramics, sewing, and task groups. In facilities identified as specializing in treating clients with physical dysfunction, the media and modality used by at least 90% or higher of respondents were focusing on activities of daily living, passive range of motion, active range of motion activities, active range of motion without activity, resistive exercise with activity, facilitation/inhibition (not qualified), facilitation/inhibition techniques with activity, homemaking training, and built-up tool handles. There was no overlap among the highest use media and modalities. Psychiatric settings used crafts activities, whereas physical dysfunction settings used exercise, facilitation or inhibition techniques, modified tools, activities of daily living, and homemaking. It is possible that the some built-up tool handles were used to facilitate craft activities, but such data were not reported in the study.

In a survey by Bissell and Mailloux (1981), respondents stated eight reasons why crafts were not used in physical disabilities or physical dysfunction programs:

- Prefer treatment techniques that can be more precisely documented
- The use of crafts is difficult to justify to patient, to the therapist, insurance company, doctors, other treatment team members and patient's family
- It is difficult to document the use of crafts (assume in some measureable unit)
- Lack of sufficient space for craft use
- Crafts give occupational therapists a poor image
- Use of crafts is insulting to the patient
- Lack of sufficient budget for craft use
- Lack of sufficient staff for craft use

However, in the same survey, respondents identified eight objectives to which craft activities could contribute:

- Improve fine-motor control
- Improve strength
- Enhance cognitive development
- Promote interests
- Improve self-esteem
- Improve decision-making capabilities
- Promote group socialization
- Facilitate prevocational training

Treatment techniques used instead of crafts included therapeutic exercise, self-care, neurodevelopment technique, home skills, role performance skills, and prevocational training without use of crafts (Bissell & Mailloux, 1981). The authors raised concerns about the use of some of the techniques, stating that other team members could address problems in strengthening and self-care, the most commonly used techniques, but there was a questions about who would address home skills, role performance skills, and prevocational training. The authors concluded that as scientific advancements and medical treatment progressed, changes occurred that emphasized a focus on use of treatment modalities that appeared more precise and were therefore substituted for craft activities. The nature of the precision appeared to move toward some idea of quantification that counting stitches, rows completed, or time spent doing a craft activity could not satisfy. The authors also suggested that "perhaps more theory should be included in the crafts skills classes in order to provide the therapists with a clearer understanding of the purposes and dimensions of craft activity" (Bissell & Mailloux, 1981, p. 374). This article was the last article on crafts to appear in the professional journal.

Drake (1992) adds another reasons for de-emphasizing crafts, stating that "in a work-oriented culture like ours, crafts have come to symbolize a leisure time activity rather than real work" (p. 3). However, she also states that "crafts are a microcosm of life." Crafts can teach many of the tools and techniques for everyday living and how to put them all together. The concept of teaching tasks and activities related to daily living makes crafts valuable therapeutic media for the modern clinical setting.

Rise of Physical Agent Modalities

In 1982, Trombly used the term adjunctive treatment to describe the use of splinting, electrical stimulation splints, exercise, biofeedback, and sensory stimulation "to enable development of motor ability needed to engage in tasks of daily life" (p. 467). Her point was that interpretations of the term purposeful activity were "limited with regard to control of parameters of gradation needed to effect an improvement in strength, range of motion, or motor control" (p. 467). She felt AOTA should legitimize the use of techniques that did not fit the definition of purposeful activity.

English, Kasch, Silverman, and Walker (1982) used the term *adjuncts* in discussing the use of "range of motion, therapeutic exercise, muscle strengthening and splinting for corrective, preventive and functional purposes" (p. 199). The authors argued that the focus on purposeful activities denied the additional skills of the restorative areas of physical disabilities practice.

Pedretti and Pasquinelli-Estrada (1985) summarized the restrictions that purposeful activity would place on practice in physical disabilities as (1) jeopardizing reimbursement, (2) negating the skills and knowledge achieved by experienced clinicians, (3) jeopardizing referrals, and (4) excluding techniques such as exercise, range of motion, splinting, and inhibition-facilitation techniques (p. 7). They concluded that the issues stemmed from an unclear or unacceptable definition of purposeful activity that excluded exercise.

Initially in 1983, the Representative Assembly adopted a policy on modalities in general (AOTA, 1983c). The Policy defines modalities as "the employment of or the method of employment of, a therapeutic agent" (p. 816). Qualifications and competencies were to be obtained through accredited education programs, specific certifications, or experience. In 1991, the policy adopted in 1983 was expanded to include the concept of using physical agent modalities, although the term physical agent modalities does not appear in the policy (AOTA, 1991). In essence, the policy states that therapists and assistants are qualified and competent to use a variety of modalities, that modalities should be used only in preparation for purposeful activity to enhance occupational performance, and that practitioners should only use modalities for which qualifications and competencies have been obtained. However, the Representative Assembly did adopt a separation motion stating "physical agent modalities may be used by occupational therapy practitioners when used as an adjunct to or in preparation for purposeful activity to enhance occupational performance and when applied by a practitioners who has documented evidence of possessing the theoretical background and technical skills for safe and competent integration of the modality into an occupational therapy intervention plan" (AOTA, 1991). The statement and the policy were to be issued together.

LEGISLATION

Legislation affecting occupational therapy is listed in Table 8-5. A few government actions deserve special mention. In 1988, the Health Care Financing Administration issued Medicare Part B medical review guidelines, which clarified occupational therapy documentation requirements (AOTA, 1988) (Table 8-6). The Veterans' Administration Bill 1989 revised standards for occupational therapy (Boyer, 1990). Two amendments to the Education of the Handicapped Act (EHA) included:

- P.L. 98-199, Education of the Handicapped Act Amendments (1983). Promoted transitional services for handicapped youth to assist in moving from public school to vocational training and competitive employment. Also encouraged states to provide services to all preschool children from birth.
- P.L. 99-457, Education of the Handicapped Act Amendments (1986). The Act spelled out related services including occupational therapy and extended special education and related services to preschoolers and handicaps, 3 through 5 years. Emphasized an early intervention

Table 8-5
LEGISLATION RELEVANT TO OCCUPATIONAL THERAPY

1980	Omnibus Reconciliation Act of 1980 (P.L. 96-1479). Lindy Boggs helped get Congress to pass a bill that would cover occupational therapy in rehabilitation facilities and independent of physical therapy and speech services in home health. The Act included outpatient rehabilitation facility and home health provisions. (a) Home health amendment: If a physician certifies that a person is homebound and an overall health care plan is established, occupational therapy services alone could qualify for Medicare. (b) Comprehensive outpatient rehabilitation facility provision: Occupational therapy covered in free-standing outpatient clinics that meet requirements. (Mallon, 1981; Reed, 1992)
1980	Social Security Amendments (P.L. 96-265). Act funded demonstration projects for developmentally disabled persons that would allow them to continue to keep Social Security benefits while working (Reed, 1992).
1981	Budget Reconciliation Act (P.L. 97-35). Removed occupational therapy as a qualifying service from home health. As a result, nursing, speech therapy, and or physical therapy must qualify the patient for skilled care before occupational therapy services can be provided (Lohman, 2014).
1982	Social Security Amendments (Katie Beckett Amendment; P.L. 97-248). Allowed disabled children to live at home and receive services. They no longer were required to live in an institution (Reed, 1992).
1982	Comprehensive Outpatient Rehabilitation Facility (CORF) Regulations. COPFs were deemed the only locations where mental health services would be covered by Medicare Part B by non-physician health professionals such as occupational therapists (Peters, 1984).
1982	Tax Equality and Fiscal Responsibility Act (P.L. 97-248). Hospice benefits were enacted on a temporary basis. Occupational Therapists started working in hospice (Lohman, 2014).
1983	Education of the Handicapped Amendment (P.L. 98-199). Facilitates transition from school to work. Established state planning grants. Preschool grants now include birth to age 5 (Reed, 1992).
1984	Developmental Disabilities Act Amendments (P.L. 98-527). Independence, integration, employment, and employment-related activities were addressed. Supported deinstitutionalization and integration into the community (Reed, 1992).
1984	Carl D. Perkins Vocational Act (P.L. 98-210). 10% is allocated for vocational education for people with disabilities (Reed, 1992).
1985	Consolidated Omnibus Budget Reconciliation Act (COBRA; P.L. 99-272). Passed to help people who are at risk for being uninsured if they change employment or have been laid off from their jobs. Hospice benefits became permanent, and occupational therapists continued to work in hospice (Lohman, 2014).
1986	Rehabilitation Act Amendments (P.L. 99-506). Act addressed employability, supportive employment, and rehabilitation engineering (Reed, 1992).
1986	Education of the Handicapped Act (P.L. 99-457). Early intervention services for children 3-5 years. Occupational therapy is a primary service. It was independent of medical, health, or other special education services (Reed, 1992; Van Slyke, 2001).
1986	Handicapped Children's Protection Act (P.L. 99-372). Parents can recover attorney fee costs if parents are the prevailing party (Reed, 1992).
1987	Developmental Disabilities Assistance and Bill of Rights Amendments (P.L. 100-146). Developmentally disabled persons receive necessary services. Monitoring system established. Supported training projects to provide services in early intervention. Effort to help people with disabilities to reach their maximum potential (Reed, 1992).
1988	Technology-Related Assistance for Individuals with Disabilities Act (P.L. 100-407). Provide funding to states to develop and distribute assistive devices and modification options allowing people with disabilities to use the services provided as a result of ADA. Assistive technology has "made it feasible to implement many provisions of ADA" (Reed, 1992; Van Slyke, 2001).

(continued)

Table 8-5 (continued)
LEGISLATION RELEVANT TO OCCUPATIONAL THERAPY

1988	Medicare Catastrophic Coverage Act (P.L. 100-360). Improve acute care benefits for the disabled and elderly. Expanding benefits to include drug coverage and limit copayments for services that were covered (Reed, 1992).
1988	Fair Housing Amendments (P.L. 100-420). Clarifies civil rights of the disabled in the arena of housing (Reed, 1992).
1988	Civil Rights Restoration Act (P.L. 100-259). Those receiving federal funds have to comply with civil rights laws in all areas, not just in the activity/area that received funding (Van Slyke, 2001).

References

Lohman, H. (2014). Payment for services in the United States. In B. A. Boyt Schell, G. Gillen, & M. E. Scaffa (Eds.), *Willard & Spackman's occupational therapy* (12th ed., pp. 1051-1067). Philadelphia, PA: Wolters Kluwer.

Mallon, F. J. (1981). History of the occupational therapy Medicare amendments. *American Journal of Occupational Therapy, 35*(4), 231-235.

Peters, M. E. (1984). Reimbursement for psychiatric occupational therapy services. *American Journal of Occupational Therapy, 38*(5), 307-312.

Reed, K. L. (1992). History of federal legislation for persons with disabilities. *American Journal of Occupational Therapy, 46*(5), 397-408.

Van Slyke, N. (2001). Legislation and policy issues. In M. Scaffa (Ed.), *Occupational therapy in community-based practice settings* (pp. 85-94). Philadelphia, PA: Davis.

Table 8-6
MEDICARE COVERAGE

PART A
<ul><li>Hospital inpatient: Occupational therapy is a covered service.</li><li>Skilled Nursing Facility: Under Part 1, occupational therapy services are reimbursed to Medicare. However, when Part A coverage is exhausted, and the person is transferred to Part B, occupational therapy services are no longer reimbursable.</li><li>Home Health Care: Medicare beneficiaries may continue to receive occupational therapy services under the home health benefit even after their need for skilled nursing, physical therapy or speech therapy ends. However, the need for occupational therapy service alone will not qualify the person for Medicare home health services.</li><li>Hospice Care: occupational therapy is covered when provided to patients receiving hospice care.</li></ul>

PART B
<ul><li>Home Health Settings: Medicare beneficiaries may continue to receive occupational therapy services under Medicare Part B even after the need for skilled nursing, physical therapy, or speech therapy ends. However, the need for occupational therapy services alone will not qualify the person for Medicare home health services.</li><li>Hospital Outpatient: In order for occupational therapy to be reimbursed for services provided to outpatients, all of the following requirements must be met.<ul><li>Service must have physician referral.</li><li>Services rendered must be by hospital personnel in the hospital or outside the hospital.</li><li>Services provided must be under the direct personal supervision of the physician who is treating the patient.</li></ul></li><li>Incident to Physician Services: Reimbursable occupational therapy service incident to physician services must meet all the following requirements:<ul><li>Service must be provided in a private physician's office or in a physician-directed clinic, and the occupational therapist must be employed full- or part-time by the physician or clinic.</li><li>Services rendered must be under the direct personal supervision of the physician, assisting the physician in the performance f his or her professional services.</li><li>Services must be directly related to the condition the physician is treating.</li><li>The physician must include in the bill the charge for occupational therapy services.</li></ul></li><li>Comprehensive Outpatient Rehabilitation Facility</li></ul>

program for handicapped infants (0 through 2 years) identifying occupational therapy as a primary early intervention service. (New law provides occupational therapy for preschoolers. AOTA, 1986b)

Revisiting the Reconstruction Aides

On July 1, 1981, the Secretary of Defense issued a memorandum stating that reconstruction aides and dieticians who served during World War I would be considered active military service personnel in the Armed Forces of the United States for purposes of all laws and services administered by the Veterans' Administration and therefore were entitled to benefits administered by the Veterans' Administration. Prior to 1981, reconstruction aides and dieticians did not qualify for veterans' benefits, including health care, because they were not technically considered to be to veterans. However, in 1978, Public Law 95-202 was enacted to allow the reconstruction aides to apply for benefits. The reason they could not previously receive benefits as military personnel was because they were women and women were not allowed to serve in the military. During World War I, the reconstruction aides had served as civilian personnel because there were no statutory provisions for women in the military, although they were required to follow, and were subject to, Army regulations. When the rules were changed to allow women to serve in the military, the retroactive status was possible.

In 1944, full military status was conferred on physical therapists and dieticians but not on occupational therapists. In 1947, the Women's Medical Specialist Corp was formed (now the Army Medical Specialist Corps). In 1981, the Department of Defense Civilian/Military Service Review Board (created by Public Law 95-202) concluded that absent the congressional restrictions against women serving in the military, the reconstruction aides and dieticians in World War I would have been considered members of the Army and would have been entitled to veterans' benefits following discharge from the service. Therefore, they were now retroactively entitled because women were now allowed to serve in the military. However, to receive veterans' benefits, reconstruction aides had to apply for and receive a discharge from the Army. Because the national records for the reconstruction aides had been destroyed in a fire in 1949, each individual aide had to supply her own records after securing the necessary forms from the local Veterans' Administration office. A more significant problem was likely that many of the reconstruction aides were well into their 80s or 90s or had already died—and, besides, where were those call to duty papers from 1918 and discharge papers from 1919 anyway? Figure 8-5 shows Lena Hitchcock at age 93, one of the few living reconstruction aides able to take advantage of the legislation.

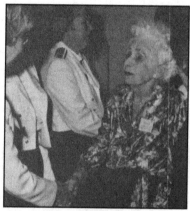

Figure 8-5. Lena Hitchcock, age 93, World War I reconstruction aide at the 35th anniversary celebration of the Army Medical Specialist Corps at the Fort McNair Officer's Club, Washington, DC, April 16, 1982. (Printed with permission from the Archive of the American Occupational Therapy Association, Inc.)

TECHNOLOGY

The Apple computer became standard equipment in many occupational therapy services (Figure 8-6). Innovations in hardware (add-on boards) and creative software programs provided opportunities to supplement other intervention programs such as perceptual motor tasks or to teach basic computer skills such as moving the mouse and clicking on a desired icon or using a simple word processing program. Other electronic devices such as electronic switches to operate battery-powered toys or robotic arms (Figure 8-7) became part of the changing technology.

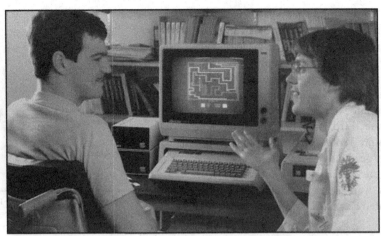

Figure 8-6. Use of an Apple computer with a client who has a head injury to assist in regaining attention, concentration, memory, and organizational skills. (Printed with permission from the Archive of the American Occupational Therapy Association, Inc.)

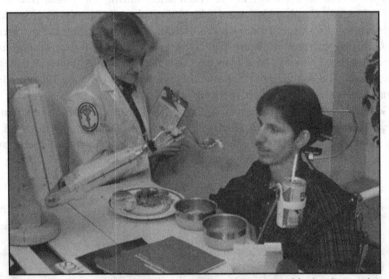

Figure 8-7. Robotic arm designed as an assistive device to enable the client with a spinal cord injury to feed himself. (Printed with permission from the Archive of the American Occupational Therapy Association, Inc.)

Assistive technology became a recognized part of occupational therapy practice. Continuing education courses were offered as the annual conference and manuals became available (Wright & Nomura, 1985).

ASSOCIATION

Headquarters

In 1980, the Association moved the national office from 6000 Executive Boulevard to 1383 Piccard Drive in Rockville, Maryland, where it would remain for 14 years. The building represented the first time the Association owned the structure in which it operated and functioned

(Figure 8-8). Previous office space had always been rented. The Association actually bought two buildings. One was a two-story building that was initially rented out and then sold. The other, a three-story structure, was the main headquarters. Initially, the Association was located on the third floor and the first two floors were rented to other organizations, but gradually Association and Foundation business increased so that all three floors were serving occupational therapy–related activities.

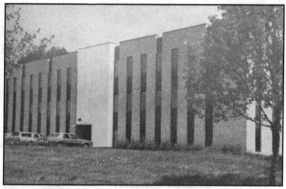

Figure 8-8. The national office from 1980 to 1994, located at 1383 Piccard Drive, Rockville, Maryland. (Printed with permission from the Archive of the American Occupational Therapy Association, Inc.)

Presidents and Executive Directors

Four people served as President of the Association during the 1980s: Mae D. Hightower-Vandamm (1978-1982), Carolyn M. Baum (1982-1983), Robert K. Bing (1983-1986), and Elnora M. Gilfoyle (1986-1989). Presidents Hightower-Vandamm, Baum, and Bing are pictured together in Figure 8-9. Gilfoyle is pictured in Figure 8-10. Table 8-7 is a review of their accomplishments during their presidencies. The long-range plan for the 1980s is listed in Table 8-8, and specific goals for 1987 are listed in Table 8-9. Important documents adopted during the 1980s are listed in Table 8-10, and publications and projects are listed in Table 8-11.

James Garibaldi continued to serve as Executive Director until his retirement in 1987. Occupational therapist Jeanette Bair (Figure 8-11) became Executive Director of AOTA after 16 years of non-therapist leadership. She would be the last occupational therapist to lead the Association in the first 100 years of its existence.

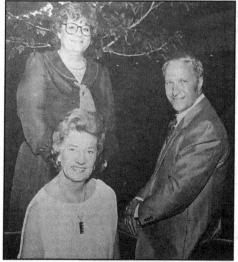

Figure 8-9. Past, present, and future Presidents in 1982: Mae Hightower-Vandamm, 1978-1982 (seated); Carolyn M. Baum, 1982-1983 (standing); and Robert K. Bing, 1983-1986. (Printed with permission from the Archive of the American Occupational Therapy Association, Inc.)

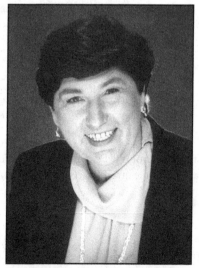

Figure 8-10. Elnora M. Gilfoyle, ScD (Hon), OTR, FAOTA, President of AOTA, 1986-1989. (Printed with permission from the Archive of the American Occupational Therapy Association, Inc.)

Table 8-7
PRESIDENTS AND THEIR ACCOMPLISHMENTS

Carolyn M. Baum, 1982-1983

Major accomplishment: She "led the transition from long-range planning to strategic planning focusing on targeted use of resources and anticipation of changing environments."

Quotation: "Our professional forebears have laid the groundwork to enable us to make an important contribution and now we need to take up that challenge and move forward."

Robert K. Bing, 1983-1986

Major accomplishment: The proposal to create the American Occupational Therapy Certification Board was adopted by the Representative Assembly.

Quotatuion: "In a world gone mad with technology, occupational therapy tenaciously clings to and advocates an immutable belief held by our professional forebears. I think of it as the poetry of the commonplace. Through work and play, the human spirit will prevail, succeed, and prolong itself in spite of biological, social, or emotional adversities."

Elnora M. Gilfoyle, 1986-1989

Major accomplishments: Promoting the concept of creative partnerships, facilitating new national office management structure, and the initial efforts to purchase *OT Week* to increase non-fee revenues.

(AOTA. (1992). AOTA's Hall of leaders. OT Week, 6(21), 40-43.)

Table 8-8
LONG-RANGE PLAN

- To provide opportunities for the expression of member concerns, to anticipate emerging issues, to facilitate decision making and to expedite the translation of those decisions into action
- To support the development of research and knowledge bases for the practice of occupational therapy, and to promote the dissemination and sharing of such information
- To facilitate and support an educational system for occupational therapy which responds to current needs, anticipates, plans for, and accommodates to change
- To promote occupational therapy as viable health profession
- To facilitate the formation of partnerships with consumers to promote optimal health conditions for the public

(August, 1980, Membership Handbook, A-3-A-4)

Table 8-9
GOALS LISTED FOR 1987

- Providing critical information resources through Association publications
- Offering new and innovative continuing education resources
- Promoting leadership in practice and quality assurance
- Representing members in key legislative and policy areas
- Providing new and streamlined service and benefit programs
- Establishing a teamwork approach to leadership and management

(Occupational Therapy News, 1987, 41(9), 16.)

Table 8-10 ASSOCIATION DOCUMENTS	
1980	• Certification Requirements • Long-Range Plan • Principles of Occupational Therapy Ethics, revised • Standards of Practice: Schools • Statement of Occupational Therapy Referral, revised
1981	• Entry-Level Role Delineation for OTRs and COTAs • Guidelines for Supervision of Occupational Therapy Personnel • Occupational Therapy as an Education-Related Service. Also called The Role of Occupational Therapy as an Education-Related Service • Occupational Therapy's Role in Independent or Alternative Living Situations • The Role of the Occupational Therapist in Home Health Care
1982	• Bylaws Revision of the AOTA • Eligibility Requirements for Foreign Graduates • Roles and functions of the Occupational Therapist in the Treatment of Sensory Integrative Dysfunction
1983	• Essentials and Guidelines of an Accredited Educational Program for the Occupational Therapist • Essentials and Guidelines of an Approved Educational Program for the Occupational Therpay Assistant • Guidelines for an Occupational Therapy Fieldwork Experience – Level II & Fieldwork Performance Report • Fieldwork Evaluation Form for Occupational Therapy Assistant Students and Raters Guide for the Fieldwork Evaluation Form • Purposeful Activities • Roles and Functions of Occupational Therapy in Long-Term Care: Programs • The Roles and Functions of Occupational Therapy Services for the Severely Disabled • Standards of Practice for Occupational Therapy
1985	• Guide for Supervision of Occupational Therapy Personnel • Guide to Classification of Occupational Therapy Personnel • Roles and Functions of Occupational Therapy in Burn Care Delivery • Roles and functions of Occupational Therapy in Hand Rehabilitation • Roles and Functions of Occupational Therapy in Mental Health • Guidelines for Occupational Therapy Documentation
1986	• Guidelines for Occupational Therapy Services in School Systems (revised, 1989) • Occupational Therapy and Hospice
1987	• Fieldwork Evaluation for the Occupational Therapist • Roles of Occupational Therapists and Occupational Therapy assistants in Schools
1988	• Occupational Therapy Services in Early Intervention and Prescho0ol Services • Reference Guide Occupational Therapy Code of Ethics
1989	• Guidelines for Occupational Therapy Services in School Systems, second edition • Human Immunodeficiency Virus • Occupational Therapy and Eating dysfunction • Occupational Therapy in the Promotion of Health and the Prevention of Disease and Disability

Table 8-11
PROJECTS AND PUBLICATIONS

- AOTA Member Handbook (1980)
- Directions for the Future: Extensive Study of Education, Practice and Research Within the Profession
- Fieldwork Evaluation form replaced the Field Work Performance Report, 1986
- Role Delineation study, 1981
- Professional and Technical Role Analysis (PATRA) project, approved by RA in 1985
- Occupational Therapy in Mental Health: A Guide to Outcomes Research (1987)
- Supervision Development of Therapeutic Competence (1987)
- Guidelines for Occupational Therapy Services in Hospice (1987)
- Guidelines for Occupational Therapy in Home Health (1987)
- The Chronically Mental Ill (proceedings) (1987)
- The Cost-Effectiveness of Rehabilitation: A Guide to Research Relevant to Occupational Therapy (1987)
- Occupation Therapy in Acute Care Settings: A Manual (1987)
- Problems With Eating: Interventions for Children and Adults With Developmental disabilities (1987)
- Learning Through Play (brochure) (1987)
- Time Traps for Parents (brochure) 1987
- Feeding and Caring for Infants and Children With Special Needs (1987)
- Quality Assurance Mentoring in Occupational Therapy (1987)
- Guide to the Archives of AOTA (1987)
- Guidelines for Occupational Therapy Services in School Systems (1987)
- Occupational Therapy News
- OT Week (1987)
- Special Interest Section Newsletters (five started in 1981: Developmental Disabilities, Gerontology, Mental Health, Physical Disabilities, Sensory Integration)

National Office Organization

In 1982, there were three major departments in the national office: Professional Services, Financial and Business Administration, and Member Services/Association Development (AOTA, 1982a). The Government and Legal Affairs Division reported directory to the Executive Director.

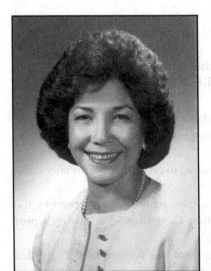

Figure 8-11. Jeanette Bair, OTR, Executive Director of AOTA, 1987-1999. (Printed with permission from the Archive of the American Occupational Therapy Association, Inc.)

The organization included the Executive Director and seven divisions: Communication, Credentialing, Education, Financial and Business Management, Government and Legal Affairs, Operations Research, and Professional Development. Two people reported directly to the Executive Director: the Editor of the American Journal of Occupational Therapy and the Conference and Meeting Section.

Occupational Therapy Directions for the Future Project (1984-1987)

In 1984, the Representative Assembly charged the Executive Board to entry-level educational preparation for professional practice (Fleming, 1987). The Board created the Entry-level Study Committee, chaired by Maureen Fleming. In addition to the Study Committee, an External Advisory Committee was created composed of agencies designated by the Representative Assembly and major groups identified by the Study Committee and national office staff that might be affected by changes in academic requirements or standards. The External Advisory Committee opposed a recommendation being considered by the Study Committee to mandate entry at the graduate level. The major reason for opposition "appeared to be the absence of an identified and generally accepted academic discipline and applied sciences of occupational therapy" (Fleming, 1987, p. v).

Special Interest Sections Added

The Administration and Management Special Interest Section (SIS) was approved in 1984, and the Work Programs SIS was approved in 1985 (AOTA, 1992). The Administrative and Management SIS addresses diverse concerns, including reimbursement, recruitment, personnel management, budgeting, staff development, supervision of certified occupational therapy assistants, fieldwork education, and ethical issues in management. A computerized network of individuals is maintained.

The Work Programs SIS provides a forum for therapists interested in work practice such as fostering worker role entry or re-entry within a variety of practice areas, including industrial rehabilitation, mental health, and physical or developmental disability.

Hightower-Vandamm (1980c) reported that 77% of AOTA members belonged to one of first five SIS in 1980. Physical Disabilities had the largest percentage (22.6%), followed by Developmental Disabilities (17.4%), Sensory Integration (15.7%), Mental Health (13%), and Gerontology (8.3%).

Professional and Technical Role Analysis Project

The Professional and Technical Role Analysis (PATRA) Project revised the Role Delineation Study to include current roles and functions of entry-level registered occupational therapists and certified occupational therapy assistants, incorporate major changes occurring in the health care delivery stem, and address the need for knowledge, skills, attitudes, and abilities to be specified for functions identified within the Role Delineation Study. The responsibility was given to the Inter-Commission Council (AOTA, 1986c).

Task Force on Occupational and Physical Therapy Issues

The task force was charged to examine documents and policies within the Association that needed clarification in relation to the practice of occupational and physical therapy. The task force made eight recommendations (Huss, 1984):

- Define purposeful activity. The document Purposeful Activities was adopted by the Representative Assembly in 1983 and published in AJOT (1983d, pp. 805-806).
- Develop documents which recognize
  - The occupational therapist who has, through available education avenues, developed additional expertise beyond the entry level. Specialty certification was started by the Association in 1984.
  - Areas of practice which require addition education leading to certification. Specialty certification was started by the Association in 1984.
  - Possibility of joint certification with specialty groups. This motion was reviewed by the Ethics Committee and Bylaws, Policies, and Procedures Committee. A follow-up report was not found but the concept was not adopted.
- Develop a policy on the use of modalities. A policy statement was adopted in 1985 entitled Occupational Therapists and Modalities and published in AJOT (1983e, pp. 815-816).
- Develop a policy regarding types of advertising accepted for publication and types of modalities displayed at conference which is consistent with documents adopted by the Association. The Executive Board was charged to study the issues of advertising.

- Recommend that the revision of the educational Essentials include the concept of purposeful activity throughout the education process. The Representative Assembly adopted the motion and referred it to the Commission on Education to implement. The 1983 Essentials and Guidelines of an Accredited Educational Program for the Occupational Therapist do include the term purposeful activities under the section on the Educational Program (Section II, E, 3, b, [1]) (AOTA, 1983f, pp. 831-840). The term also appears in the 1991 version under Section II, B, 3, b, (1).

- Recommend that the accreditation process include a more stringent review in relation to instruction in purposeful activities and their application to treat. The Representative Assembly adopted the motion and referred it to the Accreditation Committee to implement, but the degree of implementation is not stated by the Accreditation Committee in subsequent reports.

- Charge the Commission on Education to develop a mechanism for accreditation of fieldwork centers. The national office staff had been studying the issue of accrediting fieldwork sites for 20 years and included that a cost-effective mechanism was not available. The suggestion was made that educational programs establish a system of closer monitoring of fieldwork centers, including a "field work educator" category.

- Establish a program for education of members regarding the implications of the occupational therapy/physical therapy issues. The report of the task force was published (Huss, 1984).

Reimbursement for Occupational Therapy Services

Health insurance began to be available in the 1930s (Davy, 1984). Most of the coverage was for inpatient hospitalization. As services expanded beyond inpatient services, insurance coverage often did not keep pace. Insurance companies did not want to increase premiums and thus were reluctant to add new services. As a result, insurance coverage for outpatient services, home health, and hospice care did not occur without direct interaction with health insurance providers. Occupational therapy services expanded rapidly during the 1970s and early 1980s beyond inpatient settings, and thus practitioners found that reimbursement often was unavailable in the expanded service areas. Occupational therapy services were a small part of the health care delivery system, and there were few data to show that occupational therapy intervention was effective.

Separation of Certification From Membership

In 1986, the Association became a membership organization only. The American Occupational Therapy Certification Board (AOTBC) was created to manage the certification process and certification examination (AOTA, 1986a). Over the past several years, there had been increasing concern among the Association leadership that the Association was at risk of violating antitrust or noncompetition law because the Association regulated both the accreditation of occupational therapy educational programs and the credentialing of occupational therapy practitioners. The control of both accreditation and credentialing could be viewed under the antitrust law as a closed shop, which restrained potential access to the profession (restraint of trade or noncompetition). Within the profession, members were concerned about paying for both membership and recertification. They asked how much money was for membership benefits and how much money was for recertification. Furthermore, did writing a check in any way demonstrate continuing competency to practice occupational therapy? The solution to both external issues (antitrust, anticompetition laws) and internal issues (membership versus recertification) was legal separation of the certification process from the membership organization. The Association bylaws were changed in the summer of 1986, and the AOTCB formally took charge of initial certification, including administering the certification examination and maintaining records of the individuals who had passed or failed the examination.

A simultaneous change was the recommendation that the Association policy be dropped regarding lapsed certification. The policy had stated that anyone who allowed his or her certification to lapse for 5 years or more had to retake the certification examination and pass it before being reinstated. Additional payment of fees was also required. As state regulation via state licensure increased, the need for a national policy decreased. State licensure boards could make the decisions regarding continuing competency requirements such as requiring a certain number of continuing education units.

Membership Data

Although the Association was growing, the number of members in any given state was still quite small (Langwell et al., 1981). In 1980, only five states had over 1,000 therapists: California (2,887), New York (1,878), Michigan (1,363), Massachusetts (1,061), and Wisconsin (1,049). Eighteen states had less than 100 members living within the state who were members of the Association (p. 301). A graph of membership by region of the country was presented in the 1984 Annual Report (Figure 8-12). These membership numbers are in contrast to the number of therapists actually living in each state according to data collected in 1986 (AOTA, 1987). Eleven states had over 1,000 therapists living there: California, Florida, Illinois, Massachusetts, Michigan, Minnesota, New York, Ohio, Pennsylvania, Texas, and Wisconsin. The only state with more than 1,000 assistants was New York. Twelve states had less than 100 therapists living in that state. Both sets of data were collected before the separation of certification from membership.

Specialty Certification

The formal steps to create specialty certification began in 1982 when the Representative Assembly charged the Association (Resolution 581-82) to develop a voluntary advanced-level recognition program for occupational therapists (AOTA, 1982b). The major purposes were to address the need for the Association to formally acknowledge its role in the issue of continuing competency and to provide practitioners with increased recognition in a specific area of practice within the profession. The issue on continuing competency and/or quality assurance had been discussed for many years but in earnest since 1971 with Resolution 300-71. Pediatrics was chosen as the first practice area because about one-third of members worked with children. The first examination was administered in 1992, and 130 candidates passed to become Board-Certified Pediatric OTs (Javernick, 1992). The general area of pediatrics as a specialty was adopted, but specialty certification in sensory integration and school-based practice were ultimately not adopted, although they were discussed (Hightower-Vandamm, 1980b). Specialty certification was not designed to take the place of continuing education requirements for state licensure, although activities or tasks used to meet the requirements of specialty certification recognition might also be applied to requirements for continued competency required by a state regulatory board.

Uniform Terminology of Occupational Therapy, Second Edition

Revision of the Uniform Terminology document developed in 1979 began in 1983 when the Representative Assembly charged the Commission on Practice to update the document to reflect current practice (AOTA, 1989b). Input was solicited from members and from the three states that had adopted reimbursement systems based on the Product Output Reporting System developed by the AOTA in 1979 (California, Maryland, and Washington). The following guidelines for revision were established:

- To not replace the original document and to limit the revised document to defining occupational performance areas and occupational therapy performance components for occupational therapy intervention (i.e., indirect services were deleted and the Product Output Reporting System was not revised)

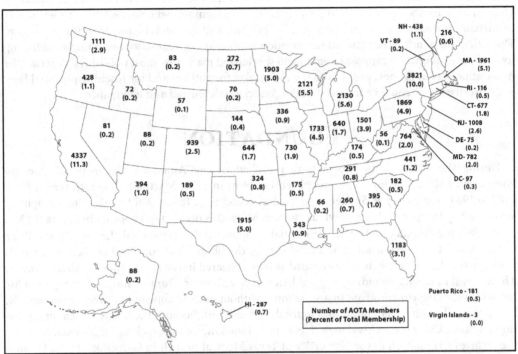

Figure 8-12. Occupational Therapy Manpower, December 1984. (Reprinted with permission from the American Occupational Therapy Association.)

- To coordinate the revision process with other current AOTA projects such as the PATRA
- To develop a document that reflected current area of practice and facilitated uniformity of definitions in the profession
- To recommend that the Association develop a companion document to define techniques, modalities, and activities used in occupational therapy intervention and a document to define specific programs that are offered by occupational therapy departments (AOTA, 1989b)

After several drafts, the revised Uniform Terminology document was expanded. The original Uniform Terminology document had included 68 terms related to direct services and 16 related to indirect services. The second edition contained 109 terms, an expansion of slightly over 50%. Major expansion of terms occurred in the areas of work activities, sensory motor components, and cognitive integration and components. Terms that were dropped included those under the heads of therapeutic adaptation and prevention, which were probably viewed as techniques or modalities. Overall, the document was reorganized into three performance areas—activities of daily living, work activities, and play or leisure activities—and three performance components—sensory motor, cognitive, and psychological. Definitions and descriptions were provided for the growing list of terms.

Publications

Although the Association had been involved in publishing occupational therapy–related manual and monographs since the 1960s, most of the early publications were proceedings of conferences or reports of committee activities. In 1982, Executive Director Garibaldi announced that a decision had been made to accelerate the Association's book publishing program (AOTA, 1982c). Costs had been a major consideration. However, discussions with publishers had resulted in the idea of having selected publishers underwrite the initial cost of typesetting, graphics, and printing and then selling copies of the book at a discount for the Association to resell to members. The emphasis for the Association to publish came from members who wanted more timely access to current information on expanding areas of practice and new developments in the profession. The article announcing the plan did not mention another major reason for becoming a publishing source. Occupational therapy was a small and specialized market by most publishers' criteria. The Association was in the best position to tap the market for authors and for reaching potential buyers. Advertisements could be included in the Association's journal and newspaper.

FOUNDATION

During the 1980s, three people were president of the American Occupational Therapy Foundation (AOTF): Wilma West completed her term in 1982, Martha S. Moersch served from 1982 to 1984, and Nancy V. Snyder completed a second term from 1986 to 1988. Photographs of West and Snyder appeared in a previous chapter. Moersch's photograph appears in Figure 8-13.

In 1980, the Foundation began to financially support the occupational therapy library. Prior to the Foundation's organization and cataloguing, the library had consisted of shelves in which books, manuals, and journals were grouped as they appeared in the Association's collective inbox. The archival materials, including original letters received by Dr. Dunton and carbon copies of his replies, were being stored offsite in a warehouse without climate control and were aging quickly. Using the collection monographs and journals was difficult because there was no real organizational system. Using the archival materials required stacking and unstacking large boxes. Initially, the archives were moved to the University of Texas Medical Branch in Galveston, Texas, because the Foundation did not have a climate control system in the Association's building. While in Texas, the archives were organized into acid-free library boxes and all materials were cataloged. The guide to the archives was prepared in 1987 by a trained librarian and continues to be updated (Bowman, 1987). An online database called OT Source was started in 1989 to make the library collection and archival materials available without having to travel to the Foundation office. The online system would be modified and updated over the coming years.

The Foundation began publishing the *Occupational Therapy Journal of Research* in April 1981, with Charles H. Christiansen at the first editor. The purposes of the new journal were to encourage dynamic dialogue between authors of published papers and discussants, thus providing a forum for research and debate; to represent a scholarly commitment to scientific research in the profession; to stimulate more research by providing an additional vehicle for publication; to further implement the research mandate to the Foundation by the Representative Assembly of AOTA; and to further strengthen relationships and joint goals of AOTA and AOTF (Llorens, 1981, p. 5) In 1983, the Foundation inaugurated the Academy of Research "to recognize researchers who have made sustained contributions toward advancing the knowledge base of the field" (AOTF, 1983, p. 3) The first three charter members were A. Jean Ayres, Mary Reilly, and Elizabeth Yerxa. Recipients received a gold pin with the logo of the Academy of Research and their name engraved on a plaque for permanent display in the AOTF office. Criteria for the award included "awards

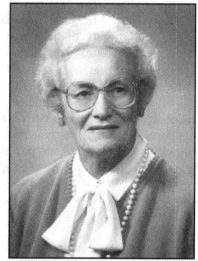

Figure 8-13. Martha S. Moersch, OTR, President of AOTF, 1982-1985. (Printed with permission from the Archive of the American Occupational Therapy Association, Inc.)

for scholarly excellence, the number and quality of publications from both within and outside the field, apparent or documented influence on the development of occupational theory and practice, and success in obtaining extramural funding for research" (AOTA, 1983h, p. 3). Initiating the journal was part of the commitment to support research activities within the profession, which had begun in earnest with the Research Seminar held in 1976 (West, 1981). Another part of the commitment was the publication of a bibliography of completed research, sponsoring a research forum at the AOTA annual conference, maintaining the regional research consultant program to assist practitioners in developing research skills, and providing funding in the form of research grants. By 1985, 182 grant requests had been received (AOTF, 1985). The largest number of grants funded were in the area of physical disabilities (18), followed by developmental disabilities (14), education (9), mental health (9), sensory integration (8), gerontology (3), and activities (1).

By 1985, the 20th anniversary of the Foundation, the total endowed scholarship funds totaled $192,000. More than 240 scholarships had been awarded (AOTF, 1985). The primary source of funds for scholarships was the state associations. In addition, the doctoral fellowship program was initiated in 1981, with funds allocated by the AOTA Representative Assembly to support a fellowship each year for 5 years so that an individual could devote time to completion of a doctoral degree. In 1984, the Foundation inaugurated a Post-Doctoral Fellowship to provide research support for a scholar each year to complete a research program.

In June 1986, the Foundation hired its first Executive Director, Martha Kirkland (AOTF, 1986). Kirkland had previously worked for the Association as Director of Continuing Education, so she was familiar with national office activities and resources.

REFLECTION

By the end of the 1980s, the professional Association had achieved the basic requirements needed to develop and maintain a profession, a professional association, a charitable foundation, and an independent agency to manage certification. Standards for education and practice had been established, a Code of Ethics was available, and mechanisms for initial certification were in place. A new journal focusing on research had been initiated by the Foundation, whereas the Association increased its commitment to publishing monographs relevant to the profession of occupational therapy. Other issues began to occupy more time and effort, such as public awareness and recognition; changing social concerns about health and wellness; accountability for services offered, including efficacy, efficiency, and scientific support; and meeting membership needs for information in a timely manner.

These years were characterized by a search for a unifying theory of occupational therapy and the development of a unique body of knowledge as the profession sought to be recognized as a true profession. The development of Gary Kielhofner's Model of Human Occupation began during this time. A number of assessment instruments and techniques created by occupational therapists were also developed during this time. There was a desire to upgrade the profession through recognition of continued competency and through recognition of those who engaged in research. There was also more emphasis on a return to authentic occupational therapy, moving out of the reductionistic paradigm. Collaboration with other disciplines, not just medicine, was accepted. This time period also saw the birth of occupational science.

REFERENCES

Acquaviva, F. A. (1985). *Occupational therapy manpower: A plan for progress.* Rockville, MD: American Occupational Therapy Association.

Acquaviva, F. A., & Presseller, S. (1983). Nationally speaking: Occupational therapy manpower. *American Journal of Occupational Therapy, 37*(2), 79-81.

American Hospital Association. (1980). *Hospital statistics, 1980 edition*. Chicago, IL: Author.

American Hospital Association. (1988). *Hospital statistics, 1988 edition*. Chicago, IL: Author.

American Occupational Therapy Association. (1980-1981). *Education programs in occupational therapy*. Rockville, MD: Author.

American Occupational Therapy Association. (1982a). *Annual report*. Rockville, MD: Author.

American Occupational Therapy Association. (1982b). The Association: 1982 Representative Assembly—62nd annual conference. *American Journal of Occupational Therapy, 36*(12), 808-820.

American Occupational Therapy Association. (1982c). WWI aides qualify for VA benefits. *Occupational Therapy Newspaper, 36*(8), 4.

American Occupational Therapy Association. (1983a). Essentials and guidelines of an accredited educational program for the occupational therapist. *American Journal of Occupational Therapy, 37*(12), 817-823.

American Occupational Therapy Association. (1983b). Essentials and guidelines of an approved educational program for the occupational therapy assistant. *American Journal of Occupational Therapy, 37*(12), 824-830.

American Occupational Therapy Association. (1983c). Policy: Occupational therapists and modalities. *American Journal of Occupational Therapy, 37*(12), 816.

American Occupational Therapy Association. (1983d). Purposeful activities. *American Journal of Occupational Therapy, 37*(12), 805-806.

American Occupational Therapy Association (1983e). Association policies. *American Journal of Occupational Therapy, 37*(12), 815-816.

American Occupational Therapy Association (1983f). Representative Assembly. *American Journal of Occupational Therapy, 37*(12), 831-840.

American Occupational Therapy Association (1983g). Essentials of an accredited educational program for the occupational therapist. *American Journal of Occupational Therapy, 37*(12), 817-823.

American Occupational Therapy Association. (1983h). Fellows invited to nominate for 1984 Academy of Research. *Occupational Therapy Newspaper, 37*(11), 3.

American Occupational Therapy Association. (1986a). AOTA certification structure changed: focus to be on membership. *Occupational Therapy News, 40*(6), 1.

American Occupational Therapy Association (1986b). New law provides occupational therapy for preschoolers. *Occupational Therapy News, 40*(12), 6.

American Occupational Therapy Association. (1986c). PATRA project: What it is and is not. *Occupational Therapy News, 40*(12), 9.

American Occupational Therapy Association. (1987). Dataline: Population ratios: A measure of supply and need for occupational therapy personnel. *Occupational Therapy News 41*(8), 6-9.

American Occupational Therapy Association. (1988). HCFA issues final Medicare Instructions for OT. Federal Report insert. *Occupational Therapy News, 42*(4), 9.

American Occupational Therapy Association. (1989a) Listing of educational programs in occupational therapy. *American Journal of Occupational Therapy, 43*(12), 833-840.

American Occupational Therapy Association. (1989b). Uniform terminology for occupational therapy, second edition. *American Journal of Occupational Therapy, 43*(12), 808-815.

American Occupational Therapy Association. (1991). Association policies: Registered occupational therapists and certified occupational therapy assistants and modalities. *American Journal of Occupational Therapy, 45*(12), 1112-1114.

American Occupational Therapy Association. (1992). An historical look at special interest sections. *OT Week*, October 16, pp. 6-7.

American Occupational Therapy Foundation. (1983). Fellows invited to nominate for 1984 Academy of Research. *Occupational Therapy Newspaper, 37*(11), 3.

American Occupational Therapy Foundation. (1985). Foundation celebrates 20th anniversary. *Occupational Therapy Newspaper, 39*(3), 8-9.

American Occupational Therapy Foundation. (1986). AOTF names first executive director. *Occupational Therapy News, 40*(8), 1.

Bair, J. (1982). Nationally speaking: Changing trends in practice. *American Journal of Occupational Therapy, 36*(11), 704-707.

Bissell, J. C., & Mailloux, Z. (1981). The use of crafts in occupational therapy for the physically disabled. *American Journal of Occupational Therapy, 35*(6), 369-374.

Blakeney, A., Strickland, L. R., & Wilkinson, J. H. (1983). Exploring sensory integrative dysfunction in process schizophrenia. *American Journal of Occupational Therapy, 37*(6), 399-406.

Bowman, I. (1987). *Guide to the archives of the American Occupational Therapy Association*. Rockville, MD: American Occupational Therapy Association.

Boyer, J. (1990). Congress passes new standards for VA OTs. *OT Week, 4*(16), 6.

Clopton, J. W. (1981). Craft use with physically disabled questioned. *American Journal of Occupational Therapy*, 35(10), 669.

Committee on Installations and Advice. (1928). Report and analysis of crafts. *Occupational Therapy & Rehabilitation*, 7, 29-43, 131-136, 211-216, 417-431.

Committee on Installations and Advice. (1929). Analysis of crafts. *Occupational Therapy & Rehabilitation*, 8, 339-352.

Davy, J. (1984). Nationally speaking: Status report on reimbursement for occupational therapy services. *American Journal of Occupational Therapy*, 38(5), 295-198.

DeGangi, G. A. (1983). Letters to the editor: Author's response. *American Journal of Occupational Therapy*, 37(12), 848-850.

DeGangi, G. A., Lurley, L., & Linscheid, T. R. (1983). Toward a methodology of the short-term effects of neurodevelopment treatment. *American Journal of Occupational Therapy*, 37(7), 479-484.

Dunton, W. R. Jr. (1950). The prescription. In W. R. Dunton, Jr. & S. Licht (Eds.), *Occupational therapy: Principles and practice* (pp. 20-44). Springfield, IL: Charles C. Thomas.

Dunton, W. R. Jr. (1957). The prescription. In W. R. Dunton, Jr. & S. Licht (Eds.), *Occupational therapy: Principles and practice* (2nd ed., pp. 29-52). Springfield, IL: Charles C. Thomas.

Drake, M. (1992). *Crafts in therapy and rehabilitation*. Thorofare, NJ: SLACK Incorporated.

Editorial. (1951). Disemphasizing crafts. *American Journal of Occupational Therapy*, 5(1), 39.

Eliason, M. L., & Gohl-Glese, A. (1979). A question of professional boundaries: Implications for educational programs. *American Journal of Occupational Therapy*, 33(3), 175-179.

English, C., Kasch, M., Silverman, P., & Walker, S. (1982). The issue: On the role of the occupational therapist in physical disabilities. *American Journal of Occupational Therapy*, 36(3), 199-200.

Fleming, M. H. (1987). *Occupational therapy: Directions for the future*. Rockville, MD: American Occupational Therapy Association.

Gilfoyle, E. (1987). AOTA at 70. *Occupational Therapy News*, 41(12), 6.

Hightower-Vandamm, M. D. (1980a). Nationally speaking: The perils of occupational therapy in several special arenas of practice. *American Journal of Occupational Therapy*, 34(5), 307-309.

Hightower-Vandamm, M. D. (1980b). National speaking. The perils of occupational therapy in several special arenas of practice (continued). *American Journal of Occupational Therapy*, 34(6), 369-371.

Hightower-Vandamm, M.D. (1980c). National speaking: - Specialty sections – A mile-high dream. *American Journal of Occupational Therapy*, 34(9), 499-502.

Huss, A. J. (1984). Nationally speaking: Whither thou goest? Report of the AOTA Task Force on OT/PT issues. *American Journal of Occupational Therapy*, 38(2), 81-84.

Javernick, J. A. (1992). 130 OTs achieve board certification. *OT Week*, 6(30), 19.

Kamenetz, H.L. (1983). *Dictionary of rehabilitation medicine*. New York, NY: Springer Publishing.

Kielhofner, G. (1980a). A model of human occupation. Part 2. Ontogenesis from the perspective of temporal adaptation. *American Journal of Occupational Therapy*, 34(10), 657-663.

Kielhofner, G. (1980b). A model of human occupation. Part 3. Benign and vicious cycles. *American Journal of Occupational Therapy*, 34(11), 731-737.

Kielhofner, G., & Burke, J. P. (1980). A model of human occupation. Part 1. Conceptual framework and content. *American Journal of Occupational Therapy*, 34(9), 572-581.

Kielhofner, G., Burke, J. P., & Igi, C. H. (1980). A model of human occupation. Part 4. Assessment and intervention. *American Journal of Occupational Therapy*, 34(12), 777-788.

Langwell, K. M., Wilson, S. D., & Deane, R. T. (1981). Geographic distribution of occupational therapists. *American Journal of Occupational Therapy*, 35(5), 299-305.

Llorens, L. A. (1981). Guest editorial: A journal of research in occupational therapy: The need, the response. *Occupational Therapy Journal of Research*, 1(1), 3-6.

Magrun, W. M., deBenabib, R. M., & Nelson, C. (1983). Letters to the editor: More criticism—Article on neurodevelopmental treatment. *American Journal of Occupational Therapy*, 37(12), 846-848.

Masagatani, G. N. (1985). Nationally speaking: AOTA's ad hoc commission on occupational therapy manpower. Part 2: Summary of recommendations. *American Journal of Occupational Therapy*, 40(8), 525-527.

Pedretti, L. W., & Pasquinelli-Estrada, S. (1985). Foundations for treatment of physical dysfunction. In L. W. Pedretti (Ed.), *Occupational therapy: Practice skills for physical dysfunction* (2nd ed., pp. 1-10). St. Louis, MO: Mosby.

Rosenthal, S. (1983). Letters to the editor: Questions cause of change. *American Journal of Occupational Therapy*, 37(12), 850.

Silvergleit, I. (1990). Employment settings of new graduates. *OT Week*, 4(10), 9.

Trombly, C. A. (1982). Letters to the editor: Include exercise in "purposeful activity." *American Journal of Occupational Therapy*, 36(7), 467-468.

Walker, J. K., Lumpkin, B., RePoserly, T., Pratt, S., Stevens, L., Wente, S., & Whitney, K. (1982). Against crafts emphasis. *American Journal of Occupational Therapy*, 36(1). 48-49.

West, W. L. (1981) Commentary: A journal of research in occupational therapy: The response, the responsibility. *Occupational Therapy Journal of Research, 1*(1), 7-12.

Wright, C., & Nomura, M. (1985). *From toys to computers: Access for the physically disabled child.* San Jose, CA: Authors.

Yerxa, E. J., Clark, F., Frank, G., Jackson, J., Parham, D., Pierce, D.,...Zemke, R. (1989). An introduction to occupational science, a foundation for occupational therapy in the 21st century. *Occupational Therapy in Health Care, 6*(4), 1-17.

BIBLIOGRAPHY

Allen, C. K. (1982). Independence through activity: The practice of occupational therapy. *American Journal of Occupational Therapy, 36*(11), 731-739.

American Occupational Therapy Association. (1981). Membership data 1980. *American Journal of Occupational Therapy, 35*(5), 301.

American Occupational Therapy Association. (1982). Data Line. *Occupational Therapy Newspaper, 36*(8), 4.

American Occupational Therapy Association. (1987). AOTA at 70: The growth of a dynamic profession. Part X: Yesterday and tomorrow. *Occupational Therapy News, 41*(12), 6-7.

American Occupational Therapy Association. (1992). Physical agent modalities? Position paper. *American Journal of Occupational Therapy, 46*(12), 1090-1091.

Ayres, A. J. (1958). Basic concepts of clinical practice in physical disabilities. *American Journal of Occupational Therapy, 12*(4), 300-302, 311.

Blakeney, A., Strickland, L. R., & Wilkinson, J. H. (1983). Letters to the editor: Author's response. *American Journal of Occupational Therapy, 37*(12), 850-951.

Grady, A. P., & Gilfoyle, E. M. (1989). The eighties: A decade of change. *OT Week, 3*(51), 2, 20.

Time of Conflict
1990s to 2000s

Key Points

- Resolution J changed the entry level for occupational therapists to post-baccalaureate level in 1999.
- The Association sold its headquarters building in Rockville, Maryland, and bought a building in Bethesda, Maryland, in 1994.
- The Accreditation Council for Occupational Therapy Education (ACOTE) formed in 1994.
- The National Board for Certification in Occupational Therapy (NBCOT) formed in 1996.
- A dispute between the Association and NBCOT over credentialing marks began in 1999.
- There was a discussion about cross-training and multiskilling personnel to perform duties or activities typically performed by others in 1997.
- The Association began a new magazine called *OT Practice* in 1996.

Highlighted Personalities

- Winnie Dunn, theorist
- Jeanette Schkade, theorist
- Sally Schultz, theorist
- Ann Patricia Grady, AOTA President, 1989-1992
- Mary Margaret Evert, AOTA President, 1992-1995
- Mary Foto, AOTA president, 1995-1998
- Karen Jacobs, AOTA president, 1998-2002
- Elizabeth Devereaux, AOTF President
- Maralynne Mitcham, AOTF President
- Jane Davis Rourk, AOTF President
- Florence Clark, researcher (well elderly project)

Andersen, L. T., & Reed, K. L.
The History of Occupational Therapy: The First Century (pp. 261-292).
© 2017 Taylor & Francis Group.

Key Places

- The national office moved to 4720 Montgomery Lane in Bethesda, Maryland.

Political Events/Issues

- 1990—Americans with Disability Act (ADA), P.L. 101-336, adopted
- 1996—Health Insurance Portability and Accountability Act (HIPAA), P.L. 104-191, adopted
- 1997—Individuals with Disabilities Education Act (IDEA), P.L. 108-446, adopted
- 1997—Balance Budget Act (BBA), P.L. 105-33, changed payment systems
- Olmstead decision by Supreme Court: States must place people with disabilities in community settings rather than institutions if appropriate.

Economic Events/Issues

- Increased governmental pressure to control costs
- Health maintenance organizations (HMOs) created
- The Balanced Budget Act extended prospective payment system to cover home health beginning in 2000, skilled nursing facilities beginning in 1999, and inpatient rehabilitation units beginning in 2006 (13 medical conditions)
- Loss of occupational therapy jobs forecasted due to effects of the Balanced Budget Act

Educational Issues

- Essentials of an Accredited Program in Occupational Therapy revised in 1965. Affiliations divided into physical and psychosocial disabilities totally 6 months and there was a de-emphasis on crafts.
- Master's degree programs started
- Increased focus on continuing education to update knowledge and skills

Key Times/Events

- Balanced Budget Act (1997) created caps on Medicare Part B outpatient rehabilitation services.
- Post-baccalaureate entry resolution was adopted in 1999 and became effective in 2007.

Sociocultural Events/Issues

- There was an increased need for occupational therapy personnel to understand and respond to the influence of political and legislative actions on occupational therapy jobs, service delivery, and payment systems.
- The marketplace for occupational therapy services grew rapidly.
- Social awareness of disability increased with passage of the Americans with Disabilities Act.

Practice Issues

- The Core Values and Attitudes of Occupational Therapy Practice document was adopted in 1993 (later integrated into the Code of Ethics).
- Uniform Terminology III was adopted in in 1994.
- Guide to Occupational Therapy Practice document was published in 1999.
- Models of practice began focusing on the concepts of person, environment, and occupation (PEO).
- Encroachment of physical therapy on concept of functional limitation.

Technological Events/Issues

- Technology Related Assistance for Individuals with Disabilities Amendments (P.L. 103-218)
- The Internet and World Wide Web expanded online capabilities to integrate graphics and text.

Association Issues

- Mission statement adopted in 1993; vision statement adopted in 1998
- Specialty certification program and board created in 1995
- Cross-training document adopted in 1997
- Human Genome Project started in 1999
- Continuation of the physical agent modality issue
- Skilled versus nonskilled services and Medicare

Foundation Issues

- Reliable Source online database started in 1994
- Centers for Scholarship and Research in Occupational Therapy established
- Mission and goal statements clarified

National Board for Certification in Occupational Therapy

- NBCOT replaced AOTCB
- Trademark dispute between NBCOT and the Association

INTRODUCTION

In 1990, U.S. President George H. W. Bush (41st President) was finishing his term. Nelson Mandela was released from a South African prison after 27 years. In 1994, he became President of South Africa. The Persian Gulf War was fought from August 1990 to April 1991. President Bill Clinton assumed office in 1992. A text-based web browser became available. In 1995, the Alfred P. Murrah Federal Building in Oklahoma City, Oklahoma, was bombed, leaving 168 people dead. The O.J. Simpson trial was held in Los Angeles, California. The Internet became a major part of many people's lives as they learned to find information at their fingertips aided by their computer.

Changes in the health care system continued as ideas and technology evolved. One change was the expansion of Diagnostic Related Groups (DRG) designed to limit health care costs, which led to a major growth in prospective payment systems in 1990s affecting home health, skilled nursing facilities, and inpatient rehabilitation facilities. Computer-based technology was advancing with the introduction of the World Wide Web, allowing graphics and text to be integrated seamlessly. Information about a wide range of topics and opinions was available via a computer with an Internet provider at any time of the day or night, and rapidly expanding the information available to clients and to occupational therapy students.

During the 1990s, many models of practice began to shift to ideas based on the interaction of occupation, person, and environment as an integrated explanation for how occupational therapy could be conceptualized. Cognitive rehabilitation through occupational therapy frames of reference became more common. Focusing adapting the task or occupation was studied more, and adapting the individual became less important.

The marketplace for occupational therapy grew rapidly. The passage of the Americans with Disabilities Act of 1990 contributed, as did the effects of more coverage under Medicare, to better reimbursement and the continued growth of practice in the school systems.

Major goals of the American Occupational Therapy Association (AOTA) were expediting political activities, helping individuals to become change agents, enhancing public awareness of occupational therapy through marketing efforts and personal action, showing value of occupational therapy outcomes, initiating group and individual advocacy of occupational therapy services, and increasing visibility of occupational therapy practitioners and leaders. The Association increased its professional autonomy as well. On January 1, 1994, the Accreditation Council for Occupational Therapy Education (ACOTE) became the accrediting agency independent of the American Medical Association (AMA). The ACOTE became responsible for accrediting both the professional (occupational therapist) and technical (occupational therapy assistant) level educational programs that were rapidly expanding across the country.

EDUCATION

Post-Baccalaureate Entry Required and Resolution J

At the Representative Assembly meeting in 1999, Resolution J was adopted and became RA 679-99 (AOTA, 1999a). Resolution J was entitled "Movement to Required Post-Baccalaureate Level of Education." The intent of the resolution was "to mandate that the entry to the professional level of practice in occupational therapy be at the post-baccalaureate degree level" and that "the official position of AOTA be one that supports post-baccalaureate education as the required level of professional entry into the field of occupational therapy" (AOTA, 1999c). The statement of intent continued, "Preparing therapists at the post-baccalaureate level means those entering the profession will be positioned to take on expanded responsibilities, assume leadership roles, and be players in areas not only where services are provided, but also where decision are made." A summary of the rationale is provided in the following statements included in the Resolution:

- Contemporary practice areas require occupational therapists, including new graduates, to demonstrate an unprecedented level of advanced clinical reasoning.
- New graduates, more than ever, need to define, demonstrate, and articulate the uniqueness and value of occupational therapy.
- New graduates need to be capable of functioning as autonomous professionals and must be encouraged to see themselves in this role.
- Practice arenas are shifting and therapists are challenged to establish programs in areas where occupational therapy services have not previously been offered.
- New graduates enter settings and are challenged to make decision and engage in a level of clinical decision making previously reserved for experienced clinicians.
- The move to the post-baccalaureate level is apt to clarify the delineation between professional and technical education.
- Movement to post-baccalaureate entry is consistent with current trends in other related professions.
- Analyses conducted by the Commission on Education Entry-Level Task Force confirm that the environment reinforces current readiness to move to this level.
- Currently, many graduates of entry-level programs have essentially been confirmed the baccalaureate degree for the equivalent of masters level education.
- Preparation of more therapists at the post-baccalaureate degree level is likely to meet the current and future needs for qualified faculty in our education programs.
- Preparation at the post-baccalaureate degree level would position occupational therapy to better meet personnel needs in emerging practice arenas, including effective and efficient staffing patterns.
- Movement to post-baccalaureate degree entry reflects and acknowledges the complexity of our knowledge base and the high degree of professional judgment required for practice.

- The preparation of occupational therapists at the post-baccalaureate level would address the needs for more outcomes research supporting the tents of occupational therapy practice, efficacy interventions and staffing models. (AOTA, 1999c, pp. RA9-RA10)

In essence, the push to move the profession to master's-level entry had finally been reacted after 40 years of talk beginning in 1958. In summary, the issues were the following:

- The curriculum content for the occupational therapist had been for many years equivalent to a master's degree in other fields.
- Therapists needed to have better skills in autonomous clinical reasoning.
- Therapists needed to be able to develop and implement new service programs in new areas of practice as new graduates.
- The profession needed more faculty trained with advanced degrees.
- Separation and clarity were needed between the levels of education for occupational therapists and assistants.
- Potential students planning on a career of working in the profession would be more likely to complete a master's-level program.
- Therapists would be better recognized as knowledgeable team members with a higher degree of education and training.
- A higher degree in some work environments equaled higher pay.
- Therapists needed to better understand the profession's body of knowledge.
- More outcomes research was needed to support the tenets and assumptions of the profession.
- The profession needed to better demonstrate its efficiency and effectiveness in delivering services.

The date for implementation to the post-baccalaureate degree was set as January 1, 2007, to give academic programs time to change the existing curriculum and program from an undergraduate-to graduate-level program (AOTA, 1999b). Universities and colleges have different requirements to granting undergraduate versus graduate degrees. Some colleges were not established to grant graduate degrees. In such colleges, the occupational therapy program had to arrange to transfer students to another university, change to offering an assistant-level program or close the program. Ultimately, six bachelor's degree programs closed because they could not transition to the post-baccalaureate requirement (AOTA, 2008, p. 2).

Doctoral Degrees

Schools began offering doctoral degrees in occupational therapy: Boston University offered a ScD in therapeutic studies, the University of Southern California offered a PhD in occupational science, and New York University offered a PhD in occupational therapy. Texas Woman's University would follow in offering a PhD, along with Nova Southeastern University.

Educational Programs

In 1992, there were 75 colleges or universities with occupational therapy programs and 74 community colleges or technical schools with occupational therapy assistant programs. Alaska, Arizona, Hawaii, Idaho, Montana, Nevada, Utah, Vermont, West Virginia, and Wyoming did not have professional educational programs. Alaska, Arizona, the District of Columbia, Idaho, Indiana, Mississippi, Nebraska, Nevada, South Dakota, Vermont, and West Virginia did not have technical education programs (Harsh, 1992). By 1999, 40 states plus the District of Columbia and Puerto Rico had occupational therapy education programs within the state boundaries, and 48 states had an assistant-level program. Only Alaska had no educational program for occupational therapy personnel at either the professional or technical level. Although the gap in Western states had decreased, there were still four states with no professional-level program within the state boundaries, including Idaho, Montana, Nevada, and Utah.

Accreditation

In 1993, the Representative Assembly approved a motion from the Executive Board to pursue recognition of the Association as an independent accrediting agency, thus ending the partnership with the AMA started in 1933 (Graves, 1994). The AMA was dissolving the Committee on Allied Health Education and Accreditation (CAHEA), and the structure and funding of an alternative umbrella organization was not yet determined (AOTA, 1993a, p. 25). Although the dissolution of CAHEA was the last straw, the issue of becoming an independent accrediting agency was under discussion by the Association. As Kyler-Hutchinson (1992) pointed out in a series of articles on the accreditation process, the profession was not totally in charge of the criteria by which the educational programs were accredited because the Essentials had to be approved by the AMA and CAHEA. Also, when a program was accredited, notification was held up until the AMA ratified the decision made by the Accreditation Committee of AOTA. Sometimes the process caused time delays that were inconvenient for all concerned. Prior to the motion being adopted, the Accreditation Council of AOTA, in collaboration with the AMA/CAHEA, accredited the occupational therapy educational programs, and the Commission on Education developed the Essentials outlining the criteria for an accepted program and curriculum, which were approved by the Representative Assembly.

The new entity formed on January 1, 1994, was called the Accreditation Council for Occupational Therapy Education (ACOTE). The ACOTE functioned as a standing committee of the Association, with the Chairperson of the Commission on Standards and Ethics serving as a liaison between the Executive Board and the ACOTE (Daigle, 1994). The ACOTE sought and secured recognition from the U.S. Department of Education (USDE) and the Commission on Recognition of Postsecondary Accreditation (CORPTA), a nongovernmental agency that basically accredits the accreditors. The ACOTE also joined the Association of Specialized and Programmed Accreditors (ASPA), the organization that carried out professional development, public relations, publications, and accreditation data collection (Daigle, 1994). Another change was that ACOTE became responsible for revising the documents known as the Essentials, which would change its title to the Standards for Establishing and Maintaining an Occupational Therapy Educational Program for Occupational Therapists or Assistants. An additional change was an added requirement for new or developing programs to submit a development plan as part of obtaining "development program status" prior to admitting students (Graves, 1994). Thus, the accreditation process for new programs had three steps as opposed to two steps under the system with the AMA. The 10-point application process was an attempt to increase the potential that the new program would actually become an accredited program. Although program development in occupational therapy had a good track record of attaining accreditation status, there was no guarantee that students would have graduated from an accredited program and would therefore become eligible to take the certification exam. By reviewing the program before students started, the ACOTE was in a better position to decrease the possibility that the first class of students would not be the last.

PRACTICE

Membership Survey

The 1990 AOTA membership survey, the last available, reported that the most common health problems or diagnoses seen by occupational therapists were stroke/hemiplegia (27.1%), developmental delay (12.9%), cerebral palsy (9.7%), hand injury (9.5%) and learning disability (7.0%). Combined diagnoses resulted in 83.4% related to physical disabilities and 16.6% related to mental health. For occupational therapy assistants, the most common diagnoses were stroke/hemiplegia (30.3%), intellectual disability (11.4%), developmental delay (8.9%), schizophrenic disorders (6.6%), and cerebral palsy (6.0%). Combining health programs resulted in 72% physical disabilities and 28% mental health. As previous membership reports had shown, occupational therapists are more likely to work with children, whereas assistants are more likely to work with older clients. However, many practitioners work equally with a wide range of client ages (AOTA, 1990).

Practice areas discussed were acute care, adults with developmental disabilities, geriatrics, graduate education, hand therapy, home health, Independent practice, industrial rehabilitation/work hardening, mental health, military, rehabilitation, school systems, technology, and vision therapy (AOTA, 1993b). Mean salary for occupational therapists was $36,470 and for assistants was $21,282. Payment for services came primarily from the patient/client directly, Medicare, Medicaid, private insurance, or workers' compensation.

To summarize, the membership survey reported the following:

- A growing proportion of occupational therapy practitioners were employed either full- or part-time.
- The proportion of practitioners working primarily with mental health problems continued to decline.
- More occupational therapists and assistants were becoming self-employed or entering private practice.
- The number of assistants working in schools systems had increased from 3.6% in 1972 to 17% in 1990, whereas the percentage of occupational therapists has rebounded over a percentage point to 18.6%.
- Salaries for practitioners increased at an average of 8% annually from 1986 to 1990.
- Occupational therapists were less likely to be certified or licensed in other fields than in the past.
- Occupational therapists were more likely to be employed in urban areas, whereas the proportion of assistants was greater in rural areas.
- More than half of occupational therapists considered themselves specialists rather than generalists.
- About a third of occupational therapists and a quarter of assistants considered consultation to be their secondary employment function.
- Most occupational therapists had a baccalaureate degree (82.3%), whereas most assistants had an associate's degree (70.8%).

The 1995 membership data showed the highest ratio of occupational therapists to population in Colorado, Massachusetts, New Hampshire, North Dakota, and Wisconsin, with ratios above 20% per 100,000 population. Sixteen states had less than 10 therapists per 100,000 population, including most of the Southern states and several Western states. Only North Dakota has a high ration of assistants per 100,000 population. States with the highest membership number of occupational therapists were California (3,520), New York (2,689), Florida (1,821), Pennsylvania (1,793), and Michigan (1,721). States with less than 80 members included South Dakota, Vermont, and West Virginia. The largest numbers of assistant members were in New York, Pennsylvania, Ohio, California, and Illinois, whereas states with less than 10 members included Alaska and Vermont.

Definitions of Occupational Therapy

Table 9-1 lists some of the definitions developed during the 1990s. The dominant phrase is *purposeful activity*, which continued to be difficult to explain to other health care professionals and the public because there was no good explanation for what constituted an activity without a purpose, or purposeless activity. How did occupational therapy practitioners know the difference between a purposeful versus purposeless activity? What were the distinguishing characteristics? Did the activity have to be purposeful to both the practitioner and the client or to just one or the other? Was there a list of purposeful activities that could be used in an occupational therapy intervention program? How was purposeful activity determined for infants, persons in a coma

Table 9-1	
DEFINITIONS OF OCCUPATIONAL THERAPY	
1990	Occupational therapy is the application of purposeful, goal-oriented activity in the evaluation, diagnosis, and/or treatment of persons whose function is impaired by physical illness or injury, emotional disorder, congenital or developmental disability, or the aging process, in order to achieve optimum functioning, to prevent disability or to maintain health. (American Medical Association. [1990]. *Allied health education directory* [14th ed., p. 112]. Chicago, IL: Author.)
1990	Occupational therapy is a vital health care service whose practitioners help to restore and sustain the highest quality of productive life to persons recovering from illnesses or injuries or coping with developmental disabilities or changes resulting from the aging process (About AOTA brochure.)
1991	Occupational therapy is the art and science of directing an individual's participation in selected tasks to restore, reinforce, and enhance performance; facilitate learning of those skills and functions essential for adaptation and productivity; diminish or correct pathology; and promote and maintain health. Reference to occupation in the title is in the context of individuals' goal-directed use of time, energy, interest, and attention. Its fundamental concern is the development and maintenance of the capacity throughout the life span to perform with satisfaction to self and orders those tasks and roles essential to productive living and to the mastery of self and the environment. (ACOTE. Essentials and Guidelines or an Accredited Educational Program for the Occupational Therapist. Modification of definition in Essentials, 1973.)
1993	Occupational therapy is the use of purposeful activity or interventions to promote health and achieve functional outcomes. Achieving functional outcomes means to develop, improve, or restore the highest possible level of independence of any individual who is limited by a physical injury or illness, a dysfunctional condition, a cognitive impairment, a psychosocial dysfunction, a mental illness, a developmental or learning disability or an adverse environmental condition. Assessment means the use of skilled observation or evaluation by the administration and interpretation of standardized or non-standardized tests and measurements to identify areas for occupational therapy services. (Resolution 542-92. *American Journal of Occupational Therapy, 47*[12], 1119-1120.)
1993	Occupational therapy is the reasoned use of occupation to assist people in adapting to the challenges that accompany disabling conditions, as well as normal growth and development. Although occupational therapy has a particularly profound effect on the lives of those with disabilities, it has an equally important role in preventing illness and promoting wellness. In all contexts occupational therapy enables people to participate in activities that give meaning to life and confer a sense of well-being. (Fine & Kirkland, Envisioning the best for occupational therapy research and education. *OT Week, 7*[8], 20.)
1995	Occupational therapy is the use of purposeful activity and interventions to achieve functional outcomes. "Achieving functional outcomes" means to maximize the independence and the maintenance of health of any individual who is limited by a physical injury or illness, a cognitive impairment, a psychosocial dysfunction, a mental illness a developmental or learning disability, or an adverse environmental condition. (American Medical Association. [1995]. *Allied health education directory* [23rd ed., p. 125]. Chicago, IL: Author.)
1999	The "Practice of Occupational Therapy" means the therapeutic use of purposeful and meaningful occupations (goal directed activities) to evaluate and treat individuals who have a disease or disorder, impairment, activity limitation, or participation restriction which interferes with their ability to function independently in daily life roles, and to promote health and wellness. (Definition of OT practice for the AOTA Model Practice Act. *OT Week, 13*[32], iii.)

or vegetative state, or others with limited communication skills? Without clarifying the term purposeful activity, the definitions seemed to lack clarity of thought. Two definitions avoided the issues of purposeful activity by focusing on other objectives. The revised Essentials (AOTA, 1991) maintained the definition from 1971, which stated that "occupational therapy is the art and science of directing an individual's participation in selected tasks" and that use of the term occupation refers to the "individuals' goal-directed use of time, energy, interest, and attention" Overall, the definition provides a concise and understandable description of occupational therapy. The other definition that avoided the term purposeful activity was created as part of a discussion of the functions of the Foundation in 1993. The phrase used to describe occupational therapy is "the reasoned use of occupation to assist people in adapting...." Use of the term reasoned focuses on the rationale or frame of reference for selecting an occupation or occupations and suggests there may be theoretical base for why and how specific occupations are selected for individual clients.

Models of Practice

Table 9-2 lists the models of practice during the 1990s. A significant change is apparent in the organization of concepts. Several of the models are organized around similar themes of person, environment, and occupation (PEO). A person may be expressed as client, patient, resident, student, worker, homemaker, retiree, or other identifier. Environment may be expressed as context, place, space, room, workplace, workstation, indoors, outdoors, or other descriptor. Occupation may be labeled as activity, activities, tasks, activities of daily living, instrumental activities of daily living, work, job, employment, homemaking, chores, play, leisure, rest and sleep, or other term specifying an occupation. The outcome from the occupational therapy perspective related to attainment or improvement in occupational role performance and/or satisfaction with quality of life. The emphasis was dependent on the focus of the model. Some models were viewed as overviews or grand models that focused on occupational therapy practice in general but provided few details on specific techniques or strategies for intervention. Other models focused on a specific area of practice of practice such as play and tended to provide more detail for intervention.

Table 9-2
EXAMPLES OF MODELS OF PRACTICE PUBLISHED FROM 1990-1999

YEAR	MODEL OF PRACTICE	REFERENCE
1991	Person–environment–occupational performance model	Christiansen, C., & Baum, C. (1990). Occupational therapy: intervention for life performance. In C. Christensen & C. Baum (Eds.), *Occupational therapy: Overcoming human performance deficits* (pp. 4-43). Thorofare, NJ: SLACK Incorporated.
1992	Occupational adaptation	Schkade, J. K., & Schulz, S. (1992). Occupational adaptation: Toward a holistic approach for contemporary practice. Part 1. *American Journal of Occupational Therapy, 46*(9), 829-837.
1992	Multicontext treatment approach	Toglia, J. P. (1992). A dynamic interactional approach to cognitive rehabilitation. In: N. Katz (Ed.), Cognitive rehabilitation: Models for intervention in occupational therapy (pp. 104-143). Boston, MA: Andover Medical Publishers.
1994	Ecology of human performance	Dunn, W., Brown, C., & McGuigan, A. (1994). The ecology of human performance: A framework for considering the effect of context. *American Journal of Occupational Therapy, 48*, 597-607.
1995	Model of occupational functioning	Trombly, C. A. (!995). Occupation: Purposefulness and meaningfulness in therapeutic mechanisms. 1995 Eleanor Clarke Slagle lecture. *American Journal of Occupational Therapy, 49*(10), 960-972.
1996	Person–environment–occupation model	Law, M., Cooper, B., Strong, S., et al. (1994). The Person–Environment–Occupational model: A transactive approach to occupational performance. *Canadian Journal of Occupational Therapy, 65*(1), 9-23.
1997	Playfulness	Bundy, A. C. (2007). Play and playfulness: What to look for. In L. D. Parham & L. S. Fazio (Eds.), *Play in occupational therapy for children* (pp. 52-66). St. Louis, MO: Mosby.

Encroachment and Licensure Laws

AOTA increased lobbying assistance to states to protect occupational therapy licensure laws, including monitoring, analysis, consultation, and development of lobbying materials.

In 1997, the American Physical Therapy Association (APTA) published the *Guide to Physical Therapist Practice* (APTA, 1997), which was revised in 1999 (APTA, 1999). The Association responded in an article in *OT Week* (AOTA, 1998c). Terminology was one issue. To physical therapy, the concept of money management meant the ability to physically manipulate coins, whereas to occupational therapy, money management included tasks such as budgeting and paying bills. Differences are explained in the white paper published in *OT Week* (Foto, 1998).

Another problem was the expansion of scope of practice to include functional training in self-care, home management, and community or work integration (APTA, 1999, pp. 1-2). The Association was concerned that the definition did not sufficiently define the limited context in which physical therapy intervention addressed patient need and could inappropriately encroach on the traditional domain of occupational therapy.

The Model Practice Act for Physical Therapy approved by the Federation of State Boards of Physical Therapy (FSBPT; APTA, 1999) included four sections: (1) examining; (2) alleviating impairment and functional limitation; (3) preventing injury, impairment, functional limitation, and disability; and (4) engaging in consultation, education, and research. The Association was primarily concerned with the second section on alleviating impairment and functional limitation, which included two statements that read "function training in self-care and home management (including activities of daily living and instrumental activities of daily living)" and "functional training in community and work (job/school/play) integration or reintegration activities (including instrumental activities of daily living, work hardening, and work conditioning)" (APTA, 1999, pp. 1-2). The Association suggested the words "in physical movement and mobility" be added after words "functional limitation" (AOTA, 1999/2000).

AOTA voiced concern about the unqualified expansion of physical therapy scope of practice because the expansion was not supported by education and training of physical therapists. A review of the educational standards for occupational and physical therapy confirmed fundamental differences in education. The occupational therapy Standards specifically require students to have a broad-based knowledge of behavioral sciences, whereas in the physical therapy Evaluative Criteria, behavioral sciences are suggested. Human development is fundamental to the entire program in occupational therapy, but there is no standard requiring study of human development in the physical Evaluative Criteria. Training in evaluation and intervention techniques is similar, but the foundation for understanding and applying the evaluations and interventions beyond the biomechanical aspects or in context of the client's roles and environment is absent (AOTA, 1999/2000).

Managed Care

Technically managed care is not a new concept but an evolving concept that integrates financial resource management with the actual cost of providing specific patient care services. Over the years, the two concepts were separate. Patients received services, and facilities received payments. The payments did not actually reflect the cost of providing the patient service because other factors such as overhead and pro bono or free care were lumped into the payment received by the facility. The real cost of providing services for a person who had had a stroke, for example, was not known nor considered important to know. As costs rose, beginning in the 1970s, insurance providers were dealing with higher costs and pressure not to raise premiums. Various techniques were tried, including prehospitalization certification, requiring second opinions before surgery, and utilization review (Christiansen, 1996). More recent techniques have been added, including preferred provider organizations (PPOs) and health maintenance organizations (HMOs). PPOs are networks of facilities with providers who discount fees in exchange for a larger volume of patient referrals because their names are listed in the insurance carrier's list of approved providers. HMOs are characterized by comprehensive benefit packages, prepaid premiums, and integrate health care delivery and insuring components (Christiansen, 1996). Rehabilitation programs were especially difficult to determine actual costs of care because the process often occurred over several months or years and may involve multiple interrelated diagnoses such as diabetes and hypertension leading to a stroke—all of which must be managed using different approaches.

LEGISLATION

Table 9-3 summarizes the legislation related to occupational therapy that was adopted during the 1990s. The most significant legislation was the adoption of the American with Disabilities Act (ADA) in 1990, the amendments to the Individuals with Disabilities Education Act (IDEA) (new name for Education for the Handicapped Act), and the Balanced Budget Act (BBA) of

| Table 9-3 |
| LEGISLATION |

1990	Americans with Disabilities Act (P.L. 101-336). Civil rights protection to persons with disabilities in all goods, services, facilities (including those that are not funded/operated by the government). Equal opportunity is the key, not equal treatment. Employers cannot discriminate. Reasonable Modifications. "Readily achievable" standard and on opportunity to help facilities and organizations achieve to become/remain ADA compliant. (Reed, 1992; Van Slyke, 2001)
1990	Individuals with Disabilities Education Act of 1990 (IDEA) (P.L. 101-476). Enforced services provided by Part H & Part B of the Education of Handicapped Act of 1986, focusing on the importance of prevention instead of remediation. Deficiencies IDEA funding exist. (Van Slyke, 2001; Cottrell, 2005)
1991	Alcohol, Drug Abuse and Mental Health Administration (ADAMHA) Re-Organization Act (P.L. 102-321). Amends the Title V of public health service Act to revise and restructure alcohol, drug, abuse, and mental health administration. (Van Slyke, 2001)
1991	Individuals with Disabilities Education Act Amendments (P.L. 102-119). Reauthorized early intervention and established the Interagency Coordinating council for each state to establish a comprehensive system of early intervention services. (Baloueff & Cohn, 2003)
1992	Rehabilitation Act Amendments (P.O. 102-569). Provides for transition planning of high school graduates including coordination of assistive technology and rehabilitation services. (Baloueff & Cohn, 2003)
1994	School-to-Work Opportunities Act (P.L. 103-239). Provides school-to-work transition systems to prepare students to move into the workforce. (Baloueff & Cohn, 2003)
1994	Head Start Reauthorization Act (P.L. 103-252). Created Early Head Start for infants and toddlers in low income families, including young children with disabilities. (Baloueff & Cohn, 2003)
1996	Health Insurance Portability and Accountability Act (P.L. 104-191). Regulates the use and disclosure of protected health information. (Lohman, 2014)
1997	Individuals with Disabilities Education Act Amendments (IDEA) (P.L. 108-446). Strength accountability for education of children with disabilities. Occupational therapy provided under this act as a related service. (Baloueff & Cohn, 2003; Lohman, 2014)

(continued)

Table 9-3 (continued)
LEGISLATION

Year	
1997	Balanced Budget Act (P.L. 105-33). Legislation to control health care costs. Reduced occupational therapy position, reduced occupational therapy applications, and several programs closed. A prospective payment system for home health was started in 2000. Medicare Part A prospective payment plan for Skilled Nursing Facilities was scheduled to begin in 1999. Caps on Part B outpatient rehabilitation services ($1500 for physical therapy and speech combined, occupational therapy separate). Established prospective payment systems in inpatient rehab units. (Lohman, 2014)
1997	Children's Health Insurance Program (CHIP) (P.L. 111-3). Provide insurance for children who do not qualify for Medicaid but cannot afford private insurance. It is jointly funded by the states and the federal government. (Lohman, 2014)
1998	Assistive Technology Act (P.L. 108-364). Provides definitions for assistive devices and clarifies the services provided. (Schoonover, Grove, & Swinth, 2010)
1999	Olmstead decision by Supreme Court. Ruled states must place clients in community settings instead of institutions if appropriate. Services and activities for persons with disabilities must be provided in the most integrated setting appropriate to needs of qualified individuals. (Cottrell, 2005)
1999	The Ticket to Work Incentives Improvement Act (P.L. 106-170). Removed disincentives to employment for people with disabilities. Program is administered by the Social Security Administration. (Cottrell, 2005)

References

Baloueff, O., & Cohn, E. S. (2003). Introduction to the infant, child and adolescent population. In E. B. Crepeau, E. S. Cohn, & B. A. Boyt Schell (Eds.), *Willard & Spackman's occupational therapy* (10th ed., pp. 691-698). Philadelphia, PA: Lippincott Williams & Wilkins.

Cottrell, R. P. F. (2005). The Olmstead decision: Landmark opportunity or platform for rhetoric? Our collective responsibility for full community participation. *American Journal of Occupational Therapy, 59*(5), 561-568.

Lohman, H. (2014). Payment for services in the United States. In B. A. Boyt Schell, G. Gillen, & M. E. Scaffa (Eds.), *Willard & Spackman's occupational therapy* (12th ed., pp. 1051-1067). Philadelphia, PA: Wolters Kluwer.

Reed, K. L. (1992). History of federal legislation for persons with disabilities. *American Journal of Occupational Therapy, 46*(5), 397-408.

Schoonover, J., Grove, R. E. A., & Swinth, Y. (2010). Influencing participation through assistive technology. In J. Case-Smith & J. C. O'Brien (Eds.), *Occupational therapy for children* (6th ed., pp. 583-619). St. Louis, MO: Mosby/Elsevier.

Van Slyke, N. (2001). Legislation and policy issues. In M. Scaffa (Ed.), *Occupational therapy in community-based practice settings* (pp. 85-94). Philadelphia, PA: Davis.

1997. One Supreme Court decision (Olmstead) is also listed because it required clients to be placed in the community rather than in institutions, further supporting the movement toward deinstitutionalization.

TECHNOLOGY

During the 1990s, technology improvements increased the use of occupational therapy services. Examples are seen here in the Figures. Figure 9-1 shows a therapists working with a client wearing an Ilizarov external fixator designed to lengthen her arm by slowly stretching her bone and tissues. The client had had an infection as a small child, which limited growth in her arm. The therapist is monitoring motion and strength as the procedure progresses. Figures 9-2 and 9-3

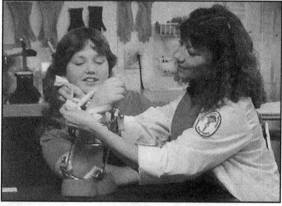

Figure 9-1. Ilizarov external fixator. (Printed with permission from the Archive of the American Occupational Therapy Association, Inc.)

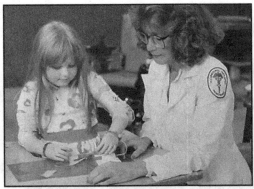

Figure 9-2. A child learning to use a prosthesis. (Printed with permission from the Archive of the American Occupational Therapy Association, Inc.)

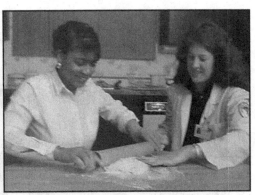

Figure 9-3. An adult learning to use a prosthesis. (Printed with permission from the Archive of the American Occupational Therapy Association, Inc.)

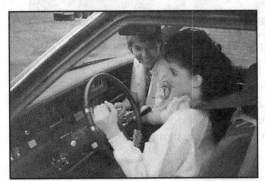

Figure 9-4. A client with a congenital amputation learning to drive. (Printed with permission from the Archive of the American Occupational Therapy Association, Inc.)

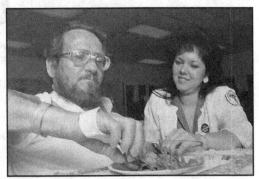

Figure 9-5. A client learning to use adapted eating devices. (Printed with permission from the Archive of the American Occupational Therapy Association, Inc.)

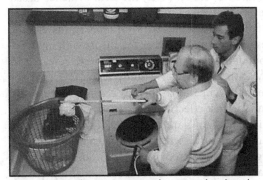

Figure 9-6. A client using a reacher to grab a laundry item. (Printed with permission from the Archive of the American Occupational Therapy Association, Inc.)

show a child and an adult with prosthetic limbs designed to look as natural as possible but still provide motion and function. Both clients are practicing using their prostheses to perform everyday occupations under the guidance of the occupational therapist. Figure 9-4 shows a client with a congenital amputation learning to manage the adaptive driving devices that will allow her drive independently.

Not all technology is high tech, requiring advanced electronics to operate the desired functions. Figure 9-5 shows a client wearing a cuff that allows devices such as a form or spoon to be inserted because the client does not have enough hand strength to hold the eating utensil without assistance. There is also a clear plastic plate guard attached to the edge of the plate to keep food from being spilled off the edge as the client scoops up the pieces of salad against the plate rail. Another low-tech device called a reacher is shown in Figure 9-6 being used to retrieve items from the laundry basket and place them in the washing machine without having to bend over or lose the support provided by the walker. Yet another low-tech device is the mouth stick shown in Figure 9-7 that allows the client to paint or draw as a leisure activity.

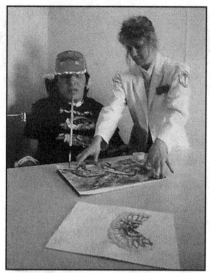

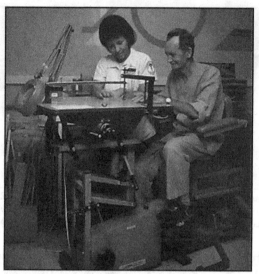

Figure 9-7. A client using a mouth stick to paint. (Printed with permission from the Archive of the American Occupational Therapy Association, Inc.)

Figure 9-8. A client using a bicycle jigsaw. (Printed with permission from the Archive of the American Occupational Therapy Association, Inc.)

Finally, not all technology is new. Figure 9-8 shows a client using a bicycle jigsaw, with which reciprocal movement of the feet power the motion of the jigsaw blade. Bicycle-powered jigsaws were used during World War I to increase motion of the lower extremities while the client guided a piece of wood to be cut by jigsaw blade.

RESEARCH

Outcomes research designed to determine the efficacy and efficiency of services such as occupational therapy became a major focus of research in 1990s. Later, the term evidence-based practice would evolve. Steib (1999) summarized several outcomes studies relevant to occupational therapy practice, including reducing the risk of falling, increasing survival rates in the elderly, reducing disability in people who have had strokes, improving outcomes for clients with hip fractures, and reducing hospitalization costs. The Foundation began funding outcomes research in 1994 (AOTF, 1996a). Among the studies funded was the Well Elderly Study at the University of Southern California. The study provided evidence that occupational therapy can improve quality of life for older individuals living independently and is cost effective. The results were published in the Journal of the American Medical Association (JAMA; Clark et al., 1997). In addition, the materials used in the study were published in a manual published by the Association (Mandel, Jackson, Zemke, Nelson, & Clark, 1999). Seven organizations were involved in funding the study, including three government and four private—a fact that speaks to the cost of conducting quality research projects.

ASSOCIATION

National Office Organization

Bair (1991) stated that there were 120 full-time employees working in the national office. Twenty-one employees were occupational therapists. The national office was reorganized into five units—professional development, finance and operations, marketing, professional resources, and professional relations—in addition to the Director's office (Bair, 1992). The national office moved from 1383 Piccard Drive in Rockville, Maryland, to 4720 Montgomery Lane in Bethesda, Maryland, in November 1994 (Figure 9-9). The building has 13 floors and allowed all Association activities to be housed under one roof. In 1998, the Association created the State Policy Department to increase the capacity to monitor and intervene in state practice act issues, especially encroachment.

Association Presidents

Four people served as President of AOTA during the 1990s: Ann P. Grady, 1989-1992 (Figure 9-10); Mary M. Evert, 1992-1995 (Figure 9-11); Mary Foto, 1995-1998 (Figure 9-12); and Karen Jacobs, 1998-2001 (Figure 9-13). Their accomplishments are summarized in Table 9-4. Biographical sketches appear in Table 9-5. Figure 9-14 shows a group photograph of past Presidents, including Ruth Brunyate-Wiemer, Robert K. Bing, Jerry A. Johnson, Florence S. Cromwell, Elnora M. Gilfoyle, Carolyn M. Baum, Ruth A. Robinson, and Wilma L. West.

Mission and Vision Statements

Figure 9-9. Association National Office, Montgomery Lane, Bethesda, Maryland. (Printed with permission from the Archive of the American Occupational Therapy Association, Inc.)

A mission statement was adopted in 1993 by the Executive Board. It reads: "The American Occupational Therapy Association advances the quality, availability, use, and support of occupational therapy through standard-setting, advocacy, education, and research on behalf of its members and the public" (AOTA, 1993a). The purpose was to guide the development of strategic planning by creating major focus areas. Examples are seen in the Strategic Plan for the years 1993 to 1996 (AOTA, 1994b).

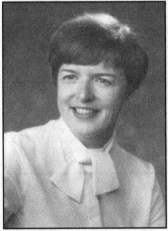

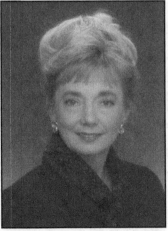

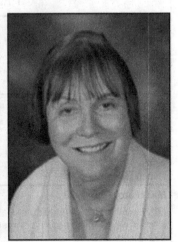

Figure 9-10. Ann P. Grady, PhD, OTR, FAOTA, President of AOTA, 1989-1992. (Printed with permission from the Archive of the American Occupational Therapy Association, Inc.)

Figure 9-11. Mary M. Evert, MBA, OTR, FAOTA, President of AOTA, 1992-1995. (Printed with permission from the Archive of the American Occupational Therapy Association, Inc.)

Figure 9-12. Mary Foto, OTR, FAOTA, President of AOTA, 1995-1998. (Printed with permission from the Archive of the American Occupational Therapy Association, Inc.)

- Goal 1: Professional Development: AOTA will promote the development and integration of occupational therapy practice, education, and research, to further enhance and promote the profession. Clarifying Statement: There is an inextricable linkage among practice, education, and research with each component interdependent and equally valued.

- Goal II: Serves the Interest of Members: AOTA will develop programs and services which address member needs and promote member recruitment and retention. Clarifying Statement: Members will perceive that they have greater access to AOTA resources which meet their needs and enable them to promote the profession.

- Goals III: Support the Professional Community: AOTA will increase mutually beneficial relationships and partnerships and state associations to enhance the professional community. Clarifying Statement: The Association must be proactive in confronting societal changes such as consumerism, education reform, health care reform, and the independent living movement.

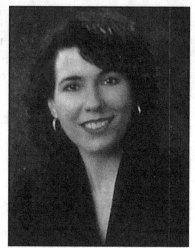

Figure 9-13. Karen Jacobs, EdD, OTR/L, CPE, FAOTA, President of AOTA, 1998-2001. (Printed with permission from the Archive of the American Occupational Therapy Association, Inc.)

- Goal IV: External Relations and Access to Occupational Therapy: AOTA will develop programs to address external factors that impact the profession and the availability of occupational therapy services to the consumer.

In 1998, the Executive Board adopted a vision statement to accompany the mission statement. The vision statement reads, "AOTA advances occupational therapy as the preeminent profession

Table 9-4
PRESIDENTIAL ACCOMPLISHMENTS

Ann P. Grady, 1989-1992

Major accomplishment: National office undertook a major reorganization to streamline operations.

Quotation: "AOTA has provided a community for OT practitioners and leadership for the profession as a whole. As we move toward our 100th anniversary, the Association and the members will play key roles in shaping health care in America." (AOTA. [1992]. AOTA's Hall of leaders. *OT Week, 6*[21], 40-43.)

Mary M. Evert, 1992-1995

Major accomplishment: Focus on building a sense of community among occupational therapy practitioners.

Quotation: "Ahead I see many OT practitioners as pivotal leaders in community-based teams of professionals and community members who advocate and implement programs for healthier life-styles and disease prevention, and for full community integration of people with functional limitations." (AOTA. [1992]. AOTA's Hall of leaders. *OT Week, 6*[21], 40-43.).

Mary Foto, 1995-1998

OT Week was discontinued due to lack of advertisers. *OT Practice* started in November 1995 to focus on practice issues. Major accomplishment during Foto's term was the focus on reimbursement for occupational therapy services.

Karen Jacobs, 1998-2001

Association retrenches as membership decreased in response to concern over implications of the Balanced Budget Act. The *American Journal of Occupational Therapy* returned to bimonthly publication. Major accomplishments during Jacobs' term were the Back Pack initiative and focus on increased consumer and public awareness of occupational therapy as a profession.

Table 9-5
PRESIDENTIAL BIOGRAPHICAL SKETCHES

ANN PATRICIA GRADY

April 28, 1935–March 18, 2012

Born in New Haven, Connecticut. She graduated from the College of New Rochelle with a bachelor's degree in sociology. She received a certificate in occupational therapy for Columbia university, a master's degree from the University of Denver and a doctoral degree in human communications from the University of Denver. She began her career at Newington Children's Hospital in Newington, Connecticut. She moved to Colorado to work as the director of the occupational Therapy Department at the Children's Hospital in Denver where she worked from 1966 to 1993. She also taught in the graduate programs at Colorado State University and the University of Colorado, Department of Pediatrics. She was president of the Association from 1989-1992, speaker of the Representative Assembly from 1977-1979, vice-president from 1987-1989 and also served as vice president of the American Occupational Therapy Foundation and was chairperson of its Research Development Committee. She received the Eleanor Clarke Slagle lectureship in 1994, the Award of Merit in 2000, and was named a Fellow in 1979 She also received the AOTF's Meritorious Service award. With Elnora Gilfoyle and Josephine C. Moore, PhD, OTR, FAOTA she coauthored two editions of *Children Adapt: A Theory of Sensorimotor Development* published by Slack, Inc. and the book *Mentoring Leaders* with Gilfoyle and Nielson published by AOTA Press. Her passion was family-centered care but she was also interest in leadership and mentoring.

MARY MARGARET KUSZEWSKI EVERT

Born February 5, 1945

A California native, Mary received her B.S. degree from the College of St. Catherine in 1967. She also has a MBA in Health Care Administration from National University in San Diego, CA, 1980 and an honorary doctor of science degree. She was a staff therapist at Rancho Los Amigo Hospital from 1968-70 and was OT Supervisor at Children's Hospital in San Diego. During the Reagan administration she worked for the federal government in the U.S. Department of Health and Human Services. . She owns a consulting business in California. She was president of the Association from 1992-95, served as Speaker of the Representative Assembly and was elected delegate to the World Federation of Occupational Therapists. She has also served as president of the California Occupational Therapy association and has been a member of California licensing board. She was named to the Roster of Fellows in 1984 and received the Award of Merit in 2000. She married Richard Evert and has a son.

MARY ELIZABETH SMITH

Born September 1, 1941

Mary was born in Iowa Falls, Iowa but her family moved to California when she was a child. She graduated from University of Southern California in 1966 with an undergraduate degree in occupational therapy. She is also a certified case manager. She serves as chief executive officer of two companies. The Foto Group, Inc. provides non-physician peer medical review and support system and Treat-it.com a software documentation and practice management package for non-physician rehabilitation and technology providers. She served as president from 1995-98 and was named to the Roster of Fellows in 1989. She has also chaired the Tri-Alliance of Therapy Professions and Coalition of Rehabilitation Therapies and has served on the AOTF Board. She is a member of the Occupational Therapy association of California in which she has held many positions and received the Award of Merit in 2008. She married Stephen Anthony Foto and has a daughter. She enjoys skiing.

KAREN JACOBS

Born January 15, 1951

Born in Massachusetts. She has a bachelor of arts in psychology from Washington University in 1973, a master's of science in occupational therapy from Boston University in 1979 and a doctorate in education in Educational Leadership in Schooling from the University of Massachusetts in 1993. She has served the Association as vice-president and president. She was named to the Roster of Fellows in 1988, received the Eleanor Clarke Slagle lectureship award in 2011 and the Award of Merit in 2003. She has also received the Award of Merit from the Canadian Association of Occupational Therapists and was a recipient of the J. William Fulbright Foreign Scholarship award in 2005. She is the founding editor of the interdisciplinary and international journal *Work: A Journal of Prevention, Assessment and Rehabilitation* and is the author of *Ergonomics for Therapists and Occupational Therapy: Work-Related Programs and Assessments* and coeditor of *Quick Reference Dictionary for Occupational Therapy, Occupational Therapy Essentials for Clinical Competence,* and *Occupational Therapy Manager,* 4th edition.

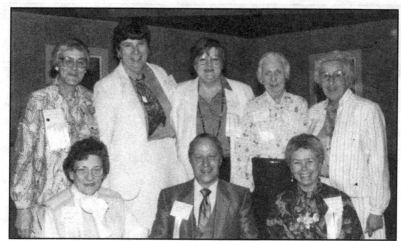

Figure 9-14. AOTA Presidents. From left to right: (standing) Florence Cromwell, Elnora Gilfoyle, Carolyn Baum, Ruth Robinson, Wilma West; (sitting) Ruth Brunyate Wiemer, Robert Bing, Jerry A. Johnson. (Printed with permission from the Archive of the American Occupational Therapy Association, Inc.)

in promoting the health, productivity, and quality of life of individuals and society through the therapeutic application of occupation" (AOTA, 1998a). This statement added criteria for developing goals.

Specialty and Board Certification Programs

The Specialty Certification Program was formalized in 1994 with a bylaws change that formed the Specialty Certification Board as a standing committee of the Executive Board (AOTA, 1995a). Specialty certification in pediatrics had begun ahead of the formal development of the Specialty Certification Board and had already developed criteria (AOTA, 1994a). The second certification was in neurorehabilitation. Initially the certification programs were for therapists but were then expanded to include assistants.

Special Interest Sections

The new Special Interest Sections (SIS) approved by Executive Board during the 1990s were the Education, Technology, Home and Community Health, and School Systems. The total number of SIS groups was now 11. The Education section provides opportunities for academicians, new faculty, fieldwork supervisors, clinicians, and students to discuss the many issues involved in occupational therapy education. This SIS provides a forum to address the art and science of teaching at all levels of occupational therapy education, as well as developments in research.

The Technology SIS provides information on the latest clinical and research technology. The section considers innovations that enhance therapy from low to high tech. It also provides a forum for continuing education and facilitates networking among all areas of practice relating to technology.

The Home and Community Health SIS provides members with networking on special clinical consideration and are advised on current legislation and regulatory and employment issues. The section conducts education programs, maintains a network of state leaders in home health, and provides an ongoing newsletter. The group also consults with academic programs on home health–specific curriculum.

The School Systems SIS is dedicated to addressing the needs of school-based practitioners to provide educationally related serves to infants, preschoolers, children, and adolescents. This SIS promotes education, research, legislation, and policy making that will enhance practice in the school systems and community (AOTA, 1994a).

Uniform Terminology for Occupational Therapy, Third Edition

In 1994, the Uniform Terminology document was revised for the third time (AOTA, 1994b). The Third Edition was expanded to reflect current practice and to incorporate contextual aspects of performance in addition to the performance areas and performance components used to organize terms in the Second Edition (AOTA, 1994c). Overall, the number of terms listed, defined, or described increased from 109 to 122. The performance areas included 37 terms, the performance components 75 terms, and the performance contexts 10 terms. The three performance areas remained essentially the same as those in the Second Edition: activities of daily living, work and productive activities, and play or leisure activities. The performance component remained the same: sensory, cognitive, and psychosocial. The performance components that were added were divided in temporal aspects and environment.

According to the President's report in 1993, the AOTA Board of Directors initially declined the invitation of the American Physical Therapy Association (APTA) to establish a joint occupational therapy/physical therapy committee to write a white paper identifying the commonalities and differences between the two professions. The focus, intent, and potential uses of the proposed paper were not clear to members of the AOTA Board, and APTA's Board of Directors was asked to provide further clarification (AOTA, 1993a, p. 3). As stated in the white paper's Preamble, the APTA House of Delegates charged the APTA Board of Directors in 1992 to develop a document with AOTA "to identify areas of commonalities and differences affecting the professions of physical therapy and occupational therapy … to include … needs of society, scope of practice, education, marketing, and reimbursement" (APTA, 1994, p. 1). The target audience was identified as members of both professions and as parties external to the two professions. The internal context of use was specifically at the chapter (physical therapy) level as an educational tool to provide basic, factual information about the two professions. The need for collaboration was acknowledged by members of both Associations as affecting four perspectives: higher education, community based practice, institution based clinical practice, and health care administration. After clarifying concerns, AOTA's Board charged the President to appoint representatives to the PT/OT Task Force, and task force members were appointed. The AOTA Executive Board reviewed the final draft of the paper in March 1994 (AOTA, 1994d). Much of the paper is a summary of issues common to both professions, including a short history, employment demographics, number and ethnicity of practitioners, education and accreditation, licensure, definitions of practice, codes of ethics, role delineation, health care reform, research, and public awareness. Two points of discussion are of special interest: physical agent modalities and the concept of function.

Under scope of practice, reference is made to a dispute between physical and occupational therapy regarding the "ownership" of "therapeutic procedures or activities," especially in relationship to the use of physical agent modalities and functional activities. A statement clarifying the issue is as follows:

Both APTA and AOTA believe that a procedure or activity is neither physical therapy nor occupational therapy in and of itself. Instead, it is the knowledge and appropriate use and integration of the procedure or activity into the therapeutic plan of care that is paramount. (APTA, 1994, p. 19)

This statement is an acknowledgement by both professions that supplies, equipment, media, and modalities are not "owned" by either profession, or any other profession. What is "owned" is the specific knowledge and skill integrated into therapeutic plan of care. The clarification helped solve disputes in preparing and revising licensure laws in which physical agent modalities were referred as a category or by specific name. Occupational therapy licensure laws could include reference to physical agent modalities also listed in physical therapy licensure laws. Education, however, was another matter. In the document, APTA's Board of Directors maintains that "all non-physical therapist providers who use physical agent modalities/electrotherapy devices should meet the same minimum educational preparation standards as physical therapists and that licensure and regulatory requirements should also take into account these competences" (APTA, 1994, p. 20). This statement does not take into account that another profession might be using the same modality with a different goal in mind, which may require a different set of knowledge and skills.

The concept of function as used within the profession of occupational therapy is described as follows:

> The capacity of individuals to engage in daily occupational of self-care, work, and play/leisure in a manner that enables them to derive satisfaction and meaning in their lives…. Function represents occupational performance, which is both a core value and a central concern of the occupational therapy profession. (APTA, 1994, p. 20)

The ideas regarding the concept of function were further refined in the position paper adopted and published the following year, which includes a historical review of the concept of function in the development of occupational therapy practice (AOTA, 1995d).

Physical Agent Modalities Issue

In 1990, Pedretti and Pasquinell proposed a solution to dilemma of whether the concept of purposeful activity is broad enough to encompass of the therapeutic potential of the profession. They suggested that occupational therapy intervention could be viewed as a continuum of four stages within an occupational performance frame of reference. At the lowest stage would be adjunctive methods, followed by enabling activities, then purposeful activities, and occupational performance and community reintegration. Adjunctive methods would include "procedures that prepare the patient for occupational performance but are preliminary to the use of the performance skills" (Pedretti & Pasquinelli, 1990, pp. 3-4). Ayres had suggested the same or similar idea in 1958. She defined purposeful motor function as follows:

> … use of the motor system as a means toward accomplishing a goal which is inherent in the nature of the activity demanding the function. These goals are separate from but vital to the therapeutic objectives involving range of motion, coordination, endurance, strength, use of the prosthetic or orthotic device, or performance of activities of daily living. (p. 300)

Pedretti and Pasquinelli (1990) suggested the procedures may include "exercise, facilitation and inhibition techniques, positioning, splinting, sensory stimulation, and selected physical modalities" (p. 4). The focus of intervention is most likely concerned with assessing and remediating performance components or skills that will be needed later for to achieve occupational performance in activities of daily living. The second stage of enabling activities is again based on Ayres and is defined as those that have "an autonomous or inherent goal beyond the motor function required to perform the task" (Pedretti & Pasquinelli, 1990, p. 4). Examples of such media are "sanding boards, stacking cones or blocks, practice boards for mastery of clothing fasteners and hardware, driving and work simulators, and tabletop activities such as pegboards for training perceptual-motor skills" (Pedretti & Pasquinelli, 1990, p. 4). Stage three includes purposeful activities that have an inherent or autonomous goal and are relevant and meaningful to the client. Examples are feeding, hygiene, dressing, mobility, communion, arts, crafts, games, sports, and work activities. Stage four includes resuming the occupational roles associated with self-care, work, education, and play or leisure performance by the client to maximum level of independence. This stage or levels approach became a workable solution to incorporating physical agent modalities into the scheme of acceptable intervention modalities within the practice of occupational therapy.

The Representative Assembly adopted a position paper on physical agent modality in 1991. The issue was controversial. Some members felt that physical agents should not be part of the modalities used by occupational therapists. The following year, two resolutions sought to rescind or modify the statement adopted in 1991. Both were rejected because members, especially in hand therapy, were already using physical agent modalities and state regulations permitted such use (Joe, 1992).

Cross-Training and Multiskilling

In 1991, the Representative Assembly initiated a charge to study issues related to personnel (other than occupational therapy practitioners) who provided occupational therapy services (Hansen, 1995). The main focus was initially on the use of aides to provide occupational therapy services. Two documents were prepared in subsequent years: Service Delivery in Occupational Therapy (AOTA, 1995c) and Use of Occupational Therapy Aides in Occupational Therapy Practice (AOTA, 1995e). At issue was the pressure by stakeholders in the health care industry for service delivery personnel to be more accountable and more cost effective. As Edward O'Neil, Executive Director of the Pew Health Professions Commission, stated in 1996, "We're not suggesting [the Pew recommendations] happen as a preemptive strike against OT to force it into cross-training" (Hettinger, 1996). However, the Pew commission was suggesting that occupational therapy practitioners and other allied health professionals would be considered more valuable to the health care system if they could carry out more functions. To that end, practitioners were being asked to provide services that might be considered outside their scope of practice, such as occupational therapy practitioners being trained to perform gait training or individuals being educated at entry level to be multiskilled practitioners capable of assuming multiple roles and duties in health care delivery, such as a person being educated as both an occupational therapist and a physical therapist (Hansen, 1995).

A white paper was written in 1995 on occupational therapy and cross-training (AOTA, 1995f). It discussed issues related to practitioners educated in occupational therapy providing services, not aides or on-the-job trained personnel. Cross-training was defined as "the preparation of an individual in one profession to perform skills (and tasks) typically associated with another profession" (AOTA, 1995f, p. 32; AOTA, 1997d, p. 854). A practitioner was defined as "an individual who is a graduate of an accredited occupational therapy preprogram and is certified" (AOTA, 1995f, p. 32). A multiskilled practitioner was defined as "an individual from one profession who has established competence in specific skills usually associated with another profession" (AOTA, 1995f, p. 32). Occupational therapy practitioners were asked to consider the following questions in relations to cross-training initiatives:

- Does the individual to be trained have the potential to achieve competency in the skill to be delegated (background knowledge and/or experience)?
- Will the trainer and the trainee be given adequate time and resources for training?
- Will appropriate supervision be available?
- Is there any state regulation or institutional policy that prohibits the assignment of this skill to another individual?
- Would participation in the proposed initiate result in a violation the profession's code of ethics or standards of practice?
- Will the trainee accept legal responsibility for performance of the skill once training is completed?
- Will the trainer accept legal responsibility of any services delegated to the trainee?

Perhaps a more important question was whether occupational therapy practitioners were seen as staff workers with a potential extra pair of hands to walk patients or change light bulbs or whether they were seen as having educated intellectual skills designed to help clients solve problems in everyday living. The hands-on nature of many aspects of occupational therapy services may lead those not trained in health care services to think the hands are the service rather than the brain that directs the hands. According to an article by Collins (1997), there was a need to clarify the terms to determine how multiskilling and cross-training would be taught in educational programs and how such personnel would be used in practice. However, the TriAlliance (1995) saw no need to study the issue further because it did not support the concept of clinical multiskilled personnel at either the professional or assistant levels. According to the TriAlliance, audiologists, occupational therapists, physical therapists, and speech-language pathologists have distinct and separate philosophical, educational, and scientific foundations. Asking them to act as multiskilled personnel at the professional or assistant level "is likely to result in unacceptable levels of risk or potential negligence that could result in harm to, or poor outcomes, for the recipient of services (TriAlliance, 1996, p. 17). Nonetheless, the Association proceeded to produce a Cross-Training Concept paper (AOTA, 1997d) outlining in detail the basic premises of cross-training; the advantages and disadvantages of cross-training for the client, occupational therapy practitioners, and administrators; factors to consider when implementing a cross-training program; and strategies for dealing with the changing health care environment. This paper seems to answer all the questions because the issue of cross-training stops appearing in the occupational therapy literature.

Skilled Versus Nonskilled Services and Medicare

The discussion of cross training and multiskilling is germane to the discussion of skilled occupational therapy services and nonskilled or caregiving services. Reimbursement under Medicare requires that skilled occupational therapy services be provided. Nonskilled services are not reimbursable. Skilled occupational therapy was defined as follows:

> ... occupational therapist modifies the specific activity by using adapted equipment, making changes in the environment and surrounding objects, altering procedures for accomplishing the task, and providing specialized assistance to meet the client's current and potential abilities. Skilled services include, but are not limited to, reasonable and necessary:
> - Evaluation of the client
> - Determination of effective goals and services with the client, family, caregiver, or other medical professional
> - Analysis and modification of functional tasks
> - Provision of task instruction(s) to the client, family, or caregiver
> - Periodic reevaluation of the client's status, with corresponding readjustment of the occupational therapy program (Health Care Financing Administration, n.d.)

Foto (1996a) quotes from a letter she received in 1992 to explain the conceptual framework that defines skilled service as those requiring the "knowledge, skills, and judgement of a therapist for the treatment and amelioration of impairment and disabilities caused by a medical condition." Knowledge involves a course of academic preparation specifically related to the services requires by the medical conditions. Skills are a specific array of technical assessment and treatment intervention appropriate to each population served that are acquired through an academic and clinical training program, followed by a supervised clinical affiliation, continuing education, and clinical experience. Judgment is the ability to apply professional practice standards to decide whether a given client requires intervention and the knowledge and skills required to appropriately treat a given condition and to decide when treatment should be discontinued. In other words, skilled occupational therapy services are:

> ... based on a formal course of occupational therapy academic and clinical preparation, are related to a medical condition and are directed toward the amelioration of impairment and disabilities for the purpose of reducing safety risks, preventing

secondary complications and facilitating a client's attainment of daily living independence that is higher than his or her existing level of independence. (Foto, 1996a, p. 169)

The focus on skilled services under Medicare is in stark contrast to the recommendations of the Pew Commission. Medicare requires hospital and facility personnel to provide skilled services acquired through a specific educational, clinical training, and/or continuing educational program, whereas the Pew Commission recommended that personnel should be educated and trained to provide services that are potentially across several disciplines of knowledge, skill, and judgment. In reality, some of both may occur. In another article, Foto (1996b) points out that one stroke rehabilitation program trained all team members to perform transfers, positioning, passive and active range of motion, dysphagia feeding techniques, stress management, and methods to facilitate and reinforcement communication. What is considered nonskilled in one setting may be considered skilled in another, depending on the degree of specialized skills available among the personnel assigned to the service unit. For example, the concept of multiskilling can be used to suggest that occupational therapists add to their basic skills set by learning to be case managers or accepted as a primary referral source (Foto, 1995). Finally, multiskilling may be seen as a step toward creating a universal therapist—a therapist who, in theory, would be capable of providing any of the therapies (physical, occupational, or speech-language). Of course, a universal therapist would likely have to obtain multiple state licenses to practice in all three disciplines, plus maintain the continuing education requirements. Such hurdles may act as barriers or disincentives to such practice.

Uniform Terminology, Third Edition

The third edition of the Uniform Terminology document was published in 1994 (AOTA, 1994b). A major change in the Third Edition was the addition of the construct of Performance Contexts to the existing constructs of Performance Areas and Performance Components. Performance Contexts are:

> … situations or factors that influence an individual engagement in desired and/or required performance areas. Performance contexts consist of temporal aspects (chronological age, developmental age, place in the life cycle, and health status) and environmental aspects (physical, social and cultural considerations). (p. 1047)

The addition of Performance Contexts completes the PEO triad discussed under Models of Practice. Performance Components are aspects of the person, Performance Contexts address the environment, and Performance Areas are the occupations.

The three constructs are listed in order as Performance Areas, Performance Components, and Performance Contexts. The Performance Areas maintain the same three subsections: activities of daily living, work activities, and play or leisure activities. The Performance Components also maintain the same three subsections: sensorimotor components, cognitive integration and cognitive components, and psychosocial skills and psychological components. A few changes were added or subtracted from the items listed under each subcategory to update understanding of items in that subcategory.

Publication and Information

OT Week and *OT Practice* combined into one publication in 1995 called *OT Practice*. Revenue from advertisements in *OT Week* had decreased from employers seeking practitioners or faculty members. Documents approved and published by the Association are listed in Table 9-6.

Table 9-6
ASSOCIATION DOCUMENTS

1990	• Entry Level Role Delineation for Registered Occupational therapists (OTRs) and Certified Occupational Therapy Assistants (COTAs). AJOT, 44(12), 1091-1102
	• Supervision Guidelines for Certified Occupational Therapy Assistants, AJOT, 44(12), 1089-1090
1991	• Essentials and Guidelines for an Accredited Education Program for the Occupational Therapist. AJOT, 45(12), 1077-1084
	• Essentials and Guidelines for an Accredited Educational Program for the Occupational Therapy Assistant. AJOT, 45(12, 1085-1092
	• Occupational Therapy and Assistive Technology. AJOT, 45(12), 1076
	• Statement: The Occupational Therapist as Case Manager. AJOT, 45(12), 1065-1066
	• Statement: Occupational Therapy Services Management of Persons with Cognitive Impairments. AJOT, 45(12), 1067-1069
	• Statement: Occupational Therapy Provision for Children with Learning Disabilities and/or Mild to Moderate Perceptual and Motor Deficits. AJOT, 45(12), 1070-1074
	• Official: AOTA Statement on Physical Agent Modalities. AJOT, 45(12), 1075
1992	• Position Paper: Physical Agent Modalities. AJOT, 46(12), 190-1091.
	• Standards of Practice for Occupational Therapy. AJOT, 46(12), 1082-1085
	• Statement: Occupational Therapy Services in Work Practice. AJOT, 46(12), 1086-1988
	• White Paper: Occupational Therapy and Long-Term Care. *OT Week, 6*(42), 24-24.
1993	• Core Values and Attitudes of Occupational therapy Practice. AJOT, 47(12), 1086-1086
	• Knowledge and Skills for Occupational Therapy Practice in the Neonatal Intensive Care Unit. AJOT, 47(12), 1100-1105
	• Occupational Therapy Roles. AJOT, 47(12), 1087-1099
	• Position Paper: Occupational Therapy and the Americans with Disabilities Act (ADA). AJOT, 47(12), 1083-1084
	• Position Paper: Purposeful Activity. AJOT, 47(12), 1081-1082
	• Statement: The Role of Occupational therapy in the Independent Living Movement. AJOT, 47(12), 1079-1080
1994	• Guide for Supervision of Occupational Therapy Personnel. AJOT, 48(11), 1045-1046
	• Occupational Therapy Code of Ethics. AJOT, 48(11), 1037-1038
	• Position Paper: Occupational Therapy and Long-Term Services and Supports. AJOT, 48(11), 1035-1036.
	• Standards of Practice for Occupational Therapy. AJOT, 48(11), 1039-1044
	• Statement of Occupational Therapy Referral. AJOT, 48(11), 1034
	• Statement: Occupational Therapy Services for Persons with Alzheimer's Disease and Other Dementias. AJOT, 48(11), 1029-1033
	• Uniform Terminology for Occupational Therapy – Third Edition. AJOT, 48(11), 1047-1055
	• Uniform Terminology- Third Edition: Application of Uniform Terminology in Practice. AJOT, 48(11), 1055-1059

(continued)

	Table 9-6 (continued) ASSOCIATION DOCUMENTS
1995	• Concept Paper: Service Delivery in Occupational Therapy. AJOT, 49(10), 1029-1031. • Elements of clinical Documentation (Revision). AJOT, 49(10), 1032-1035 • Position Paper: Broadening the Construct of Independence. AJOT, 49(10), 1014 • Position Paper: Occupation. AJOT, 49(10), 1015-1018 • Position Paper: Occupational Performance: Occupational Therapy's definition of Function. AJOT, 49(10), 1019-1020 • Position Paper: The Psychosocial Core within Occupational Therapy. AJOT, 49(10), 1021-1022 • Position Paper: Use of Occupational Therapy Aides in Occupational Therapy Practice. AJOT, 59(10), 1023-1028 • Statement: Nondiscrimination and Inclusion Regarding Members of the Occupational Therapy Professional Community. AJOT, 49(10), 1009-1010 • Statement: Psychosocial Concerns within Occupational Therapy Practice. AJOT, 49(10), 1011-1013 • White Paper: Occupational Therapy and Cross-Training Initiatives. *OT Week, 9*(10), 31-33
1996	• Enforcement Procedures for Occupational Therapy Code of Ethics. AJOT, 50(10), 848-852. • Occupational Therapy: A Profession in Support of Full Inclusion. AJOT, 50(10), 855 • Position Paper: Eating Dysfunction. AJOT, 50(10), 847-848 • Position Paper: Providing Services for Persons with HIV/AIDS and Their Caregivers. AJOT, 50(10), 853-854 • Statement: Purpose and Value of Occupational Therapy Fieldwork Education. AJOT, 50(10), 845 • White Paper: The Role of the Occupational Therapy Practitioner in the Implementation of Full Inclusion. AJOT, 50(10), 856-857
1997	• A Guide to Self-Appraisal. *OT Week, 11*(25), 27-34. • Cross Training Concept Paper. AJOT, 51(10), 853-860 • Statement: Fundamental Concepts of Occupational Therapy: Occupation, Purposeful Activity, and Function. AJOT, 51(10), 864-966 • Position Paper: Physical Agent Modality (Edited). AJOT, 51(10), 870-871 • Philosophy of Education, replaces 1980. AJOT, 51(10), 867 • Statement: Sensory Integration Evaluation and Intervention in School Based Occupational Therapy. AJOT, 51(10), 861-863. • Position Paper: The Psychosocial Core of Occupational Therapy, edited. AJOT, 51(10), 868-869 • White paper: AOTA and Development of Standards of Practice for the Profession of Occupational Therapy. *OT Week, 11*(47), 16-17.
1998	• Guidelines to the Occupational Therapy Code of Ethics. AJOT, 52(10), 881-884 • Position Paper: The Use of General Information and Assistive Technology Within Occupational Therapy Practice. AJOT, 52(10), 870-871 • Standards of Practice for Occupational Therapy. AJOT, 52(10), 866-869 • Statement: Occupational Therapy and Hospice. AJOT, 52(10), 872-873 • Statement: Occupational Therapy for Individuals with Learning Disabilities, AJOT, 52(10), 874-880 • White paper: Professional evolution: Should health care environmental changes force OT and PT practice into a new delivery model? *OT Week, 12*(15), 17-19.

(continued)

Table 9-6 (continued)	
ASSOCIATION DOCUMENTS	
1999	• Definition of OT Practice for the AOTA Model Practice Act. AJOT, 53(6), 608
	• Guide for Supervision of Occupational Therapy Personnel in the Delivery of Occupational Therapy Services. AJOT, 53(6), 592-594
	• Guidelines for the Use of Aides in Occupational Therapy. AJOT, 53(6), 595-597
	• Statement: Management of Occupational Therapy Services for Persons with Cognitive Impairment. AJOT, 53(6), 601-608
	• Position Paper: Occupational Therapy's Commitment to Nondiscrimination and Inclusion. AJOT, 53(6), 598
	• Standards for an Accredited Educational Program for the Occupational Therapist. AJOT, 53(6), 575-582
	• Standards for an Accredited Educational Program for the Occupational Therapy Assistant. AJOT, 53(6), 583-589
	• Glossary: Standards for an Accredited Education Program for the Occupational Therapist and the Occupational Therapy Assistant. AJOT, 53(6), 590-591
	• Standards for Continuing Competence. AJOT, 63(6), 599-600

FOUNDATION

In 1995, the Foundation was 30 years old. Major activities continued to focus on fellowships, scholarships, education of faculty, and research grant support. The Foundation managed 37 named scholarships (24 state or district and 13 organizational) and awarded 67 scholarships. Three Centers for Scholarship and Research in Occupational Therapy continued to be supported (Boston University, University of Illinois at Chicago, and University of Southern California). Seventy occupational therapy faculty members participated in workshops designed to promote transition from clinical activities to an academic career. Support for research included awarding nine outcomes research projects, three innovative studies related to development of assessments, and eight student research projects. The Wilma L. West Library received approximately 4,400 requests for information (AOTF, 1996a).

Presidents of the Foundation

Three people served as president of the AOTF during the 1990s: Elizabeth B. Devereaux, 1989-1993 (Figure 9-15); Maralynne Mitcham, 1994-1996 (Figure 9-16); and Jane Davis Rourk, 1997-2002 (Figure 9-17).

Mission and Goals

In 1996, the mission statement was restated to read: Through the use of fiscal and human resources, AOTF expands and refines the body of knowledge of occupational therapy and promotes the understanding of the value of occupation in the interest of the public good (AOTF, 1996b). The goals focused on research, education, and securing financial resources and were stated as follows:

- Fund scientific and scholarly inquiry relevant to occupational therapy research, practice, and education to develop new knowledge, test and refine existing knowledge, and validate theories.

- Promote excellence in education about occupation and occupational therapy by providing resources to develop the corps of skilled faculty; educating practitioners about the relevance

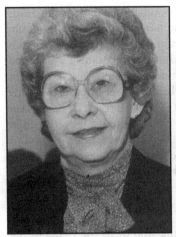
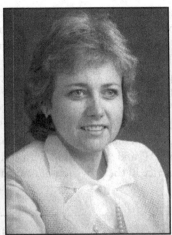
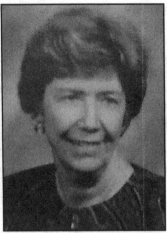

Figure 9-15. Elizabeth B. Devereaux, MSW, OTR, FAOTA, President of the AOTF, 1989-1993. (Printed with permission from the Archive of the American Occupational Therapy Association, Inc.)

Figure 9-16. Maralynne Mitcham, PhD, OTR/L, FAOTA, President of the AOTF, 1994-1996. (Printed with permission from the Archive of the American Occupational Therapy Association, Inc.)

Figure 9-17. Jane Davis Rourk, OTR/L, BCP, FAOTA, President of the AOTF, 1997-2002. (Printed with permission from the Archive of the American Occupational Therapy Association, Inc.)

of research to practice; recognizing students who demonstrate excellence; and organizing the disseminating information from scientific and scholarly inquiry.

- Secure financial resources to support programs and operations annually and to build the endowment to ensure long-term viability.

Reliable Source

The database Reliable Source was initiated in 1994 to replace the original OT Source. The database was overseen by the AOTF. Reliable Source was built on new software. It was designed to be the most extensive collection of occupational therapy literature in existence (AOTA, 1995b).

NATIONAL BOARD FOR CERTIFICATION IN OCCUPATIONAL THERAPY

Formation and Purpose

The National Board for Certification in Occupational Therapy (NBCOT) was the new name given to the American Occupational Therapy Certification Board (AOTCB) in 1996. The name was changed to reflect a broader mission to access the competency of occupational therapy practitioners over the lifetime of the professional, not just the initial certification process and continued listing of active practitioners over the years through payment of fees. At the time NBCOT was formed, about 66,500 therapists had been certified (original term was registered) since the process began in 1931, and about 23,000 assistants had been certified since the process for assistants began in 1977 (NBCOT, 1996).

The NBCOT functions as an independent national credentialing agency that certifies eligible persons as occupational therapists registered (OTR) and certified occupational therapy assistants (COTA). Both OTR and COTA are registered marks. The mission of the NBCOT is "to serve the public interest by providing high standards for the certification of occupational therapy practitioners" (NBCOT, 1996). To accomplish its mission, the NBCOT maintains a certification program, a certification renewal program, and a disciplinary action program. The certification program develops and administers the initial certification program. The renewal program is concerned with continuing competency to practice, and the disciplinary action program is responsible for disciplinary action against practitioners who do not maintain the behaviors specified in the Code of Ethics developed by the NBCOT. Other activities of the NBCOT involve research on current practice trends to update the certification examination focus and content, credential verification for anyone interested in determining whether a practitioner has passed initial certification and/or maintained certification with NBCOT, and partnership with state regulatory agencies to protect the public and support quality practice in the provision of occupational therapy services.

Trademark Dispute Between NBCOT and AOTA

On March 2, 1999, a settlement agreement was signed regarding who owns the rights to the trademarks OTR and COTA (NBCOT, 1999). The rights go with the initial certification exam and thus belong to NBCOT. The signed agreement ended a 2-year dispute between the Association and NBCOT over who owned the trademarks.

In March 1997, AOTA started legal proceedings against the NBCOT over the trademarks. AOTA argued that the credentialing marks were generic and not unique to the profession of occupational therapy. The NBCOT argued that the marks provided credibility and mobility to the profession (NBCOT, 1997). The problem arose when the NBCOT started a certification renewal program that was mandatory if the therapist or assistant wanted to continue to use the marks OTR or COTA after their name (Foto, 1997).

The dispute began in October 1996, when AOTA became aware of two major issues: the NBCOT's use of the trademarks and the NBCOT's alleged noncompliance with contracts between the two organizations (Foto et al., 1997). Attempts in January 1997 to settle differences were not successful. The NBCOT responded by sending state association presidents, members of the AOTA Representative Assembly, and state licensure board members a publication outlining the certification renewal program it had developed (AOTA, 1997b). On March 11, 1997, the Association filed petitions with the U.S. Patent and Trademark Office to cancel federal registration of the trademarks Occupational Therapist Registered, OTR and Certified Occupational Therapy Association, COTA claimed by the NBCOT (AOTA, 1997c). Another meeting was scheduled for March 17, but NBCOT members refused to meet with AOTA members unless AOTA withdrew the petition filed on March 11. On March 17, 1997, the NBCOT file a lawsuit in federal court in Maryland against AOTA and its members for "injunctive relief and damages in connection with violation of Section 2 of the Sherman Act" (Steib, 1997, p. 7). The suit charged AOTA with breaching its October 1995 Licensing Agreement with the NBCOT by challenging NBCOT's ownership of the certification marks. The suit also alleged that AOTA and its members were conspiring to engage in an unlawful group boycott of the NBCOT in violation of the Sherman Antitrust Act of 1890 by attempting to recapture certification authority from the NBCOT and thus monopolize trade (Steib, 1997).

At issue was the right of therapists to use the title Occupational Therapist, Registered and initials OTR and of assistants to use the title Certified Occupational Therapist Assistant and initials COTA. Under the NBCOT proposed renewal plan, only therapists and assistants who recertified with the NBCOT would be allowed to use the title and initials. Therapists had been using the title and initials since 1943, and assistants had been using the title and initials since 1958. In addition, many state licensure laws and regulations incorporated the initials into approved signatures such as OTR/L, LOTR, or COTA/L. Under the certification renewal program outlined by the NBCOT, such use would not be permitted, and AOTA was concerned that some practitioners might lose their employment if they could not use the title or initials (Steib, 1997). A second issue was the development of the continuing certification program itself, what policies would be adopted, how the program would be administered, and by whom. The announcement by the NBCOT of their certification renewal program was the catalyst for the dispute in the first place (Foto et al., 1997). A third issue was that the NBCOT was a fee-for-service organization responsible to the public, not a membership organization responsive to the needs and concerns of occupational therapy members. The issue was "about who speaks for practitioners and how important policy matters affecting practitioners ought to be decided" (AOTA, 1998c, p. 23). The NBCOT was functioning in 1997 as a self-selected 15-member Board of Directors to whom its activities were responsible.

At the April 1997 meeting of the Representative Assembly, six principles for resolving the differences between the two organizations were adopted (AOTA, 1997a, p. 900). AOTA President Mary Foto made attempts to use the principles in negotiating with NBCOT President Diana Ramsey with little success.

- A clear distinction must be maintained between entry-level certification and continued competency assessment.
- Any continuing competency assessment program should not imperil the practice or the livelihood of qualified occupational therapy practitioners.
- The NBCOT should explore ways to become more representative of and accountable to the occupational therapy profession.
- The current legal dimensions of the dispute should promptly be eliminated by NBCOT withdrawing the trademark registrations relating to occupational therapist registered OTR and certified occupational therapy assistant COTA, AOTA withdrawing its petitions to cancel the registration of those marks and NBCOT dismissing its lawsuit against AOTA and its members.
  ○ When the steps in number 4 are accomplished, AOTA and the NBCOT will jointly develop a collegial task force or commission to address the appropriate use of the designations OTR and COTA.
- Establish by consensus standards and role delineations for competency assessment that reflect appropriate professional expertise and roles for AOTA, NBCOT, AOTF, state regulatory bodies, and practitioners.
- If these steps are not taken, the Executive Board is to seek negotiations with the NBCOT with the assistance of a neutral mediator.

In February 1998, AOTA made four new proposals:
- Create a new joint AOTA and NBCOT entity to own the OTR and COTA marks
- Reformulate the NBCOT Board of Directors selection progress to be accountable to the public and certificants according to National Commission on Certifying Agencies (NCCA) standards
- Amicably renegotiate the license agreement
- Establish new designations for practitioners or have the NBCOT simply give up the use of the OTR and CORA marks for renewed certification so that the marks could continue to signify initial certification (AOTA, 1998f)

The NBCOT's negotiating members agreed to reformulate the Board of Directors to meet the NCCA standards but did not agree to any attempts to modify the lawsuit claiming sole ownership of the titles or initials. Although President Foto wrote four letters to President Ramsey, no other progress was made during the rest of the year (AOTA, 1998f). Finally, on March 1, 1999, AOTA's Executive Board voted to settle the dispute, and the agreement ending the lawsuit was signed on March 2, 1999, by President Karen Jacobs for AOTA and President Diana Ramsey for the NBCOT (AOTA, 1998d; Ramsey, 1999). The settlement acknowledged the ruling by Judge Andre Davis that the NBCOT owned the trademarks OTR and COTA, which it registered with the U.S. Patent and Trademark Office in December 1995 and January 1996. Judge Davis ruled on September 30, 1998, that AOTA automatically transferred the trademarks when it created AOTCB, the predecessor to NBCOT, in 1986 (AOTA, 1998b). As part of the settlement, the NBCOT agreed not to initiate proceedings against any individuals who used the certification marks without meeting the certification requirements during the time of the dispute. Judge Davis also ruled that AOTA had breached the License Agreement of 1995 by challenging the ownership and validity of trademarks and by distributing pins and patches bearing the trademarks. However, AOTA did not wrongfully interfere with the NBCOT's voluntary certification program or disparage the NBCOT, as had been claimed in the lawsuit (AOTA, 1998b).

Thereafter, NBCOT proceeded with the recertification program and restricted the use of the titles and initials to those would recertified with NBCOT. State licensing boards had to change their rules to eliminate titles and initials containing the trademarks. Instead, the titles had to be restricted to licensed occupational therapist; OT, occupational therapy assistant licensed; OTA; or similar designations. In addition, all AOTA documents that used the titles or initials had to be revised or rescinded to eliminate use of the titles or initials to comply with the intent of the settlement.

The cost of the dispute is difficult to calculate because some costs are not provided. AOTA's business liability insurance covered most of the legal expenses (AOTA, 1998c). However, AOTA reported that over 50,000 pages of copy were provided to the court to fulfill requests for information (AOTA, 1998f). The cost of paper and staff time is not recorded.

REFLECTION

Conflict, highs, and lows characterized this decade. There was an increased need for occupational therapists and growth in the number of educational programs. There was healthy competition between schools. The educational entry level was upgraded to master's level with the AOTA Representative Assembly passing Resolution J at the 1997 annual conference in Indianapolis. As quickly as the need for occupational therapists grew in the early 1990s, it crashed in the late 1990s with the passing of the Balanced Budget Act in 1997. Many occupational therapists lost jobs, and school enrollments declined for the next several years. Many educational programs closed for occupational therapy assistants because of low enrollment and poor employment outlook. The end of the 1990s saw the battle between AOTA and the NBCOT for the professions' trademarks, a battle brought on by the age-old discussion on accountability and measures of continued competence.

REFERENCES

American Occupational Therapy Association. (1990). *Membership data*. Rockville, MD: Author

American Occupational Therapy Association. (1991). Essentials and guidelines for an accredited education program for the occupational therapist. *American Journal of Occupational Therapy, 45*(12), 1077-1084.

American Occupational Therapy Association. (1993a). *73rd annual business meeting*. Seattle, WA: Author.

American Occupational Therapy Association. (1993b, April 23). A variety of settings under a unifying philosophy. *OT Week*, Spring Student Edition, pp. 14-28.

American Occupational Therapy Association. (1994a). *74th annual business meeting*. Bethesda, MD: Author.

American Occupational Therapy Association. (1994b). *Building for the profession in the 21st century. 1994 annual report*. Boston, MA: Author.

American Occupational Therapy Association. (1994c). SIS variety reflex practice variety. *OT Week's Today's Student*, Spring, pp. 8-9.

American Occupational Therapy Association. (1994d). Uniform terminology for occupational therapy, third edition. *American Journal of Occupational Therapy, 48*(11), 1047-1054.

American Occupational Therapy Association. (1995a). *75th annual business meeting*. Bethesda, MD: Author.

American Occupational Therapy Association. (1995b). AOTA's reliable research tool. *OT Week, 9*(1), 22.

American Occupational Therapy Association. (1995c). Concept paper: Service delivery in occupational therapy. *American Journal of Occupational Therapy, 49*(10), 1029-1031.

American Occupational Therapy Association. (1995d). Position paper: Occupational performance: Occupational therapy's definition of function. *American Journal of Occupational Therapy, 49*(10), 1019-1020.

American Occupational Therapy Association. (1995e). Position paper: Use of occupational therapy aides in occupational therapy practice. *American Journal of Occupational therapy, 49*(10), 1023-1025.

American Occupational Therapy Association. (1995f). White paper: Occupational therapy and cross-training initiatives. *OT Week, 9*(10), 32-33.

American Occupational Therapy Association. (1997a). The 1997 Representative Assembly Summary of minutes. *American Journal of Occupational Therapy, 51*(10), 898-901.

American Occupational Therapy Association. (1997b). AOTA board says NBCOT program raises questions about future of the profession. *OT Week, 11*(12), 27-30.

American Occupational Therapy Association. (1997c). AOTA challenges certification board's trademark registration. *OT Week, 11*(12), 28-29.

American Occupational Therapy Association. (1997d). Cross-training concept paper. *American Journal of Occupational Therapy, 51*(10), 853-860.

American Occupational Therapy Association. (1998a). *78th annual business meeting.* Baltimore, MD: Author.

American Occupational Therapy Association. (1998b). News this week: Court issues split decision in NBCOT lawsuit. *OT Week, 12*(42), 5.

American Occupational Therapy Association. (1998c). Questions and answers on the AOTA/NBCOT dispute. *OT Week, 12*(11), 23-25.

American Occupational Therapy Association. (1998f). Update on the AOTA-NBCOT dispute. *OT Week, 12*(24), A1.

American Occupational Therapy Association. (1999a). The 1999 Representative Assembly summary of minutes. *American Journal of Occupational Therapy, 53*(6), 628-630.

American Occupational Therapy Association. (1999b). ACOTE sets timeline for post baccalaureate degree programs. *OT Week, 13*(33), i-iii.

American Occupational Therapy Association. (1999c). AOTA's 1999 Representative Assembly proposed business agenda. *OT Week, 13*(5), RA1-RA24.

American Occupational Therapy Association. (1999d). Questions and answers regarding the AOTA and NBCOT settlement agreement. *OT Week, 13*(11), iii-iv.

American Occupational Therapy Association. (1999/2000). Challenging PT scope of practice expansion. *State Policy Department News, 1*(4), 1-3.

American Occupational Therapy Association. (2008). *Academic programs annual data report: Academic year 2007-2008.* Bethesda, MD: Author.

American Occupational Therapy Foundation. (1996a). 1995 annual report. *OT Week, 10*(11), A1-A12.

American Occupational Therapy Foundation. (1996b). *1996 annual report of the American Occupational Therapy Foundation.* Bethesda, MD: Author.

American Physical Therapy Association. (1994). *Commonalities and differences between the professions of physical therapy and occupational therapy: An American Physical Therapy Association white paper.* Alexandria, VA: Author.

American Physical Therapy Association. (1997a). Guide to physical therapy practice. *Physical Therapy, 77*, 1163-1650.

American Physical Therapy Association. (1999). *Guide to physical therapy practice, Revised.* Alexandria, VA: Author

Bair, J. (1991). From my office. *OT Week, 5*(42), 2.

Bair, J. (1992). From my office. *OT Week, 6*(6), 2.

Christiansen, C. (1996). Nationally speaking: Managed care: Opportunities and challenges for occupational therapy in the emerging systems of the 21st century. *American Journal of Occupational Therapy, 50*(6), 409-412.

Clark, F., Azen, S. P., Zemke, R., Jackson, J., Carlson, M., Mandel, D.,...Lipson, L. (1997). Occupational therapy for independent-living older adults: A randomized controlled trial. *Journal of the American Medical Association, 278*(16), 1321-1326.

Collins, A. L. (1997). Multiskilling: a survey of occupational therapy practitioners' attitudes. *American Journal of Occupational Therapy, 51*(9), 748-753.

Daigle, W. W. (1994). Accreditation Council for Occupational Therapy Education. In *American Occupational Therapy Association 74th annual business meeting* (pp. 56-57). Bethesda, MD: AOTA.

Foto, M. (1995). National speaking: New president's address: The future—challenges, choices, and changes. *American Journal of Occupational Therapy, 49*(10), 955-959.

Foto, M. (1996a). Nationally speaking: Delineating skilled versus nonskilled services: A defining point in our professional evolution. *American Journal of Occupational Therapy, 50*(3), 168-170.

Foto, M. (1996b). Nationally speaking: Multiskilling: Who, how, when, and why? *American Journal of Occupational Therapy, 50*(1), 7-9.

Foto, M. (1997). Dear AOTA member [Letter]. *OT Week, 11*(15), 15.

Foto, M. (1998). White paper: Professional evolution: Should health care environmental changes force OT and PT practice into a new delivery model? *OT Week, 12*(15), 17-19.

Foto, M., Jacobs, K., Knox, S. H., Ethridge, D. B., Barnes, L. C., Clerico, C.,...Boyt Schell, B. A. (1997). An open letter to the members from the executive board about NBCOT's certification renewal program. *OT Week, 11*(1), 1, 7.

Graves, S. (1994). Independent. *OT Week, 8*(18), 20-22.

Hansen, R. (1995). For the record: Task force on cross-training. *OT Week, 9*(5), 6.

Harsh, C. (1992). Program development: Balancing quantity with quality. *OT Week, 6*(46), 16-17.

Health Care Financing Administration. (n.d.). Medical hospital manual 10 (HCFA Publication 13-3, Section 3906). Bethesda, MD: Department of Health and Human Services.

Hettinger, J. (1996). Pew Commission: What is it, and why should OTs care? *OT Week, 10*(8), 18-20.

Joe, B. E. (1992). Efficiency pervades 1992 RA Meeting: Physical agent modality position stands. *OT Week, 6*(15), 14.

Kyler-Hutchison, P. (1992). Issues in accreditation. *OT Week, 6*(29), 7.

Mandel, D. R., Jackson, J. M., Zemke, R., Nelson, L., & Clark, F. A. (1999). *Lifestyle redesign: Implementing the well elderly program.* Bethesda, MD: AOTA.

National Board for Certification of Occupational Therapy. (1996). *National Board for Certification of Occupational Therapy: What it is. What it does* [Brochure]. Gaithersburg, MD: Author.

National Board for Certification of Occupational Therapy. (1997). NBCOT responds to AOTA legal action. [Letter]. Gaithersburg, MD: Author.

National Board for Certification in Occupational Therapy. (1999). NBCOT and AOTA sign agreement establishing collaborative task force. *Report to the Profession, 4*(1), 1-2.

Pedretti, L. W., & Pasquinell, S. (1990). A frame of reference for occupational therapy in physical dysfunction. In. L. W. Pedretti & B. Zoltan (Eds.), *Occupational therapy skills for physical dysfunction* (3rd ed., pp. 1-17). St. Louis, MO: Mosby.

Ramsey, D. L. (1999). Dear colleague. *Report to the profession, 4*(1), 1.

Steib, P. A. (1997). News this week: NBCOT sues AOTA and its members. *OT Week, 11*(14), 7.

Steib, P. A. (1999). Occupational therapy works: The studies say so. *OT Week, 13*(37), 8-9.

TriAlliance of Health and Rehabilitation Professionals. (1995). Use of multiskilled personnel. *OT Week, 10*(78), 17.

BIBLIOGRAPHY

American Occupational Therapy Association. (1993). AOTA's 1993 Representative Assembly approved business agenda. *OT Week, 7*(11), 1-32.

American Occupational Therapy Association. (1994). Uniform terminology, third edition: Application to practice. *American Journal of Occupational Therapy, 48*(11), 1055-1059.

American Occupational Therapy Association. (1997). News this week: NBCOT refuses to negotiate. *OT Week, 11*(13), 7.

American Occupational Therapy Association. (1997). News this week: NBCOT sues AOTA and its members. *OT Week, 11*(14), 7.

American Occupational Therapy Association. (1998). AOTA responds to APTA practice guidelines. *OT Week, 12*(35), 9.

American Occupational Therapy Association. (1998). News this week: NBCOT-AOTA litigation update. *OT Week, 12*(39), 5.

American Occupational Therapy Association. (1999). NBCOT and AOTA sign settlement agreement: Collaborative tasks. *OT Week, 13*(10), i-iii.

American Occupational Therapy Association. (1999). *Physical therapy profession: Scope of practice.* Bethesda, MD: Author.

American Occupational Therapy Association. (1999). Settlement proposed in the NBCOT-AOTA lawsuit. *OT Week, 13*(5), i-iii.

American Physical Therapy Association. (1997). Model definition of physical therapy for state practice acts. In *Guide to physical therapist practice* (pp. 1-2). Alexandria, VA: Author.

Foto, M. (1998). A message from AOTA president Mary Foto. *OT Week, 12*(11), 22.

Hansen, R. (1996). The task force on cross-training. *OT Week, 10*(14), 15.

Nielson, C. S. (1997). NBCOT action usurps our democratic tradition. *OT Week, 11*(16), 61-52.

10

Looking to the Future
2000s to 2010s

Key Points

- The Centennial Vision Statement was created with eight elements in 2006.
- The Occupational Therapy Practice Framework was adopted in 2002 and revised in 2008.
- Living Life to Its Fullest was adopted as the brand in 2008.
- The Association was reorganized to stress financial accountability.

Highlighted Personalities

- Barbara L. Kornblau, AOTA President, 2001-2004
- Carolyn M. Baum, AOTA President, 2004-2007
- Penelope Moyers Cleveland, AOTA President, 2007-2010
- Joseph Isaacs, AOTA Executive Director
- Frederick Somers, AOTA Executive Director
- Martha Kirkland, AOTF Executive Director
- Charles Christiansen, AOTF Executive Director
- Ruth Ann Watkins, AOTF President

Key Places

- The national office was still located in Bethesda, Maryland.

Andersen, L. T., & Reed, K. L.
The History of Occupational Therapy: The First Century (pp. 293-323).
© 2017 Taylor & Francis Group.

Key Times/Events

- The World Federation of Occupational Therapists was 50 years old in 2002.

Political Events/Issues

- No Child Left Behind (NCLB; P.L. 107-110) adopted in 2001
- Medicare Prescription Drug Improvement and Modernization Act (P.L. 108-173) adopted in 2003
- Individual with Disabilities Improvement Act (P.L. 108-446) adopted in 2004
- Deficit Reduction Act (P.L. 109-171) adopted in 2006

Economic Events/Issues

- AOTA published a workforce survey in 2006 based on membership and non-membership data.
- AOTA published a compensation survey in 2000 based on membership data.

Educational Issues*

- Educational Standards and Guidelines Revised, 2006
- Value and Purpose of Field Work
- Model Education Curriculum created
- Philosophy of Professional Education
- Scholarship
- Specialized Knowledge and Skills of Occupational Therapy Educators

Sociocultural Events/Issues

- The AOTA Societal Statement started in 2006 and included topics on health disparities, stress, posttraumatic stress disorder, youth violence, nondiscrimination, and inclusion.

Practice Issues*

- Promotion of Health and Prevention of Disease and Disability
- Providing Occupational Therapy Using Sensory Integration Theory and Methods
- Occupational Therapy and Hospice (replaced in 2011 by end-of-life document)
- Occupational Therapy Services in Facilitating Work Performance (revised 2011)
- Occupational Therapy Services in Early Childhood and School-Based Settings (revised 2011)
- Scope of Services for Individuals With Autism (revised 2010)
- Occupational Therapy Services for Individuals Who Have Experienced Domestic Violence (revised 2011)
- Guidelines for Supervision, Roles, and Responsibilities During Delivery of Occupational Therapy Services
- Occupational Therapy Services in Promotion of Psychological and Social Aspects of Mental Health
- Role of Occupational Therapy in Wound Management (revised 2013)
- Physical Agent Modalities (revised 2012)

Technological Events/Issues

- The use of social media begins.

---

* Adapted from AOTA, 2010c.

Association Issues

- The Association initiated the Centennial Vision program in 2003.
- Eight elements were adopted for Centennial Vision in 2006.
- The Code of Ethics was revised in 2005.
- Fact Sheets began being published in 2001.

Foundation Issues

- Reinstated support for dissertation research
- 25th anniversary of Wilma L. West library
- Research priorities adopted

National Board for Certification in Occupational Therapy

- Development of Continuing Certification Program
- Second practice analysis study completed

"Living Life to Its Fullest"

–AOTA branding statement
(2008c, p. 7)

INTRODUCTION

George W. Bush was President of the United States from 2000 to 2008. The war in Afghanistan continued, and the war in Iraq began. Barack Obama became the first Black president of the United States in 2008. The economy went into a severe depression beginning in 2008, resulting in the loss of jobs and reducing the savings accounts of many families. Hurricane Katrina in Louisiana and Mississippi and Hurricanes Rita and Ike in Texas ravaged the Gulf Coast region, adding to the economic decline.

Occupational therapy as a profession was influenced by the revision of the World Health Organization's (WHO's) publication of the International Classification of Impairments, Disabilities and Handicaps (ICIDH), originally published in 1980. The revision was given a new name: the International Classification of Functioning, Disability and Health and abbreviated ICF (WHO, 2001). Health and disability are described as interrelated concepts, and disability occurs to most people over a lifetime, not to just a few people with specifically named diseases or disorders. The issue, however, is not the label but the degree to which disability results in body structure (anatomical) or body function (physiological) impairments, activity restriction, and participation restrictions in life situations. In addition, the document acknowledges that disability occurs as a result of contextual or environmental factors, not just medically diagnosed conditions and biological factors. The term *activity* now had a working definition in relation to a person's health status: "the execution of a task or action by an individual" (WHO, 2001, p. 10). In contrast, activity limitations are "difficulties an individual may have in executing activities" (WHO, 2001, p. 10). Participation is defined as "involvement in a life situation," and participation restrictions are defined as "problems an individual may experience in involvement in life situations" (WHO, 2001, p. 10). Contextual factors include both environmental and personal factors (WHO, 2001, p. 11). Environmental factors "make up the physical, social and attitudinal environment in which people live and conduct their lives" (WHO, 2001, p. 10). These changes and clarifications in terminology appeared in many definitions and descriptions of occupational therapy practice and services as the effects of the ICF were integrated in published works.

The Association felt the effects of the 1997 Balanced Budget Act (BBA) as practitioners continued to lose jobs through the early years of the 21st century. Membership dropped significantly, and the loss of revenue required several budget adjustments, including reducing the number of issues of the American Journal of Occupational Therapy (AJOT) from 12 to six per year. A turnaround did not begin to occur until 2005, but membership numbers continue lag behind the benchmark of 1996.

Occupational therapy was listed in a chart in U.S. News & World Report as a best career choice for the years 2007 and 2008 (Nemko, 2007, 2008). In both years, the job market outlook was considered excellent. Median pay was listed as $60,855 in 2007 and $63,900 in 2008. Recognition of the profession by the public media was beginning to occur.

EDUCATION

Blueprint for Entry-Level Education and Occupational Therapy Model Curricula

The committees for the two documents were appointed by President Penelope Moyers Cleveland (LaGrossa, 2008). The committees were appointed in response to motion adopted by the Board of Directors in 2006 which included priorities established by a Zoomerang survey (AOTA, 2006b). The Blueprint for Entry-Level Education was published (AOTA, 2010b). The Model Curricula for occupational therapists and for assistants were not published.

The purpose of the Blueprint was to "identify the content knowledge that occupational therapists and occupational therapy assistants should receive in their educational program" and make the information available as a content guide (AOTA, 2010b, p. 186). Content considered important addressed persons who were healthy, persons at risk for disability, and persons with chronic disabilities. Four sections were created: (1) person-centered factors, (2) environment-centered factors, (3) occupation-centered factors, and (4) professional and interpersonal factors. Key concepts, scientific rationale, and skills to be developed were included, as well as the areas of practice related to the concepts. The conceptual model used to organize the ideas was occupational performance. The person was viewed in terms of cognitive, psychological, physiological, sensory, perceptual, motor and spiritual aspects or skills. The environment was organized into social, cultural, natural, design and technology, environmental support (assistive technology), and environment for occupational performance. The concept of occupation-centered factors was organized into doing at the person level, doing at the organization and population level, classification of occupational activity, and core occupational therapy outcomes. Professional and interpersonal factors were divided into ethics and advocacy, communication, culture, professional development, evidence-based practice, and business fundamentals.

The Blueprint illustrates the change in thinking from the Curriculum Guide originally published in 1950 and updated in 1958 (AOTA, 1958). The four organization themes were sciences, clinical conditions, occupational therapy media, and application to occupational therapy practice. The sciences were anatomy and physiology, kinesiology and growth, and development and gaining. The clinical conditions related to psychiatry, neurology, orthopedics, cerebral palsy, general medical and surgical conditions, tuberculosis, cardiac conditions and rheumatic fever, and visual and auditory sensory disturbances. Media included art and design, block printing, ceramics, general crafts, leatherwork, metal work, needlecrafts plastics, printing, recreational activities, silk screening, stenciling, weaving, wood carving, woodworking and methods of instruction. Application to occupational therapy included orientation to occupational therapy, organization and administration, pediatric conditions, geriatric conditions, psychiatric conditions, mentally deficient, physical disabilities, general medicine and surgery, tuberculosis and cardiac conditions, and sensory disabilities.

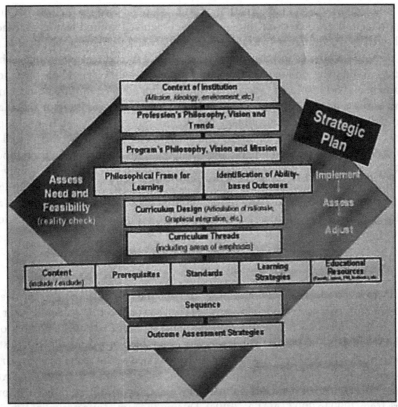

Figure 10-1. Design and development of a model curriculum. (Printed with permission from the Archive of the American Occupational Therapy Association, Inc.)

The change in thinking is consistent with the changes seen in the accreditation documents over the years. There is shift away from medical conditions and medical specialties to a focus on the person performing occupations in the environment under a variety of conditions from healthy and able to those with health conditions resulting in disability. The disease itself is no longer the focus. Instead, the focus is on the disability that may disrupt occupational performance.

According to LaGrossa, the purpose of the model curricula documents was to raise the bar in education to meet 21st century health care needs and ensure more consistency in the education and training of occupational therapy and assistant-level students. The Model Curricula Guides provide information of the issues that must be considered in creating or revising a course of study or curriculum within an institution of higher learning (AOTA, 2009a, 2009b). Some issues are the profession's philosophy, vision, and trends; the program's philosophy, mission, and vision within the institution; curriculum design and threads of ideas; suitable prerequisite courses; course content; learning strategies; sequence of courses; and outcomes assessment. Figure 10-1 illustrates the strategic plan for designing and developing a curriculum. Of particular importance is the overall philosophy. As the model curriculum for the occupational therapist states, a curriculum "may be organized according to the major diagnostic areas that occupational therapy addresses in practice" (AOTA, 2009b, p. 4). The course sequence is then structured according to physical and mental dysfunctions and the treatment strategies viewed as most effective in reducing the consequence of identified dysfunction. Such a curriculum is actually stressing reductionistic ideology and reinforcing a perspective that disability occurs as a result of the individual's biology while ignoring the environmental factors that may contribute to the dysfunction, including social stigma, which may act as a restraint on achieving successful community living. Course content tends to focused on courses that resemble a medical curriculum. In contrast, a philosophy could focus on health, wellbeing, and participation as a philosophy based on the concept of emergence rather than reductionism. The curriculum could be organized around factors that facilitate successful and satisfying community living, methods to decrease or prevent the effect of factors that may act to restrict such living and the role of occupational therapy in promoting such living patterns. Courses would focus on how healthy living supports well-being and participation and how the environment and occupational tasks can be modified or adapted to support a person's abilities and minimize effects of disability. As changes occur over the person's lifespan and changes occur in the socio-politico-economic environment and preferred occupations, additional modifications and changes can occur. Successful and satisfying living is viewed as an interactive and transactive process between the person, environment, and occupation in support of maximum occupational performance. Course content focuses on the unique aspects of occupational therapy as a health promotion and prevention profession and the role of occupational therapy in providing leadership to advocate for successful and satisfying living for all people. Within the document, a version of such a philosophical view is stated as an example based on the concept of "occupational needs" (AOTA, 2008e, p. 136).

Educational Programs

The number of accredited educational programs for the occupational therapists at the entry level was 146 (four entry-level doctoral and 142 master's) for the academic year 2009-2010 (AOTA, 2010a). Relatively few new programs were being developed; thus the number of programs remained fairly constant since 2004. There were 131 accredited programs for the assistant, but 15 programs were in the developmental stage and 29 had applied as the job market began to open up again following the loss of job opportunities due to the effects of the BBA of 1997. Sixty assistant programs had closed during the turndown in employment opportunities for occupational therapy practitioners from 2000 to 2007 (AOTA, 2010a). During the same time period of time, there were no reported closures of occupational therapist programs as a result of reduced employment opportunities, although there were closures due to the change in requirements for post-baccalaureate entry, which began January 1, 2007. The data suggest that assistant-level programs are more sensitive to employment trends than occupational therapist–level programs. If the employment market for practitioners is reduced due to legislation, the economy, or other factors, educational programs for the assistant are likely to close, whereas those for the occupational therapist are likely to continue.

The distribution of education programs continued to be unequal between the two levels of education. Entry-level programs for the occupational therapist were most available in the Northeast (48) and Midwest (39), followed by the South (36), West (15), and Southwest (13). In contrast, educational programs for the assistant were most available in the Midwest (43) and South (51), followed by the Northeast (31), Southwest (19), and West (9). The difference is not explained by employment trends or attitudes toward assistants. The last listing of educational programs in AJOT was in 2008. At that time, educational programs for the occupational therapist were available in 44 states, the District of Columbia, and Puerto Rico (AOTA, 2008a). Six states had no accredited educational program listed at the professional level: Alaska, Delaware, Hawaii, Rhode Island, Montana, and Vermont. A program is listed in the developing stage for Alaska as an extension campus from Creighton University in Nebraska. Occupational therapy assistant-level programs were available in 42 states, not including Alaska, Arkansas, Delaware, Idaho, Montana, Nebraska, Oregon, and Vermont. The goal still has not been reached of having educational programs in each state for both the occupational therapist and assistant to provide a steady and ready source of practitioners to work in occupational therapy service programs.

Education Standards Revision

The Standards were revised in 2006, published in 2007 in AJOT, and set to take effect in January 2008. Each of three sets of Standards included a list of expected outcomes in the Preamble, which are summarized in Table 10-1. A major issue in the revision concerned the qualifications and degree level earned by the program director and faculty members. In essence, the program director was expected to have a doctoral degree at both the master's and doctoral program levels, although programs offering a master's degree had until July 1, 2012, to install such a person. At the doctoral level, the director was expected to have 8 years of experience in the profession, including 3 years in an academic setting, whereas for the master's level program, 6 years of experience was considered

Table 10-1
ACCREDITATION STANDARDS EXPECTED OUTCOMES FOR THE OCCUPATIONAL THERAPIST
A graduate from an AOTE-Accredited master's-degree-level occupational therapy program must
• Have acquired, as a foundation for professional study, a breadth and depth of knowledge in the liberal arts and sciences and an understanding of issues related to diversity
• Be educated as a generalist with a broad exposure to the delivery models and systems used in setting where occupational therapy is currently practiced and where it is emerging as a service
• Have achieved entry-level competence through a combination of academic and fieldwork education
• Be prepared to articulate and apply occupational therapy theory and evidence-based evaluations and interventions to achieve expected outcomes as related to occupation.
• Be prepared to be a lifelong learner and keep current with evidence-based professional practice
• Uphold the ethical standards, values, and attitudes of the occupational therapy profession
• Understand the distinct roles and responsibilities of the occupational therapist and occupational therapy assistant in the supervisory process
• Be prepared to advocate as a professional from the occupational therapy services offered and for the recipients of those services
• Be prepared to be an effective consumer of the latest research and knowledge bases that support practice and contribute to the growth and dissemination of research and knowledge.
(Note: Additional requires apply to doctoral-degree-level programs. The occupational therapy assistance is expected to achieve the first eight statements but not the ninth.)
ACOTE (2007). Accreditation standards for a master's-degree-level education program for the occupational therapist. *American Journal of Occupational Therapy, 61*(6), 652.

minimum, including 2 years in academia. All full-time faculty teaching in the doctoral program must hold doctorates. By July 1, 2012, the majority of full-time faculty teaching in the master's-level program must hold a doctoral degree. The date of 2012 was an extension of 2 years from the draft published in 2005 (Olson, 2005).

Continuing Education Program

In 2002, the Representative Assembly adopted a motion to establish the Commission on Continuing Competence and Professional Development (CCCPD or 3CPD), and the bylaws were amended to include the CCCPD as a standing commission. The purpose of CCCPD was to recommend standards for continuing competence and develop strategies for communicating information about continuing competency to stakeholders. The purpose of the Association's involvement in promoting continuing competence was to foster the objective of promoting high professional standards, a role the Association had maintained since adopting the Minimum Standards for

Courses in Training of Occupational Therapists in 1923 (AOTA, 1924). Actually, the first Standards for Continuing Competence were adopted in 1999 (AOTA, 1999).

In 2006, 42 states or jurisdictions required continuing education or continuing competence requirements for licensure renewal for occupational therapy practitioners (AOTA, 2007b, p. 2)

PRACTICE

Definitions of Occupational Therapy

Definitions began to focus on occupation as the core or unique concept of occupational therapy rather than the vague terms of purposeful, meaningful, or goal-directed activity (Table 10-2). Occupation meant "everyday life activities" in which people participated as they engaged in roles and situation in their home, school, workplace, community, or other setting. The focus of occupational therapy was directed was described in terms of health, wellness, participation, and quality of life. Evaluation included instrumental activities of living for the first time as a category separate from activities of daily living (AOTA, 2004a). Social participation was added reflecting the influence of the ICF. Intervention might focus on one or more of the following depending on the client's needs:

- Establishment, remediation, or restoration of a skills or ability that has not yet developed or is impaired
- Compensation, modification, or adaptation of activity or environment to enhance performance
- Maintenance and enhancement of capabilities without which performance in everyday life activities would decline
- Health promotion and wellness to enable or enhance performance in everyday life activities
- Prevention of barriers to performance, including disability prevention (AOTA, 2004a)

Table 10-2
OCCUPATIONAL THERAPY DEFINITIONS

2002	Occupational therapy: The art and science of applying occupation as a means to effect positive measurable change in the health status and functional outcomes of the client by a qualified occupational therapist and/or occupational therapy assistant (as appropriate). (AOTA. Glossary: Standards for an accredited education program for the occupational therapists and occupational therapy assistant. AJOT, 56(6), 667-668.)
2004	The practice of occupational therapy means the therapeutic use of everyday life activities (occupations) with individuals or groups for the purpose of participation in roles and situations in home, school, workplace, community, and other settings. Occupational therapy services are provided for the purpose of promoting health and wellness and to those who have or are at risk for developing an illness, injury, disease, disorder, condition, impairment, disability, activity limitation, or participation restriction. Occupational therapy addresses the physical, cognitive, psychosocial, sensory, and other aspects of performance in a variety of contexts to support engagement in everyday life activities that affect health, well-being, and quality of life. (AOTA, (2004). Policy 5.3.1. AJOT, 58(6), 694-695.)
2008	The Occupational Therapist Registered (OTR) is a professional who works with clients whose occupational performance is impaired or at risk of impairment to facilitate engagement in meaningful occupations across the lifespan. The OTR uses collaborative, client-centered strategies to obtain information regarding personal and environmental factors that impact occupational performance and formulates conclusions to develop an intervention plan. The OTR selects and implements interventions to support participation in basic and instrumental activities f daily living, education, work, plan, leisure, and social participation. The OTR engages in professional development activities to maintain competence and uphold standards of practice. (NBCOT 2008 Practice Analysis, p. 10)
2009	Occupational therapy is essentially an educative profession. (AOTA. (2009). Specialized knowledge and skills of occupational therapy educators of the future. AJOT, 63(6), 804.)

Practice Patterns

A survey initiated by the Association to determine participation in the Association's activities also collected some data about practice (AOTA, 2009a). The data are based on 2,130 practitioners but are not separated by occupational therapist or assistant. The three major work settings continue to be schools and early intervention programs, hospital settings except for mental health, and long-term care or skilled nursing facilities. These three settings plus academia account for 75% of work settings. The percentages are listed in Table 10-3. Work time allocation is presented in Table 10-4. Because people working in academia are included, the percentages probably do not accurately represent the amount of time practitioners work with clients. Rather, the percentages reflect the total effort in time of all types of occupational therapy personnel whether they work with clients, students, research subjects, or other stakeholders.

Evidence-Based Practice

The concept of evidence-based practice developed from evidence-based medicine. The concept of evidence-based medicine was an attempt to increase the use of information collected from research studies, especially studies in basic sciences, and translate the data into clinical practice as opposed to practitioners relying on rote routines developed by other practitioners who were regarded as experts but may have little scientific basis for their protocols

Table 10-3
PRIMARY WORK SETTING

SETTING	PERCENTAGE
Schools/early intervention	24.7%
Hospital (non-mental health)	21.2%
Long-term care/skilled nursing	18.7%
Academia	11/2%
Freestanding outpatient	09.6%
Home health	05.7%
Mental health	03.0%
Community	02.6%
Other (not specified)	03.3%

AOTA. (2009). Member participation survey. Bethesda, MD: Author.

Table 10-4
WORK TIME ALLOCATION

SETTING	PERCENTAGE
Direct client intervention	55.8%
Indirect client work/administration	22.4%
Education	11.3%
Consultation	07.0%
Research	03.3%

AOTA. (2009). Member participation survey. Bethesda, MD: Author.

(Sackett, Straus, Richardson, Rosenberg, & Hayes, 2000). Law (2000) paraphrased the definition used by Sackett et al. (2000) in the first edition of their book as "conscientious, explicit and judicious use of current best evidence in making decision about the care of individual patients. The practice of evidence-based medicine means integrating individual clinical expertise with the best available external clinical evidence from systematic research" (Sackett, Richardson, Rosenberg, & Haynes, 1997, p. 2). In the second edition, Sackett et al. (2000) expand on the concept of evidence-based (medicine) practice, stating that it is the "integration of best research evidence with clinical experience and patient values" (p. 1). Of importance is the addition of patient values. In other words, there are three factors to consider in evidence-based practice: research evidence, clinical expertise, and patient/client values. Best research evidence means "clinically relevant research … into the accuracy and precision of diagnostic tests (including the clinical examination), the power of prognostic markers, and the efficacy and safety of therapeutic, rehabilitative, and prevention regiments." Clinical expertise means the "ability to use clinical skills and past experience to identify each patient's unique health state and diagnosis their individual risks and benefits of potential interventions and their personal values and expectations." Values mean the "unique preferences, concerns and expectation each patient brings to a clinical encounter and which must be integrated into clinical decision if they are to serve the patient" (Sackett et al., 2000, p. 1).

Law (2000) summarizes four stages for the application to occupational therapy practice: (1) ask a clinical question about a specific client's problem, (2) search for information or evidence about the problem, (3) critically appraise the evidence to determine whether it is useful, and (4) apply the findings. To assist practitioners in evaluating research studies, the Association began publishing an online series called AOTA Evidence Briefs. Topics ranged from stroke and substance abuse to massage therapy and music therapy for infants and children (Lieberman, Scheer, & Erby, 2003). Peterson (2003) reports that students could learn to apply the principles of evidence-based practice in an article about working with older individuals at risk for falls.

Reimbursement and the Prospective Payment System

The prospective payment system (PPS) was part of the BBA of 1997 that caused a significant reduction in employment opportunities and failure to renew membership in the Association. The PPS changed the mechanisms for reimbursing facilities for services to Medicare clients, including services provided by occupational therapy practitioners. Medicare had originally been set up as a "cost-based reimbursement system" (Boerkoel, 2004). In other words, the Medicare program reimbursed facilities for the cost of providing all covered services, including therapy, to Medicare recipients. The more services needed, the more reimbursement provided. There was little, if any, incentive to limit costs, and the budget for Medicare services was growing every year. The PPS was designed to put some parameters on what services would be reimbursed. Boerkoel (2004) outlines six minimum requirements:

- A competent, trained provider of these services (i.e., licensed provider)
- Ethical and moral standards (i.e., recognized standard of care)
- A limitation of the services (i.e., services could not be provided indefinitely)
- A demonstrated justification based on outcomes (i.e., evidence-based practice)
- Record keeping of the services provided
- A quality assurance process (i.e., review process)

Initially, facility managers were concerned that the PPS would reduce reimbursement significantly and negatively impact their bottom line. As the PPS went into effect, facility managers learned how to use the PPS and comply with the requirements. Practitioners also had to learn new methods of justifying their services and demonstrating that services were outcome based with support from published literature.

Encroachment and Turf Wars With Other Professions Regarding Scope of Practice

In a memorandum to the state association presidents and legislative chairs in 2000, Fred Somers, Karen Smith, and Charles Willmarth outlined four areas of concern: physical therapy, orthotics and prosthetics, vision therapy, and psychological testing (Somers, Smith, & Willmarth, 2000). The issue with physical therapy continued to be the definition of physical therapy practice in the Model Practice Act for Physical Therapy approved by the Federation of State Boards of Physical Therapy. The issue in orthotics and prosthetics was laws that might exclude occupational therapists in the design and fit of orthotic devices. The same issue applied to vision therapy; in the state of New York, the practice of vision therapy was limited to those with a license as a vision rehabilitation therapist. Of particular concern were restrictions on who could work with patients on safety-related training activities. Psychologists in Indiana distributed a list of over 3,000 tests and instruments that they proposed to restrict for use by psychologists only. Three of the tests were authored by occupational therapists: FirstSTEP: Screening Test for Evaluation Preschoolers by Miller; the Miller Assessment of Preschoolers (MAP) by Miller; and the Sensory Integration and Praxis Test by Ayres. Recreational therapy also encroached by defining itself in a bill before the Iowa Senate in 2007 as "a treatment service designed to restore, remediate, or rehabilitate a patient's or client's level of functioning and independence in life activities, or to reduce or eliminate the life activity restriction caused by an illness or disability condition" (AOTA, 2007a). Other professions' practitioners who have proposed legislation that encroaches upon or limits occupational therapy practice include athletic trainers, developmental therapists, optometrists, speech-language pathologists, and wheelchair suppliers and manufacturers (AOTA, 2007a). Audiology is also mentioned (AOTA, 2007a) regarding who can treat balance disorders and engage in fall prevention. A bill introduced to the Colorado legislature defined athletic training to include "serves appropriate for the prevention, recognition, assessment, management, treatment, rehabilitation and reconditioning of injuries and illnesses that are sustained in sports, recreation, games or exercise or might affect an individual's participation in those activities" (AOTA, 2006a). Athletic trainers attempted to expand their scope of practice (AOTA, 2006a). The ICF (WHO, 2001) popularized the words *participation* and *activities*, whereas Medicare popularized the word *function* (*functional* or *functioning*).

Other professions are not the only threat to scope of practice. Occupational therapy practitioners may be their own worst enemies. As job opportunities decreased, the possibly of finding employment elsewhere may have encouraged practitioners to try new or different assessment or intervention strategies that may or may not have fit within the occupational therapy scope of practice. Legal and ethics concerns led to the publication of two articles in *OT Practice* reviewing questionable examples of scope of practice and suggesting a decision-making process for determining whether the action, practice, or intervention was within the occupational therapy scope of practice (Slater, 2004; Slater & Willmarth, 2006) (Table 10-5).

Table 10-5
FRAMEWORK FOR DECISIONS ABOUT SCOPE OF PRACTICE

- Was this body of knowledge or skill part of my educational coursework or curriculum?

- Am I competent (and is it baseline or advanced competence) to perform this skill or provide this intervention based on my past education, continuing or ongoing education, and experience?

- Is my knowledge current (evidence-based, meets accepted practice standards, AOTA standards, and what most people consider accepted practice) and state of the art to provide competent service?

- Would most practitioners agree that this intervention qualifies as "usual and customary" practice? Does it meet widely held standards?

- Have I sought clarification from the state licensure board (or other regulatory body) in interpreting less-well-defined areas of the occupational therapy scope of practice?

- Have I sought resources like AOTA position papers or official documents relating to this area of practice, or done a literature search to provide evidence for my intervention or practice?

- How does this intervention or practice relate to the philosophy of occupational therapy? Am I using occupation to promote engagement in meaningful activities and participation in life roles?

Adapted from Slater, E. Y. (2004). Legal and ethical practice: A professional responsibility. *OT Practice, 9*(16), 13-16 and Slater, D. Y., & Willmarth, C. (2006). Understanding and asserting the occupational therapy scope of practice. *OT Practice, 10*(10), CE-1-CE-8.

Impact of Balanced Budget Act of 1997

The BBA (P.L. 105-33) of 1997 changed the method for reimbursement of inpatient rehabilitation facilities, skilled nursing facilities, and home health agencies under Medicare Part A from a retrospective to a PPS. In addition, the BBA imposed a cap on the dollar amount for outpatient therapy services incurred in a calendar year for services furnished in skilled nursing facilities, physician's offices, and home health agencies under Medicare Part B. The limit on expenses applied to all three rehabilitation services—occupational therapy, physical therapy, and speech-language pathology—but the impact was felt most by occupational and physical therapy. Rehabilitation facilities began laying off therapists, and hiring freezes occurred because managers were concerned about future financial reimbursement. Reliance on Medicare had become widespread, and regulations adopted by a major government program were often adopted by private insurance companies. The financial status of the rehabilitation health care market was potentially unstable. The long-term effects of managed care and changes in Medicare reimbursement were difficult to calculate, and managers responded by cutting expenses, especially personnel. Unlike previous changes in government policies, the restriction of therapy services hit hard as the job market for therapists collapsed. Occupational therapy assistants were affected more than occupational therapists because more assistants worked in skilled nursing homes (Fisher & Cooksey, 2002).

The impact of changing reimbursement rules and procedures was felt throughout the occupational therapy community, including Association membership. In 1997, before the impact occurred, membership in the Association had grown to 59,371. Growth in Association membership had been a given since the Association was formed in 1917. Even during the Great Depression years of the 1930s, membership in the Association grew. But by January 2004, the lowest point, membership had fallen for 7 straight years to a low of 34,303 (AOTA, 2004b). The reduction in membership and income to the Association resulted in restricting the Association journal. Instead of 12 issues a year, the journal was reduced to six, although the page number remained the same (Hasselkus, 1999). Student enrollment was also affected. Potential students were told there were no jobs available, so do not apply to an occupational therapy educational program. The highest number of students enrolled in the occupational therapist programs occurred in 1999 (11,746), but by 2004, the number had dropped to 10,117, a 42% decrease. For occupational therapy assistants, the high point was 1998 (7,610) and the low point was 2002 (3,350, a 56% decrease). Educational programs for the occupational therapist did not close as a result of the decreased enrollment. Five closures were due to the change in degree requirements mandated by 2007 to move to a master's degree (AOTA, 2007/2008). However, occupational therapy assistant educational programs were affected. In 2002, there were 172 programs, but by 2007, there were 128, a drop of 44 programs (AOTA, 2007/2008). Actually, a total of 60 occupational therapy assistant programs closed between 2000 and 2007, but the totals do not reflect the openings and closings within each time period.

The job market began to stabilize in 2001 (Fisher & Cooksey, 2002). Over the years, a variety of legislation has reduced the impact of the therapy cap by initiating repeals or by placing moratoriums on the implementation, and the managers of rehabilitation facilities began to adjust their budgets to the changes in reimbursement procedures. The initial repeal on Medicare Part B Outpatient occupational therapy became effective on January 1, 2000, after the Association lobbied effectively against blending the three therapy services (occupational therapy/physical therapy/speech-language pathology) into one generic rehabilitation benefit. Money was also restored to the skilled nursing facility funding, the home health rate reductions were postponed and the reimbursement rates were increased. In response, numbers in the occupational therapy world began to improve. By 2005, Association membership began to increase again, due in part to membership recruitment efforts. By 2007, the educational programs were on the increase in response to growing demands for practitioners (AOTA, 2008/2009). In 2009, membership had reached 38,894. The number of accredited occupational therapist programs was 142 with 3 applicants, whereas the number of assistant programs was 129 with six developing and 23 applicants.

So what was learned from a severe blow to the existence and psyche of occupational therapy as a profession? One lesson was the characteristics employers wanted from therapists. Fisher and Cooksy (2002) stated that desirable qualities included "the ability to promote and 'sell' occupational therapy, strong communication skills, sufficient experience and initiative to require little supervision, flexibility, effective problem-solving ability, innovation, good documentation skills, and professionalism" (p. 1). A second lesson was that new and expanding job markets were available, such as ergonomics consulting to reduce workplace injuries, home modification and accessibility consulting, older driver assessment, assisted living facility consulting, technology development and consulting, health and wellness consulting, low-vision rehabilitation, and caregiver training for Alzheimer's disease (Brachtesende, 2005). Expanding opportunities for school-based practice also helped ease the job market shortage. A third lesson was to broaden the scope of services and products available through the Association at reduced rates for members.

Numbers of Licensed or Regulated Therapists and Assistants

The five states with the largest number of therapists and assistants in 2009 were New York (13,641), California (12,358), Texas (9,185), Pennsylvania (8,948), and Florida (7,340) (AOTA, 2009b). Earlier, in 2006, the states with the largest number of employed practitioners had been California, New York, Ohio, and Pennsylvania (AOTA, 2006a). Geographically, the South Atlantic, North Central, and South Central regions of the country had seen the largest growth in the number of practitioners, averaging 4% growth per year. The Mountain region had experience the slowest growth, averaging 2.3% per year.

Workforce and Compensation

According to the 2006 AOTA Workforce and Compensation Survey, occupational therapists were 95% female and 5% male; assistants were 97% female and 3% male. Median age of occupational therapists was 42 years, up from 36 years in 1990; for assistants, median age was 45 years, up from 33 years in 1990 (AOTA, 2006c). The number of practitioners between the ages of 50 and 59 years was at its highest level ever, whereas the percentage of practitioners younger than 30 years was 7.9%, compared with 23% in 1997. A major concern was that if the trend continued, the field could experience a significant shortage of practitioners due to retirement. As the workforce aged, the median years of professional experience increased to 13 years, up from 9.5 in 2000. Ten percent of practitioners had at least 30 years of professional experience, and 3.2% had achieved advanced practice certification or recognition, up from 15.4% in 2000. The median salary for a full-time occupational therapist increased 24%, from $45,000 to $55,800 in 2006. For assistants, the salary had increase 26.7% from $30,000 in 2000 to $38,000 in 2006.

LEGISLATION

A Model Practice Act to provide a guide for state licensure legislation was first written in 1989 by the State Policy Department (AOTA, 2000). The Model Practice Act was revised in 1999, 2004, and 2011 to update the definition of occupational therapy and other technical and legal changes. Significant federal legislation is summarized in Table 10-6.

TECHNOLOGY

A useful development in technology was the creation of the certification program in assistive technology (Lenker, 2000). Although the certification program was developed outside the profession, it provided a benchmark for practitioners to identify their skill level in using assistive technology. The certification program was developed by the Rehabilitation Engineering Society of North America (RESNA) in 1996 but took a while to be accepted in the occupational therapy field. There are two certifications: assistive technology practitioner (ATP) and assistive technology supplier (ATS). To administer the programs, RESNA created a separate entity called the Professional Standards Board (PSB).

	Table 10-6 LEGISLATION
2001	No Child Left Behind (NCLB) (P.L. 107-110). Schools were to test students in reading and math at grades 3 and 8 and once in high school. All schools in the state education system were to meet a certain proficiency level. (Bazyk & Case-Smith, 2010)
2003	Medicare Prescription Drug Improvement and Modernization Act (P.L. 108-173). Law to support consumer-driven health care and lowering health care expenditures. Decision making is shifted from the insurance company to the consumer. High-deductible health plans and consumer-directed health plans are examples. These plans provide incentive not to spend health care dollars, so occupational therapists need to educate people on the benefits of services. (Lohman, 2014)
2004	Individuals with Disabilities Education Improvement Act (IDEIA or IDEA) (P.L. 108-446). Reauthorized and updated the 1997 IDEA Increased emphasis on accountability and outcomes. Supports response to intervention (RtI) and early intervention services (EIS). (Bazyk & Case-Smith, 2010)
2006	The Deficit Reduction Act (P.L. 109-171). Allows for temporary exemption of the therapy cap for certain condition in hospital and nonhospital-based clinics. If continued interventions are "reasonable and medically necessary," exemptions can be granted. If client has "qualifying condition or complexity," an automatic exemption process exists. (Lohman, 2014)
2010	Patient Protection and Affordable Care Act (PPACA) (P.L. 111-148). Attempts to provide affordable medical insurance to persons with no health insurance or who are uninsured. (Lohman, 2014)

References

Bazyk, S., & Case-Smith, J. (2010). School-based occupational therapy. In J. Case-Smith & J. C. O'Brien (Eds.), *Occupational therapy for children* (6th ed., pp. 713-743). St. Louis, MO: Mosby/Elsevier.

Lohman, H. (2014). Payment for services in the United States. In B. A. Boyt Schell, G. Gillen, & M. E. Scaffa (Eds.), *Willard & Spackman's occupational therapy* (12th ed., pp. 1051-1067). Philadelphia, PA: Wolters Kluwer.

RESEARCH

In 2004, a joint task group from both the Association and the Foundation developed a set of research priorities for the profession (Table 10-7).

The Evidence-Based Literature Review Project began in 1998 as "a feasibility study to assess the use fullness of a standardized format to code selected occupational therapy outcome literature" in the online search system (Lieberman & Scheer, 2002). As the project evolved through three phases, a format was developed to separate levels of evidence regarding outcomes research. The format included four levels: evidence for design, evidence for sample size, evidenced for internal validity, and evidence for external validity. There were five levels of evidence for design: randomized control trial (I), non-randomized control trail—two groups (experimental and control) (II), nonrandomized control trial—one group, one treatment (pretest and posttest) (III), single-subject design (IV), and not applicable (NA), which included narratives, case studies, expert opinion, literature reviews, consensus statements, and other nonquantifiable designs. Sample size was divided into two levels, internal validity into three levels, and external validity into three levels. In essence, the research study was evaluated on design + sample size + internal validity + external validity. Although the format was not formally adopted by AJOT, it provided a useful method for teaching practitioners and students to evaluate research studies on a scale. Studies using randomized, controlled trial design with a larger number of subjects (20 or more per cognition) and high internal and external validity should be given greater weight or consideration in translating the information from research to practice.

The Association has developed additional tools to help translate research into clinical practice called Critically Appraised Topics (CATs) or Critically Appraised Papers (CAPs). CATs are designed to provide evidence-based information on a specific clinical situation and provide a brief, easy-to-read summary of results of a systematic review of the literature (Arbesman, Scheer,

Table 10-7
TEN RESEARCH PRIORITIES
1. Are occupational therapy interventions effective in achieving targeted activity and participation outcomes and preventing/reducing secondary conditions?
2. To what extent does occupation-based intervention promote learning adaptation, self-organization, adjustment to life situations, and self-determination across the life span?
3. Are environmental interventions that support occupation effective in preventing impairment and promoting activity and participation in the individual, community, and societal levels?
4. When, when, how, and at what level (body structure/body function, activity, participation, and environmental) should an occupational therapy intervention occur to maximize activity and participation, as well as cost-effectiveness of services?
5. What measures/measurement systems reflect the domain of occupational therapy and identify factors (body structure/body function, activity, participation, and environment) or document the impact of occupational therapy on these factors?
6. How do activity patterns and choices (occupations), both in everyday life and across the lifespan, influence the health and participation of individuals?
7. What is the impact of activity patterns and choices (occupations), both in everyday life and across the lifespan, on society?
8. What are the conceptual models that explain the relationship among body structure/body function, activity, environment, and participation? What is the role of occupational therapy within these models?
9. What factors contribute to effective partnerships between customers and practitioners that foster and enhance participation in individuals with or at risk for disabling conditions?
10. What factors support occupational therapy practitioners' capacities to maximize the occupational performance of the persons they serve?
AOTF/AOTA. (2004). Research priorities and the parameters of practice for occupational therapy. *OT Practice, 9*(4), 20-21.

& Lieberman, 2008). CAT authors develop a focused question to delineate the systematic review of literature; identify studies on a topic under consideration using specific inclusion and exclusion criteria; select a group of the highest quality and most relevant articles, ranked according to the standardized criteria for study design as described in the previous paragraph; critically appraise and evaluate the design and methods used in the study; present the findings in the articles; and synthesize the findings. CAPs summarize individual studies using a standardized format. CAPs may be grouped together to develop a CAT. The Association maintains both CAPs and CATs on its website. Information from the CAPs and CATs has also been included in the Practice Guideline series of topics developed over several years.

ASSOCIATION

Centennial Vision Project

The Board of Directors endorsed the development of a Centennial Vision project to act as road map for the future of the profession. The goal was to:

> … ensure that individuals, policy-makers, populations, and society value and promote occupational therapy's practice of enabling people to prevent and overcome obstacles to participation in the activities they value, to prevent health-related issues, improve their physical and mental health, secure well-being and enjoy a higher quality of life. (Christiansen, 2004, p. 10)

The eight elements developed were the following:

1. Expanded collaboration for success

2. Power to influence

3. Membership equals professional responsibility

4. Well-prepared, diverse workforce

5. Clear, compelling public image

6. Customers demand occupational therapy

7. Evidence-based decision making

8. Science-fostered innovation in occupational therapy practice

The Centennial Vision statement was as follows: "We envision that occupational therapy is a powerful, widely recognized, science-driven, and evidence-based profession with a globally connected and diverse workforce meeting society's occupational needs." The statement was adopted by the Association Board of Directors in October 2003 and was posted to the Association website, but was first published in 2007 (Corcoran, 2007, p. 267). The Centennial Vision project was envisioned "to be a road map for the future of the profession to commemorate the Association's 100th anniversary in 2017" (AOTA, 2007c, p. 613). Charles Christiansen and Florence Clark were Vice Presidents whose job was to track and record the developments toward the goals of the Centennial Vision statement (Sidebar 10-1).

Corcoran (2007) states that the Centennial Vision project involved a "synchronized set of strategies, imperatives, and priorities for advancing our profession" (p. 267). Four strategic directs were identified at a retreat in 2006:

1. Build the capacity to fulfill the profession's potential and mission

2. Demonstrate and articulate our value to individuals, organizations and communities

3. Build an inclusive community of members

4. Link education, research, and practice (AOTA, 2007c, pp. 613-614)

Branding Statement

"Occupational Therapy: Living Life to Its Fullest" was adopted as the new brand phrase in April 2008 by the Representative Assembly at the meeting in Long Beach, California, and reported to the membership by President Penelope Moyers Cleveland (2008). The new brand replaced "Occupational Therapy: Skills for the Job of Living," which had been used as an advertising message for several years. In explaining the new brand, Cleveland (2008) gave several examples:

- When occupational therapy says the impossible is possible, we are helping people live life to its fullest.

- When occupation therapy works with a person with mental illness to set meaningful occupational goals thought to be beyond reach, we are helping that person live life to its fullest.

- When occupational therapy helps a wounded soldier learn to regain the balance and vision and perception to ride a bike again, we are helping him or her live life to its fullest.

- When occupational therapy inspires people to reach for the summit, no matter what, we are helping them live life to its fullest.

- When occupational therapy helps adults stay active in their own homes and communities, we are helping them live life to its fullest.

- When occupational therapy helps a child control negative behaviors and engage in positive socialization, we are helping him or her live life to its fullest (p. 742).

Sidebar 10-1

AOTA Celebrates Century of Service

Prior to the adoption of the Centennial Vision, AOTA President Carolyn Baum developed a plan to set a strategic vision for the future of the profession. She distributed this press release envisioning AOTA celebrating the accomplishments at the end of a century of service.

FOR IMMEDIATE RELEASE   **CONTACT: John Q. Spokesperson**
April 28, 2017   **301-652-6611   praota@aota.org**

AOTA CELEBRATES CENTURY OF SERVICE

(Washington, DC) – Membership in the American Occupational Therapy Association has reached record numbers as the profession of occupational therapy celebrates its centennial.

"Since the profession's genesis one hundred years ago, practice, education, research and society have changed and grown," said AOTA's President. "Today occupational therapy is a powerful, widely recognized, science-driven, and evidence-based profession that is globally connected and employs a diverse workforce. We have come far in meeting the needs of society. Occupational therapy practitioners have made much progress for:

Elderly Citizens

OT has been essential to the redesign of services and advocated for programs and funding—changing Medicare as well as private services—to enable our elderly to stay active and safe in their own homes and communities.

Young Children

OTs have been elected to local school boards across the country and now OT is available to any child in school to help them acquire the learning, coping, and developmental skills to be successful in school and transition to adult life.

People With Mental Illness

OT research has guided successful strategies that have put OT into the mental health mainstream, helping clinicians meet the needs of individuals with mental illness to enable them to lead independent and productive lives.

The Workforce

OT has become integral to the development of safe and productive workplaces, providing interventions in manufacturing, service, sales and other industries so all workers can avoid injury and older, disabled and all workers are valued and valuable.

People with Disabilities

OT has been the driving force behind a 'Second Wave' ADA effort to finally and fully remove barriers that limit the full participation of people with disabilities in society.

Education

Doctorally prepared faculty are educating record numbers of OT students to use their knowledge to enhance the lives of people with chronic disease and disability. Occupational Therapy is established as an academic discipline. Five faculty currently are Fulbright scholars studying services in developing countries for people with disabilities.

Research

Record numbers of occupational therapy scientists have received funding from NIH and NIDRR and are contributing knowledge to improve the lives of individuals with disabilities and ways to prevent disease resulting in improved health and well-being.

The American Occupational Therapy Association, established in 1917, represents nearly 75,000 members. AOTA is an active advocate for the profession and for individuals who can benefit from occupational therapy services."

Reprinted with permission from Baum, C. (2006). Presidential Address, 2006: Centennial challenges, millennium opportunities. *American Journal of Occupational Therapy, 60*(6), 609-616.

Presidents, Executive Directors, and Association Priorities

Three people served as President of AOTA from 2001 to 2010: Barbara L. Kornblau, 2001-2004 (Figure 10-2); Carolyn M. Baum, 2004-2007 (Figure 10-3); and Penelope Moyers-Cleveland, 2007-2010 (Figure 10-4). Table 10-8 summarizes their accomplishments. Biographical sketches are included in Table 10-9. Joseph Isaacs served as Executive Director from 2000 to 2003 (Johansson, 2000) (Figure 10-5), and Frederick Somers began serving as Executive Director in 2004 (Figure 10-6). Examples of goals and objectives appear in Table 10-10, and documents adopted by the Representative Assembly appear in Table 10-11 (Figure 10-7).

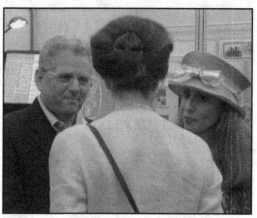

Figure 10-2. Barbara L. Kornblau, JD, OT/L, FAOTA, President of AOTA, 2001-2004, (right) and her husband Larry Sherry (left) meeting Princess Anne in July 2001 at the 25th Annual Conference of the College of Occupational Therapists, held at the University of Wales, Swansea. (Reprinted with permission from Barbara L. Kornblau.)

Finances

In 2000, the Association faced a serious loss of income and had to revise Association priorities. All volunteer bodies were asked to make do with less. Layoffs continued in the national office. Departments were consolidated; such the Conferences and Meetings Departments were merged to form a new Continuing Education and Events Department. Full-time staff were reduced from 143 in 1998 to 94. Members were given the option to choose not to receive the a mailed copy of AJOT to save postage. Some committees, such as the Recognitions Committee, were asked to conduct business via technology, such as email and conference calls, rather than face-to-face meetings (AOTA, 2000).

Primary sources of income in fiscal year 2001 were member fees, conference, books and publications, subscriptions, and building rental income. Major expenses were administration, periodical publication, continuing education, and building maintenance (AOTA, 2001).

Continuing Competence and Competency

In 2002, the Representative Assembly voted, and the membership approved, to establish the CCCPD to "address the growing awareness of and need within the profession for continuing competence" (AOTA, 2002b, p. 7). The specific purposes were to promote high professional standards and continuing competence and to foster success in both existing and emerging practice settings (AOTA, 2002b, p. 7). The CCCPD has no

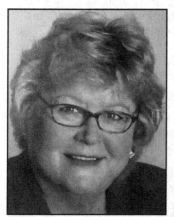

Figure 10-3. Carolyn M. Baum, PhD, OTR/L, FAOTA, President of AOTA, 2004-2007. (Printed with permission from the Archive of the American Occupational Therapy Association, Inc.)

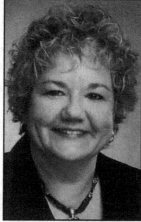

Figure 10-4. Penelope Moyers Cleveland, EdD, OTR/L, BCMH, FAOTA, President of AOTA, 2007-2010. (Printed with permission from the Archive of the American Occupational Therapy Association, Inc.)

Table 10-8
PRESIDENTIAL ACCOMPLISHMENTS
Barbara L. Kornblau, 2001-2004
Reorganization of the Association stressing financial accountability and overseeing initiation of the centennial vision
Carolyn Baum, 2004-2007
Development of the Model Education Curriculum
Penelope Moyers-Cleveland, 2007-2010
Overseeing creation of a new brand phrase

Table 10-9
BIOGRAPHICAL SKETCHES
BARBARA L. KORNBLAU
Born August 17, 1956
Born in Flushing, New York. She has a bachelor of science degree from the University of Wisconsin-Madison and a doctorate in jurisprudence from the University of Miami. She holds certifications in case management, disability management, and pain management and is credentialed in disability analysis and pain management. She is member of the Florida Bar and the United States Supreme Court Bar. She became a Fellow in 1996, received the Award of Merit in 2009, and served as President from 2001 to 2004. She had held positions as Professor of Occupational Therapy and Public Health in the Colleges of Allied Health and Osteopathic Medicine and Adjunct Professor in the Sheppard Board Law Centre at Nova Southeastern University. She has been a Professor and Former Dean of the School of Health Professions and Studies at the University of Michigan-Flint. She is Professor of Occupational Therapy, School of Allied Health Science, Florida A&M University, and Executive Director of the Society for Participatory Medicine and Founder and CEO of the Coalition for Disability Health Equity. Her research interests include health and disability policy, disability health, disparities, and health equity. She is the co-author of the book *Ethics in Rehabilitation: A Clinical Approach.*
CAROLYN M. BAUM
(See Chapter 9)
PENELOPE A. MOYERS CLEVELAND
Born September 7, 1955
Lived in Indianapolis. Her bachelor's degree in occupational therapy is from the University of Missouri in 1977, her master's degree in community development is from the University of Louisville, and her doctoral degree is in adult education with a major in public administration from Ball State University. She served as President from 2007 to 2010. Her work career includes working at the Central State Hospital in Louisville, Kentucky and Plastic Surgery Associates in Indianapolis, Indiana. She has served as Dean of the School of Occupational Therapy at the University of Indianapolis, professor and Chair of the Occupational Therapy Department at the University of Alabama-Birmingham, and Dean of the College of St. Catherine in Minneapolis. She is Board certified in mental health from the Association. She received the Award of Merit in 2013 and was named a Fellow in 1997. She has published on substance use disorders, continuing competence, and professional development. Prior to becoming President, she was chair of the Commission on Continuing Competence and Professional Development.

regulatory authority to remove a practitioner's license to practice; rather, the focus is on setting model standards, tools, and guidelines to assist practitioners in their professional development. An example is the Model of Continuing Competence Guidelines for the Occupational Therapist and Occupational Therapy Assistant: A Resource for State Regulatory Boards approved by the Representative Assembly in 2002 (AOTA, 2002d). The Association had originally approved Standards for Continuing Competence in 1999, but revisions of the document would become the responsibility of CCCPD, including the revision in 2006 (AOTA, 1999, 2005).

According to Moyers, competence refers to an individual's capacity to preform job (profession) responsibilities. "Capacity is most clearly related to ongoing professional develop or life-long learning" (Moyers, 2002, p. 19). Competence, in contrast, "focuses on an individual's actual performance in a particular situation. Competency implies a determination of whether one is competent to perform a behavior or task as measured against a specific criterion" (Moyers, 2002, p. 19). Continuing competence "is a process involving the examination of current competence and the development of capacity for the future (AOTA, 2005, p. 661). The

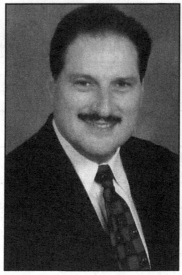

Figure 10-5. Joseph Isaacs, Executive Director of AOTA, 2000-2003. (Printed with permission from the Archive of the American Occupational Therapy Association, Inc.)

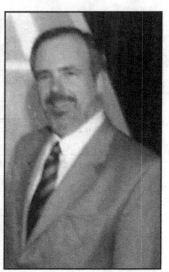

Figure 10-6. Frederick Somers, Executive Director of AOTA, 2004-present. (Printed with permission from the Archive of the American Occupational Therapy Association, Inc.)

role of competence, competency, and continued competence would become major issues as the state regulatory boards reviewed the process of renewing licenses to practice.

The CCCPD also oversees the development and administration of the Board and specialty certification. The Board for Advanced and Specialty Certification (BASC) is responsible for the ongoing activities. These programs are voluntary but are designed to allow practitioners to demonstrate expertise in a particular area of practice or a specific technique used as an intervention in occupational therapy practice. There are four areas of Board Certification with recognized credentials: Gerontology (BCG), Mental Health (BCMH), Pediatrics (BCP), and Physical Rehabilitation (BCPR). There are five Specialty Certification programs available for either the occupational therapist or the assistant: Driving and Community Mobility, Feeding, Eating and Swallowing, Environmental Modification, Low Vision, and School Systems.

Table 10-10
STRATEGIC PLAN GOALS AND OBJECTIVES 2000-2004

- To ensure a member-centered focus
- To advance excellence in practice, education and research
- To represent and advocate for the profession
- To pursue strategic alliances
- To remain a viable and financially sound organization
- To improve governance and management effectiveness

Reference Manual 10th ed.

Fund to Promote Awareness of Occupational Therapy

The Fund was created in 2002 in response to a membership survey that indicated that the number one priority was to raise awareness about occupational therapy services and their potential contribution to society both inside and outside the profession. The Fund was created as a 501(c)(3) charitable organization with the goal of building corporate

	Table 10-11
	DOCUMENTS OF THE ASSOCIATION
2000	• Occupational therapy Code of Ethics (2000). AJOT, 54(6), 614-616.
	• Enforcement Procedure for Occupational Therapy Code of Ethics. AJOT, 54(6), 617-621.
	• Occupational Therapy and the Americans with Disabilities Act (ADA). AJOT, 54(6), 622-625.
	• Specialized Knowledge and Skills in Eating and Feeding for Occupational Therapy Practice. AJOT, 54(6), 629-641.
	• Specialized Knowledge and Skills for Occupational Therapy Practice in the NICU. AJOT, 54(6), 641-648.
	• Statement: Occupational Therapy Services in Facilitating Work Performance. AJOT, 54(6), 626-628
2001	• Occupational Therapy in the Promotion of Health and Prevention of Disease and Disability (replaced 1989 document). AJOT, 55(6), 656-660
	• Specialized Knowledge and Skills in Adult Vestibular Rehabilitation of Occupational Therapy Practice. AJOT, 55(6), 661-665.
2002	• Position Paper: Broadening the construct of Independence. AJOT, 56(6), 660
	• Enforcement Procedure for Occupational Therapy Code of Ethics. AJOT, 56(6), 661-666
	• Glossary: Standards for an Accredited Education Program for the Occupational Therapists and Occupational Therapy Assistant. AJOT, 56(6), 667-668.
	• Occupational Therapy Practice Framework: Domain and Process. AJOT, 56(6), 609-639
2003	• Concept Paper: Scholarship and Occupational Therapy. AJOT, 57(6), 641-643
	• Guidelines for Documentation of Occupational Therapy, AJOT, 57(6), 646-649.
	• Position Paper: Physical Agent Modalities. AJOT, 57(6), 650-651.
	• Statement: Applying Sensory Integration Framework in Educationally Related Occupational Therapy Practice. AJOT, 57(6), 652-659. (replaces 1997 Sensory Integration Evaluation and Intervention in School-Based Occupational Therapy)
	• Statement: Philosophy of Professional Education (revised 2007). AJOT, 57(6), 640
	• Statement: The Purpose and Value of Occupational Therapy Fieldwork Education (replaces 1996). AJOT, 57(6), 644
	• Statement: The Viability of Occupational Therapy Assistant Education. AJOT, 67(6), 645
	• Specialized Knowledge and Skills for Eating and feeding in Occupational Therapy Practice. AJOT, 57(6), 660-678.
2004	• Academic Terminal Degree. AJOT, 58(6), 648
	• Assistive Technology within Occupational Therapy Practice. AJOT, 58(6), 678-680
	• Enforcement Procedures for Occupational Therapy code of Ethics. AJOT, 58(6), 655-662/
	• Guidelines for Supervision, Roles, and Responsibilities During the Delivery of Occupational Therapy Services. AJOT, 58(6), 663-667.
	• Occupational Therapy Services in Early Childhood and School-based Settings. AJOT, 58(6), 681-685
	• Occupational therapy's Commitment to Nondiscrimination and Inclusion, AJOT, 58(6), 668.
	• Psychosocial Aspects of Occupational Therapy. AJOT, 58(6), 669-672
	• Role Competencies for an Academic Fieldwork Coordinator. AJOT, 58(6), 653-654
	• Role Competencies for a Professional-Level Occupational Therapist Faculty Member in an Academic Setting. AJOT, 58(6), 649-650.
	• Role Competencies for a Professional-Level Program Director in an Academic Setting. AJOT, 58(6), 651-652.
	• Scope of Practice. AJOT, 58(6), 673-677.
	(continued)

Table 10-11 (continued)
DOCUMENTS OF THE ASSOCIATION

2005	• Occupational Therapy and Hospice. AJOT, 59(6), 671-675
	• Occupational Therapy Code of Ethics. AJOT, 59(6), 739-642
	• Enforcement Procedures for the Occupational Therapy Coe of Ethics. AJOT, 59(6), 643-652
	• Occupational Therapy Services in Facilitating Work Performance. AJOT, 59(6), 676-679
	• Position Paper: Complementary and Alternative Medicine (CAM) (replaces 2003 White paper).
	• Role Competencies for a Faculty Member in an Occupational Therapy Assistant Academic Setting. AJOT, 59(6), 635-636.
	• Role Competencies for a Program Director in an Occupational Therapy Academic Setting. AJOT, 59(6), 637-638
	• Standards for Continuing Competence (replaces 1999 document). AJOT, 59(6), 661-662
	• Standards of Practice for Occupational Therapy (replaces 1998 document). AJOT, 59(6), 663-665
	• Statement: Driving and Community Mobility. AJOT, 59(6), 666-670.
	• The scope of occupational therapy service for individuals with autism spectrum disorders across the life span. AJOT, 59(6), 6800683
	• Telerehabilitation. AJOT, 59(6), 656-660
2006	• AOTA's Statement on Health Disparities. AJOT, 60(6), 679
	• AOTA's Statement on Obesity. AJOT, 60(6), 680
	• Bylaws: The American Occupational Therapy Foundation, Inc. (Delaware)
	• Guidelines to the Occupational Therapy Code of Ethics. AJOT, 60(6), 652-658.
	• Role Competencies for a Fieldwork Educator. AJOT, 60(6), 650-651.
	• Specialized Knowledge and Skills for Occupational Therapy Practice in the Neonatal Intensive Care Unit (replaces 2000 document). AJOT, 60(6), 659-668.
	• Specialized Knowledge and Skills in Adult Vestibular Rehabilitation for Occupational Therapy Practice (replaces 2000 document). AJOT, 60(6), 669-678.
	• The Role of Occupational Therapy in Disaster Preparedness, Response, and Recovery. AJOT, 60(6), 642-549.
2007	• A descriptive review of occupational therapy education, AJOT, 61(6), 672-677.
	• Accreditation Standards for a Doctoral-Degree-Level Educational Program for the Occupational Therapist. AJOT, 61(6), 641-651
	• Accreditation Standards for a Master's-Degree-Level Educational Program for the Occupational Therapist. AJOT, 61(6), 652-661
	• Accreditation Standards for tan Educational Program for the Occupational Therapy Assistant. AJOT, 61(6), 662-671
	• AOTA's Statement on Family Caregivers. AJOT, 61(6), 710
	• AOTA's Statement on Stress and Stress Disorders. AJOT, 61(6), 711
	• Enforcement Procedures for the Occupational Therapy Code of Ethics (edited 2007). AJOT, 61(6), 679-685.
	• Occupational therapy services for individuals who have experienced domestic violence. AJOT, 61(6), 704-709
	• Philosophy of Occupational Therapy Education. AJOT, 61(6), 678
	• Position Paper: Obesity and Occupational Therapy. AJOT, 61(6), 701703.
	• Specialized Knowledge and Skills in Feeding, Eating, and Swallowing for Occupational Therapy Practice. AJOT, 61(6), 686-700

(continued)

Table 10-11 (continued) DOCUMENTS OF THE ASSOCIATION	
2008	• Academic Terminal Degree. AJOT, 62(6), 704 • AOTA's Societal Statement on Play. AJOT, 62(6), 707-708 • AOTA's Societal Statement on Youth Violence. AJOT, 62(6), 709 • Guidelines for Documentation of Occupational Therapy. AJOT, 62(6), 684-690. • Occupational Therapy Practice Framework: Domain and Process. 2nd edition. (AJOT, 62(6), 625-683 • Occupational Therapy Services in the Promotion o Health and the Prevention of Disease and Disability. AJOT, 62(6), 694-703 • Position Paper: Physical Agent Modalities. AJOT, 62(6), 691-693 • The Importance of Occupational Therapy Assistant Education to the Profession. AJOT, 62(6), 705-706 • White Paper: Wound management. OT Practive13(7), 17-18
2009	• AOTA's Societal Statement on Autism Spectrum Disorders. AJOT, 63(6), 843-844 • AOTA's Societal Statement on Combat-Related Posttraumatic Stress. AJOT, 63(6), 845-846 • AOTA's Societal Statement on Livable Communities. AJOT, 63(6), 847-848 • Guidelines for Supervision, roles and responsibilities during the delivery of occupational therapy services. AJOT, 63(6), 797-803 • Occupational Therapy Fieldwork Education: Value and Purpose. AJOT, 63(6), 821-822 • Occupational Therapy's Commitment to Nondiscrimination and Inclusion. AJOT, 63(6), 819-820 • Providing Occupational Therapy Using Sensory Integration Theory and Methods in "School-Based Practice. AJOT, 63(6), 823-842. • Scholarship in Occupational Therapy. AJOT, 63(6), 790 • Specialized Knowledge and Skills of Occupational Therapy Educators of the Future. AJOT, 63(6), 804-818.

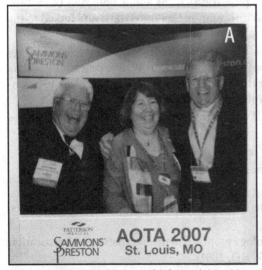
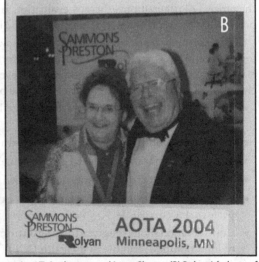

Figure 10-7. (A) Polaroid photo of (left to right) Fred Sammons, Lori T. Andersen, and Larry Sherry. (B) Polaroid photo of Kitty Reed (left) and Fred Sammons (right). Fred Sammons is one of AOTA's treasured members and benefactors. Early in his occupational therapy career, he started an adaptive equipment company. He is well known for taking Polaroid photos with conference-goers at his exhibitor booth at AOTA conferences. Many occupational therapy practitioners still have these photos in personal scrapbooks. This tradition continued until Polaroid film was no longer available. (Reprinted with permission from Fred Sammons.)

funding to support projects designed to promote recognition and visibility of occupational therapy as a profession. The mission is to achieve greater understanding, availability, and use of occupational therapy and to promote the profession's contribution to health, wellness, participation, productivity, and quality of life in society (Fund to Promote Occupational Therapy, 2014). Its purposes are to serve as the message hub and dissemination arm of the profession, help practitioners tell their own stories more effectively, and focus on high-impact communication aimed at the general public (Glomstand, 2003). One of the first projects was a commissioned survey conducted by the Gallup Organization in March/April 2003 to assess the understanding of older adults as what occupational therapy could do to meet their needs (Gallop Organization, 2003). Survey results indicated that awareness of occupational therapy was low; only 32% of respondents considered themselves to be very knowledgeable about occupational therapy, compared with 44% for physical therapy and 58% for nurses. Home health aides and nursing assistants are perceived as similar in function to occupational therapists. The Gallup Organization recommended that occupational therapy needed to be defined based on training and professional knowledge to help distinguish occupational therapy practitioners from home health aides and nursing assistants.

Another project underwritten by the Fund is National School Backpack Awareness Day, which is an annual campaign to promote awareness of occupational therapy's role in the health and well-being of children. In addition, the Fund in involved in Occupational Therapy Month which supports occupational therapy as a career choice and celebrates the work of practitioners in their practice settings. The Fund has also partnered with Rebuilding Together, a national organization that works to preserve and renew houses in communities.

Occupational Therapy Practice Framework

The Occupational Therapy Practice Framework was developed in response to current practice needs to more clearly "affirm and articulate" the focus of occupational therapy on occupation, activities of daily living, and the application of an intervention process that facilitates engagement in occupation to support participation in life (AOTA, 2002c, p. 609). The purpose was to (1) describe the domain that centers and grounds the profession's focus and actions and (2) outline the process of occupational therapy evaluation and intervention that is dynamic and linked to the profession's focus on and use of occupation (AOTA, 2002c, p. 609).

The Commission on Practice had begun reviewing the document entitled Uniform Terminology for Occupational Therapy, Third Edition (Uniform Terminology III) in 1998 to potentially update it (AOTA, 1994). During the review process, several problems became apparent, leading to a conclusion that another approach was needed. The problems identified were the following:

- Terms defined in the Uniform Terminology III document were unclear, inaccurate, or categorized improperly.
- Terms that should have been in the Uniform Terminology III document were missing.
- Too much emphasis was placed on performance components.
- The concept of occupation was not included.
- Terms were used that were unfamiliar to external audiences (i.e., performance components, performance areas).
- Consideration should be given to using terminology proposed in the International Classification of Functioning Disability and Health (ICF) (WHO, 2001).
- The Uniform Terminology III document was being used inappropriately to design curricula.
- The role of theory application in clinical reasoning is being minimized by using the Uniform Terminology III document as a recipe for practice.
- The practice environment had changed significantly since the last revision.
- The understanding had evolved within the profession of core constructs and service delivery process. (AOTA, 2002c, p. 637)

As a result of the review, changes were made to create a new document designed to replace Uniform Terminology III. The new document was called the Occupational Therapy Practice Framework: Domain & Practice (OTPF) and was adopted by the Representative Assembly in 2002 as Motion 29 (AOTA, 2002a). The document separated discussion of the domain of concern from the process of service delivery. The domain of concern presented the "areas of human experience in which practitioners of the profession offer assistance to others" (Mosey, 1981, p. 51). The domain was described as being concerned with "assisting people to engage in daily life activities that they find meaningful and purposeful" that stemmed from the professional "interest in human beings' ability to engage in everyday life activities" called occupation (AOTA, 2002c, p. 610). The domain included six major aspects: performance in areas of occupation, performance skills, performance patterns, context, activity demands, and client factors.

The process of occupational therapy was descripted in three aspects focusing on occupation: evaluation, intervention, and outcome. The process began by evaluating a client's occupational needs, problems, and concerns. Intervention focused on efforts to foster improved engagement in occupation. Outcome focused on the success in reaching the targeted goals or objectives.

The glossary to the OTPF lists 109 terms, which is less than the number defined in the Uniform Terminology III document (122 terms). However, additional terms appear in the document text that are not listed in the glossary. Whether some changes in terminology are due to consolidation of synonyms or elimination because they were not needed is not discussed. The discussion of changes in terminology from the Uniform Terminology III to the OTPF only covers the six major aspects but not the terms listed under the major headings (AOTA, 2002c).

2008 Revision of the Occupational Therapy Practice Framework

The OTPF was reviewed in 2007 as part of the 5-year review cycle established for all documents of the Association to determine whether a document needs revision, can remain unchanged, or should be rescinded because it is out of date or no longer useful. In general, the OTPF was found to be useful, but some reorganization, additions, and clarification of definitions were needed (AOTA, 2008b). For example, the concept of spirituality was moved from the section on Context to the section on Client Factors because feedback from members suggested that individuals considered spiritually to reside within the client rather than as part of a context. Context itself was expanded to include the concept of environment to acknowledge that the two are different ideas, but the term environment is used more often in the general literature. The concept of rest and sleep was separated from the concept of activities of daily living because all people need rest and/or sleep following occupation throughout their lifespan, as Adolf Meyer suggested in his 1921 lecture (Meyer, 1922). The concept of performance skills was broadened to include the concepts of abilities and capacities. The category of outcomes was expanded to include occupational justice and self-advocacy as legitimate outcomes of occupational therapy intervention. The term *client* was expanded to include person, organization, and population as opposed to being restricted to an individual only. The role of research in support of practice was emphasized by adding the concept of evidence-based practice. In general, the changes did not alter the overall structure of the OTPF but rather increased the consistency of the concept s with the current practice and delivery of occupational therapy services. A summary of the changes appears in AJOT (2008, pp. 605-667).

FOUNDATION

During the years 2000 to 2010, there were changes in personnel when three key people retired: Martha Kirkland, who had served as Executive Director of the American Occupational Therapy Foundation (AOTF) since 1986 (Figure 10-8); Nedra Gillette, who had been in charge of research efforts; and Mary Binderman, librarian of the Wilma L. West Library. Charles Christiansen

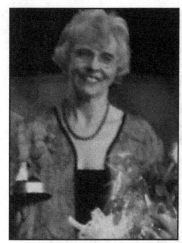
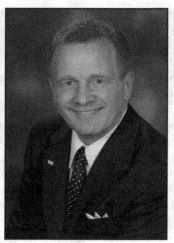
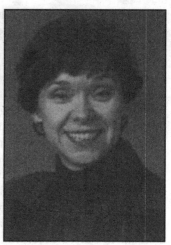

Figure 10-8. Martha Kirkland, OTR, FAOTA, Executive Director of the AOTF, 2006-2015. (Printed with permission from the Archive of the American Occupational Therapy Association, Inc.)

Figure 10-9. Charles H. Christiansen, EdD, OTR, FAOTA, Executive Director of the AOTF, 2006-2015. (Printed with permission from the Archive of the American Occupational Therapy Association, Inc.)

Figure 10-10. Ruth Ann Watkins, OTR, President of the AOTF, 2003-2007. (Printed with permission from the Archive of the American Occupational Therapy Association, Inc.)

become Executive Director in 2006 (Figure 10-9). Ruth Ann Watkins (Figure 10-10) served as President of the Foundation for 6 years, following Jane Davis Rourk.

In 2001, the Association and Foundation were involved in a serious dispute over the relationship between the two entities. The Association was experiencing financial hardship due to loss of membership revenue and was realigning priorities. Fiduciary responsibilities to the Association to operate as a business were viewed as top priorities (AOTA, 2001; Rourk, 2001). The Executive Board voted on three motions:

- Investigate the legal obligations to continue the 2% of each individual's annual Association membership feeds designated as a contribution to the AOTF in support of the Foundation's mission (approximately $120,000)
- Create a charitable 401(c)(3) organization to receive tax-deductible gifts separate from the Foundation (Fund to Promote Awareness of Occupational Therapy)
- Formulate an agreement to eliminate and/or reduce significant subsides from AOTA to the AOTF related to rented space, utilities, and other operating agreements which had totaled approximately $100,000 annually

The result of the motions would have been to (1) end direct member support of the Foundation and its educational, research, and public awareness activities; (2) establish a new charitable organization that would compete directly with the Foundation for private- and public-sector funding; and (3) alter the collaborative relationship between the Association and Foundation that had jointly supported initiatives to broaden and strengthen the knowledge base of the profession and its practitioners. On the other hand, the Foundation was fiscally sound and could pay the going rate for office space rent. A more important point was that the relationship established in 1965 would be substantially changed. The Foundation was created to take advantage of the IRS tax code that allowed certain activities, such as education, research, and public awareness, to be considered charity and thus not taxable or taxed at a reduced rate from activities considered business related. The separation of functions between the Association and Foundation was never intended to create two free-standing organizations with no interrelation except an agreement to cooperate on projects of mutual interest. There were no federal laws or guidelines adopted between 1965 and

2001 that required the Foundation to become a free-standing organization without any subsidy from the Association.

In September 2002, an AOTA/AOTF Collaboration Task Force developed a set of principles to guide collaboration between the Boards of three organizations (AOTA, AOTF, and National Board for Certification in Occupational Therapy [NBCOT]). In essence, the guidelines allowed each organization to seek charitable contributions but to communicate what each organization was doing to the others (Rourk & Kirkland, 2003). In addition, the Association agreed to continue to transfer the 2% of membership dues to the Foundation. Financial arrangements regarding rental space and other operating expenses were to be reviewed annually. Budgeting for joint projects was to be developed by the Association staff first, and then Foundation staff would be approached to determine what assistance the Foundation could provide to avoid conflicts regarding who was doing what with which money.

NATIONAL BOARD FOR CERTIFICATION IN OCCUPATIONAL THERAPY

Continuing Certification Program

NBCOT began phasing in a continuing certification program on July 1, 2002, and completed the initial phase on January 1, 2005, as part of program of accountability to the public (NBCOT, 2000a). Continuing certification must be renewed every 3 years and required obtaining 36 Professional Development Units (PDUs) during the 3-year period to continue using the terms occupational therapy registered or certified occupational therapy assistant or the use of the initials OTR or COTA after an individual's name. PDUs could be acquired through any of 23 activities, none which involved retaking the certification examination. Examples include attending workshops, making presentations, completing requirements for specialty certification, publishing an article or chapter, mentoring a colleague, guest lecturing, writing a report about an peer-reviewed article, supervising Level II students, participating in a study group, completing a self-assessment and professional development plan, completing an independent study course, or taking a college course. A chart of activities and their PDU values appeared in the spring issue of the newsletter (NBCOT, 2002a). At least 50% (18) of the required PDUs must be directly related to the delivery of occupational therapy services: "Directly related ... included models, theorie,s or frameworks that related to client/patient care in preventing or minimizing impairment, or enabling function within the person/environment or community context" (NBCOT, 2002b). In general, activities accepted as continuing education requirements for state licensure were accepted as PDUs for continuing certification. Although practitioners do not have to maintain certification with NBCOT, many choose to do so. States with the highest number of OTRs are California, New York, Pennsylvania, Texas, and Florida. States with the highest number of COTAs are New York, Pennsylvania, California, and Texas. Florida and Illinois are tied for fifth place (NBCOT, 2003, p. 5).

Practice Analysis Studies

NBCOT conducted its second practice analysis in 2003 (the first was in 1998) to obtain a detailed description of practice or what an occupational therapy or assistant does. The results were used to guide the development and content of the certification examination to ensure that the examination reflects current roles and responsibilities of entry-level practitioners. Each level of practice is divided into major performance domains. Each performance domain in turn is delineated in terms of its major tasks. Each task was then divided into a series of knowledge and skills statement (NBCOT, 2003). Table 10-12 shows the blueprint for the examinations, based on

Table 10-12
BLUEPRINTS FOR 2005 INITIAL CERTIFICATION EXAMINATIONS

	OTR	COTA
Evaluate individual/group to identify needs/priorities	25%	12%
Develop intervention plan addressing occupational needs	21%	22%
Implement occupationally meaningful interventions	41%	50%
Provide occupational therapy services addressing needs of populations	06%	09%
Manage/organize/promote occupational therapy services	07%	07%

the results of the 2003 practice analysis. Survey results of practitioners renewing the certification with NBCOT during the time period of 2003/2004 found that disorders most commonly seen by both OTRs and COTAs were, in order, neurological, orthopedic, developmental, psychosocial, musculoskeletal, cardiopulmonary, and systemic. The first three diagnostic groups accounted for approximately 60% of clients seen (NBCOT, 2004).

REFLECTION

The development and implementation of activities to support the Centennial Vision took center stage during this decade. Mid-decade, the profession began to recover from the effects of the BBA. There was further distancing from the medical model and sponsorship by the medical profession. The profession continued to develop new strategic partnerships. The profession also increased advocacy efforts and initiated efforts to mentor/develop leaders. Not everything was serious business. Figure 10-11 shows Florence Clark and Virgil Mathiowetz dancing in the aisle at the opening session of the 2005 annual conference in Long Beach, California.

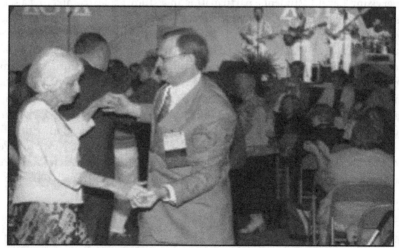

Figure 10-11. Dancing in the aisle: Florence Clark and Virgil Mathiowetz at the 2005 annual conference dancing in the aisle at the opening ceremony. (Printed with permission from the Archive of the American Occupational Therapy Association, Inc.)

REFERENCES

American Occupational Therapy Association. (1924). Minimum standards for courses of training in occupational therapy. *Archives of Occupational Therapy, 3*(4), 295-298.

American Occupational Therapy Association. (1958). *Curriculum guide for occupational therapy.* New York, NY: Author.

American Occupational Therapy Association. (1994). Uniform terminology for occupational therapy, third edition. *American Journal of Occupational, 48*(11), 1047-1054.

American Occupational Therapy Association. (1999). Standards for continuing competence. *American Journal of Occupational Therapy, 53*(6), 559-560.

American Occupational Therapy Association. (2000). Summary of AOTA's Executive Board actions: June 2000. Retrieved from www.aota.org

American Occupational Therapy Association. (2001). AOTA Board of Directors October 2001 meeting summary. Retrieved from www.aota.org

American Occupational Therapy Association. (2002a). 2002 Representative Assembly summary of minutes. *American Journal of Occupational Therapy, 56*(6), 695-696.

American Occupational Therapy Association. (2002b). CCCPD background and purpose. *OT Practice, 7*(18), 7.

American Occupational Therapy Association. (2002c). Occupational therapy practice framework: Domain & process. *American Journal of Occupational Therapy, 56*(6), 609-639.

American Occupational Therapy Association. (2002d). RA approves model continuing competence guidelines. *State Affairs Group News, 4*(2), 1, 6.

American Occupational Therapy Association. (2004a). *AOTA management report to the Representative Assembly.* Bethesda, MD: Author.

American Occupational Therapy Association. (2004b). Association policies: Definition of occupational therapy practice for state regulation (Policy 5.3.1). *American Journal of Occupational Therapy, 58*(6), 694-695.

American Occupational Therapy Association. (2005). Standards for continuing competence. *American Journal of Occupational Therapy, 59*(6), 661-662.

American Occupational Therapy Association. (2006a). Athletic trainers aim to expand their scope. *AOTA State Affairs Group News, 8*(2), 3.

American Occupational Therapy Association (2006b). Board of directors meeting minutes. Bethesda, MD: Author.

American Occupational Therapy Association (2006c). Workforce and Compensation Survey. Bethesda, MD: AOTA Press.

American Occupational Therapy Association. (2007a). State scope of practice challenges. *AOTA State Policy Update, 9*(4), p. 3.

American Occupational Therapy Association. (2007b). AOTA's APP recognized in state regulation. *State Affairs Group News, 9*(4), p. 2.

American Occupational Therapy Association. (2007c). AOTA's centennial vision and executive summary. *American Journal of Occupational Therapy, 61*(6), 613-614.

American Occupational Therapy Association. (2007/2008). *Annual data report.* Bethesda, MD: Author.

American Occupational Therapy Association. (2008a). Listing of educational programs in occupational therapy. *American Journal of Occupational Therapy, 62*(6), 721-732.

American Occupational Therapy Association. (2008b). Occupational therapy practice framework: Domain & process, second edition. *American Journal of Occupational Therapy, 62*(6), 625-683.

American Occupational Therapy Association. (2008c). New OT brand "Living life to its fullest." *OT Practice, 13*(6), 7.

American Occupational Therapy Association. (2008d). Occupational therapy practice framework: Domain & Process, 2nd ed. *American Journal of Occupational Therapy, 62*(6), 625-668.

American Occupational Therapy Association (2008e). *Occupational therapy model curriculum.* Bethesda, MD: Author.

American Occupational Therapy Association. (2008/2009). *Annual data report.* Bethesda, MD: Author.

American Occupational Therapy Association. (2009a). AOTA member participation survey: Overview report. Bethesda, MD: Author.

American Occupational Therapy Association. (2009b). Number of licensed/regulated OTs and OTAs. *State Policy Update, 11*(2), 4.

American Occupational Therapy Association. (2010a). *Academic programs annual data report.* Bethesda, MD: Author.

American Occupational Therapy Association. (2010b). Blueprint for entry-level education. *American Journal of Occupational Therapy, 64*(1), 186-203.

American Occupational Therapy Association (2010c). *The reference manual of the official documents of the American Occupational Therapy Association, Inc.*, 15th ed. Bethesda, MD: AOTA Press.

Arbesman, M., Scheer, J., & Lieberman, D. (2008). Using the AOTA's critically appraised topic (CAT) and critically appraised paper (CAP) series to link evidence to practice. *OT Practice, 13*(5), 18-22.

Boerkoel, D. (2004). Thriving with PPS. *OT Practice, 9*(20), 9-12.

Brachtesende, A. (2005, January). New markets emerge from society's needs. *OT Practice, 24*, 5-6.

Christiansen, C. (2004). AOTA's centennial vision: A map for the future. *OT Practice, 9*(17), 10.

Cleveland, P. M. (2008). Presidential address, 2008: Be unreasonable. Knock on the big doors. Knock loudly! *American Journal of Occupational Therapy, 62*(6), 737-742.

Corcoran, M. (2007). From the desk of the editor: AJOT and the AOTA Centennial Vision. *American Journal of Occupational Therapy, 61*(3), 267-268.

Fisher, G., & Cooksey, J. A. (2002). The occupational therapy workforce. Part two: Impact and action. *Administration & Management Special Interest Section Quarterly, 18*(3), 1-3

Fund to Promote Occupational Therapy. (2014). About the Fund to Promote Occupational Therapy. Retrieved from www.aota.org

Gallup Organization. (2003). Forging connections: A national public awareness survey of occupational therapy's role in helping independent-living older adults: Preliminary report. Retrieved from www.aota.org

Glomstad, J. (2003). The Fund to Promote Awareness of Occupational Therapy. *Advance for Occupational Therapy Practitioners, 19*(19), 13.

Hasselkus, B. R. (1999). From the desk of the editor: Incentives for change. *American Journal of Occupational Therapy, 53*(1), 7-8.

Johansson, C. (2000). Meet Joe Isaacs, AOTA's new captain. *OT Practice, 5*(16), 7-8.

LaGrossa, J. (2008). AOTA's model curriculum. *Advance for Occupational Therapy Practitioners, 24*(18), 22.

LaGrossa, J. (2008). AOTA's model curriculum: Raising the bar in education to meet 21st century health care needs. *Advance for Occupational Therapy Practitioners, 24*(18), 232-235.

Law, M. (2000). Evidence-based practice: What can it mean for me? *OT Practice, 5*(17), 16-18.

Lenker, J. A. (2000). Certification in assistive technology. *OT Practice, 5*(16), 12-15.

Lieberman, D., & Sheer, J. (2002). AOTA's evidence-based literature review project: An overview. *American Journal of Occupational Therapy, 56*(3), 344-349.

Lieberman, D., Scheer, J., & Erby, K. (2003). In the clinic: AOTA offers evidence-based reviews. *OT Practice, 8*(3), 19-21.

Meyer, A. (1922). Philosophy of occupation therapy. *Archives of Occupational Therapy, 1*(1), 1-10.

Mosey, A. C. (1981). Definition of a model. In *Occupational therapy: Configuration of a profession* (pp. 49-57). New York, NY: Raven Press.

Moyers, P. A. (2002). Continuing competence and competency: What you need to know. *OT Practice, 7*(17), 18-22.

National Board for Certification in Occupational Therapy. (2002a). Five easy steps to renewing your certification as an OTR or COTA. *Report to the Profession, Spring Newsletter,* 4-5.

National Board for Certification in Occupational Therapy. (2002b). Frequently asked questions (FAWS) about the New Guidelines for Certification Renewal. *Report to the Profession, Spring Newsletter,* 6.

National Board for Certification in Occupational Therapy. (2003). Practice analysis ensures valid examination. *Report to the Profession, Spring Newsletter,* 3.

National Board for Certification in Occupational Therapy. (2004). Results from NBCOT practice metrics survey. *Report to the Profession, Fall Newsletter,* 1.

Nemko, M. (2007). Career guide 2007: The best job for you. *U.S. News & World Report, 142*(10), 36-40.

Nemko, M. (2008). Career guide 2008: Best careers. *U.S. News & World Report, 144*(9), 60-61.

Olson, J. (2005). Call for comment on the ACOTE educational draft standards. *OT Practice, 10*(3), 23-24.

Peterson, E. W. (2003). Evidence-based practice: Case example: A matter of balance. *OT Practice, 8*(3), 12-14.

Rourk, J. D. (2001). *Foundation's perspective on the AOTA/AOTF relationship.* Bethesda, MD: AOTF.

Rourk, J. D., & Kirkland, M. (2003). Report of the AOTF President to the Representative Assembly. Retrieved from www.aota.org

Sackett, D. L., Richardson, W. S., Rosenberg, W., & Haynes, R. B. (1997). *Evidence-based medicine: How to practice and teach EBM.* London, UK: Churchill Livingstone.

Sackett, D. L., Straus, S. E., Richardson, W. S., Rosenberg, W., & Haynes, R. B. (2000). *Evidence-based medicine: How to practice and teach EBM* (2nd ed.). London, UK: Churchill Livingstone.

Slater, D. Y., & Willmarth, C. (2006). Understanding and asserting the occupational therapy scope of practice. *OT Practice, 10*(10), CE1-CE8.

Slater, E. Y. (2004). Legal and ethical practice: A professional responsibility. *OT Practice, 9*(16), 13-16.

Somers, F., Smith, K., & Willmarth, C. (2000). *Key issues for the 2000 state legislative sessions.* Bethesda, MD: AOTA.

World Health Organization. (2001). *International classification of functioning, disability and health.* Geneva, Switzerland: Author.

BIBLIOGRAPHY

American Occupational Therapy Association. (2002). Glossary: Standards for an accredited education program for the occupational therapists and occupational therapy assistant. *American Journal of Occupational Therapy, 56*(6), 667-668.

American Occupational Therapy Association. (2007). 2006 AOTA workforce and compensation survey. *AOTA State Affairs Group News, 9*(4), 4-6.

OT Model Curriculum Ad Hoc Committee. (2009). Occupational therapy model curriculum. Bethesda, MD: AOTA.

11

On the Road to
the Centennial Vision
and Beyond

Key Points

- Licensure achieved in all 50 states and three jurisdictions (DC, Guam, and Puerto Rico)
- Value statement adopted in 2015
- Occupational Therapy Practice Framework, Third Edition (2014)
- Discussion of moving to doctorate-level entry
- Focus on increasing awareness of politicians of occupational therapy role in mental health and behavioral management
- Communicating to all stakeholders that occupational therapy is a scientific-based profession with research to support practice approaches
- Defining the role of occupational therapy as an autonomous profession concerned with health, well-being, and participation.

Highlighted Personalities

- Florence Clark, AOTA President, 2010-2013
- Virginia Stoffel, AOTA President, 2013-2016
- Amy Lamb, AOTA President, 2016-2019
- Diana Ramsey, AOTF President
- Scott Campbell, AOTF Executive Director

Key Places

- The national office remains in Bethesda, Maryland.

Key Times/Events

- Centennial conference in Philadelphia

Andersen, L. T., & Reed, K. L.
The History of Occupational Therapy: The First Century (pp. 325-358).
© 2017 Taylor & Francis Group.

Political Events/Issues

- State licensure achieved in all 50 states in 2014 for therapists and in 2015 for assistants
- 2010 Patient Protection and Affordable Care Act (ACA; P.L. 111-148)
- 2011 OT Mental Health Act (HR3752) introduced at 112th Congress to include occupational therapists as behavioral and mental health professionals in National Health Service Corps (NHSC). Not adopted.

Economic Events/Issues

- AOTA published Salary & Workforce Surveys

Educational Issues*

- Availability: Options for education such as online courses, home study, downloading
- Affordability: Reducing costs and increasing funding through scholarships, grants, loans, sponsorships
- Competency-based model curriculum
- Continuing education: measuring effectiveness
- Interprofessional Education in Occupational Therapy
- Education Standards and Guidelines Revised, 2011
- Fieldwork Level II
- Philosophy of Occupational Therapy Education
- Value of Occupational Therapy Assistant Education

Technological Events/Issues

- Telehealth and telerehabilitation are viewed as methods to reduce costs and expand services.
- Technology and Environmental Interventions in Occupational Therapy Practice (AOTA document)

Sociocultural Events/Issues*

- Changing health care problems caused by lifestyle factors (obesity, living conditions, violence, stress, health literacy)
- Occupational Therapy's Perspective on the Use of Environments and Contexts to Facilitate Health, Well-Being, and Participation in Occupations
- Societal Statement on Health Literacy
- Role of Occupational Therapy in Disaster Preparedness, Response, and Recovery: A Concept Paper
- Complex Environmental Modifications
- Promotion of Health and Well-Being
- Nondiscrimination and Inclusion.

Practice Issues*

- Driving and Community Mobility
- Guidelines for Re-Entry Into the Field of Occupational Therapy
- Scope of Practice
- Standards for Continuing Competence
- Documentation of Occupational Therapy Services
- Supervision, Roles, and Responsibilities During Delivery of Occupational Therapy Services
- Mental Health Promotion, Prevention, and Intervention
- Role of Occupational Therapy in Wound Management
- Cognition and Cognitive Rehabilitation
- Occupational Therapy Services in Early Childhood Education and School-Based Practice
- Role of Occupational Therapy on End-of-Life Care
- Scope of Occupational Therapy Services for Individuals With Autism Across the Life Span
- Role of Occupational Therapy in Primary Care

---

* Adapted from AOTA, 2010c.

Association Issues

- Strategies and goals to keep the Association a strong and viable membership organization
- Communication formats to keep members informed on relevant issues and opportunities for leadership and participation
- Developing leaders
- Revision of the Occupational Therapy Code of Ethics and enforcement procedures, 2015

Foundation Issues

- Celebrated 50th anniversary in 2015
- Created the Leaders and Legacies Society but has since become an independent group
- Continue to increase support for scholarships and research grants
- Continue support and development of the Wilma L. West Library

National Board for Certification in Occupational Therapy

- Practice analysis of entry-level practice data and trends to keep certification examination current
- Practice analysis to evaluate state of occupational therapy practice

> *Occupational therapy's distinct value is to improve health and quality of life through facilitating participation and engagement in occupations, the meaningful, necessary, and familiar activities of everyday life. Occupational therapy is client-centered, achieves positive outcomes, and is cost-effective.* (AOTA, 2015b)

> *Occupational therapy maximizes health, well-being, and quality of life for all people, populations, and communities through effective solutions that facilitate participation in everyday living.* (AOTA Vision 2025)

INTRODUCTION

Barack Obama was reelected President of the United States for a second term in 2012. The wars in Afghanistan and Iraq ended, but new crises arose in Syria and throughout the Middle East. Immigration, both legal and illegal, became a hot topic of discussion. Concern was expressed that immigrants were taking away jobs Americans needed and were making use of social benefits such as welfare programs designed to help American citizens in time of need. Mass shootings involving injury or death of four or more persons tended to dominate the news, along with rhetoric about whether gun control would have any effect in reducing the incidents. Most states responded by permitting more guns and permitting guns to be openly displayed (open carry). Civil liberties were challenged by states demanding that voters present a valid (defined as government issued) identification (ID) card with a photograph to prevent perceived voter fraud. Those most likely not to have a photo ID were those who did not drive or have a passport. The economy, although growing, was not improving everyone's lives. Manufacturing jobs requiring minimum skills or education continued to disappear or were replaced by jobs requiring more advanced skills, such as using a computerized control system to operate machinery. Reflecting back on 100 years provides an opportunity to pose some issues, questions, and comments regarding the profession that transcend the years.

CRITERIA FOR RECOGNITION AS A PROFESSION

Addressing a group of occupational therapists at a workshop on graduate education, Brandenburg (1963) offered that he felt there were eight characteristics of a discipline that qualified as a profession:

- A body of knowledge
- Education required
- Practical application (to society)
- Standardized qualification and admission to membership in the profession
- Widely recognized organization for the profession
- Ethical and altruistic behavior by its members
- Commonly recognized status
- Emphasis on the need for continuing education

The question is: Has occupational therapy fulfilled the requirements to be recognized as a profession? The answer appears to be yes, although some characteristics may be demonstrated to a greater degree than others. Occupational therapy has developed and will continue to develop its own knowledge base. Models of practice and intervention approaches are published that address the occupational nature of humans based on best available literature, current trends, values systems, and research. Research techniques will expand to better facilitate the heterogeneous practice of occupational therapy as it interacts with humans and their many activities and tasks. Computer programs, including apps, will facilitate the collecting and sharing of information, whereas safeguarding privacy is a challenge to assist data management and analysis.

Education is and has been required for many years. Originally, the national Association published its own educational standards and conducted its own accreditation process. Beginning in 1935, the process of developing standards was shared jointly with the American Medical Association (AMA), and the first list of jointly accredited programs was published in 1938. Beginning in 1992, the national Association again took over sole responsibility for setting educational standards and accrediting educational programs. Educational programs at the professional and technical level are increasingly available in most, but not all, states. Since 2007, the requirement has been at the post-baccalaureate level.

Practical application has been documented for many years, but perhaps the recognition of the discipline as a reimbursable therapy in the national Medicare program is the most public acknowledgement of its practical application to society. Qualifications to become a registered (now certified) practitioner initially required the person to submit proof that the individual had work experience as an occupational therapist in a hospital or other specialized work setting, or had graduated from a training school meeting AOTA minimum standards starting in 1932 but the qualifications were changed in 1947 to require passing a written examination after graduating from an accredited educational program in occupational therapy. Licensure was obtained in all 50 states and three other jurisdictions for occupational therapists in 2014 and for occupational therapy assistants in 2015.

A formal organization has been available to occupational therapy personnel since 1917. The national Association has functioned continuously since its founding, with only one change of name in 1921, from the National Society of the Promotion of Occupational Therapy to the American Occupational Therapy Association (AOTA). The location of the national office head-quarters was originally in New York City but has been in the Washington, DC, area since 1973.

Ethical and altruistic behavior was originally integrated in the constitution and bylaws of the national organization. A separate document formalizing the Code of Ethics was adopted in 1977. The Code of Ethics and enforcement procedures have been revised and updated in an attempt to keep the ethical standards for behavior current with changes in social points of view and legal opinion.

Status may the most problematic characteristic. Although occupational therapy is well rec-ognized within the rehabilitation field, it may be less recognized in other fields concerned with health, well-being, and education. More consumers are familiar with the name but may be unable to give a working definition or description of services. Status in the community continues to be a work in progress. However, occupational therapy personnel are able to consult and work with a variety of other professions, including educators, architects, politicians, engineers, computer pro-grammers, dieticians, physical therapists, speech-language pathologists, psychologists, and others and are beginning to be recognized as autonomous practitioners in their own right beyond the concept of medical extenders.

Finally, continuing education and lifelong learning are accepted values within occupa-tional therapy. Many state licensure laws require continuing education for license renewal. The Association has offered an annual conference yearly, except during World War II, to present information through presentations and opportunities to gain skills through workshops and dem-onstrations. The Association also offers publications and online seminars to help therapists and assistants gain new knowledge and skills or relearn existing knowledge and skills for those return-ing to the field after an absence.

This chapter includes both current, past, and future ideas about occupational therapy as a profession and discipline within society. Looking forward to plan ahead and looking back to see whether useful knowledge and skills already exist are equally important. Planning ahead allows strategies to be developed in advance to be implemented in a timely fashion. Using what is already known and learned saves time and energy to deal with new situations for which current knowledge and skill may be useful but not sufficient. Resources should always be used wisely to both conserve and expend at the most appropriate time and situation.

EDUCATION

2011 Educational Standards

The Accreditation Council for Occupational Therapy Education (ACOTE) Educational Standards documents for accreditation were revised for the eleventh time in 2011 for the profes-sional level (original in 1923 and one revision by AOTA in 1930, seven revisions by AMA/AOTA, and three revisions by ACOTE). For assistants, the 2011 revision was the ninth since the original document in 1958 (six by AOTA and three by ACOTE). A major change in the 2011 revision was the requirement for psychological factors, social factors, and psychosocial factors content in fieldwork (practicum experience). Section C of the Educational Standards covers fieldwork. Item C.1.7 states that the educational programs at all levels (assistant, master's, doctorate) must "ensure that at least one fieldwork experience (either Level I or Level II) has as its focus psycho-logical and social factors that influence engagement in occupation" (ACOTE, 2011, p. 34). Item C.1.12 states that "in all settings, psychosocial factors influencing engagement in occupation must be understood and integrated for the development of client-centered, meaningful, occupation-based outcomes" (ACOTE, 2011, p. 35). The requirement is the first since the Essentials of 1965 to specify field work in a setting that focuses on "psychological and social factors" or psychosocial factors. Brown (2012a) quotes Neil Harvison, then Director of Accreditation and Academic Affairs in the national office, as saying that "the basic rationale was that programs were not adequately addressing psychosocial needs" and that employers were looking for people with psychosocial skills (p. 13).

Doctoral-Level Single-Entry Education

As the knowledge base expands, the level of education for entry into the profession has increased. A post-baccalaureate degree for initial entry was accepted in 1999 and implemented in 2007. Post-baccalaureate can mean either a master's or a doctoral degree. A doctoral degree at the initial level of entry may be warranted, especially because other team members have chosen to select the doctorate as the minimum entry point. In 2014, the Association Board of Directors issued a position statement on doctoral-level single point of entry for occupational therapists (AOTA, 2014). The Board members were responding to advisory committee reports recommending that the Board consider the issue of doctoral-level entry. In addition to aligning educational requirements with other health care team members, the doctoral degree also supports the need to more academic faculty and provides the training for research studies need by an autonomous profession. Although doctoral-level entry may be viewed as increasing cost of service, such increase should be offset by improved quality of service in education of personnel, practice, and research.

A related question is the status of the assistant. If the entry level for the occupational therapist is a doctoral degree, should the entry level for the assistant be a baccalaureate degree? These questions of entry level and the status they may provide continue to be discussed within the professional community of occupational therapy.

At the same time, educational institutions continue to be challenged to teach more content in less time. As a result, students will need to take more responsibility for self-learning and peer teaching away from traditional classrooms. Online and Internet content can facilitate learning useful material, but the quality must be carefully measured and evaluated because it may be of poor or questionable accuracy or simply wrong. Faculty need to evaluate content before directing students to access the sites and/or develop criteria students can use to determine content quality for themselves. Faculty can also continue to improve online content by adding useful material, revising existing content, and recommending that poor-quality or inaccurate content be labeled as such or removed.

Our knowledge base needs to continue to expand. For example, techniques in imaging the body have continued to improve so that the techniques are less invasive and potentially harmful while improving the quality of the image. As a result, imaging of fetuses and newborns is rapidly expanding our knowledge of both fetal development and disorders occurring before birth. This improved knowledge can help better direct practice to maximize therapy time. For example, if imaging techniques determine that functional connections in the brain, such as the corticospinal tract, did not develop and are not working, time spent on attempting remediation can be redirected to compensatory and adaptive techniques. The result may be better occupational performance for the individual and less frustration practicing skills that have a low probability of becoming effective in everyday life.

PRACTICE

Sponsorship of Occupational Therapy

Sponsorship occurs between professions when one profession takes responsibility for supporting and promoting activities of another or allowing its influence and prestige to be used by another profession. As stated by Maxwell and Maxwell (1984), who studied the development of occupational therapy in Canada:

> ... sponsorship has significance for the study of professionalization. An occupation may create and sponsor another occupation in the status struggle within a differentiating occupational structure. Such sponsorship will likely have a different effect on the recipient group that if that group were to struggle on its own under conditions of "pure" competition. It may also have certain benefits as well as costs for the sponsoring occupation in the struggle for power. Like professionalization, sponsorship may occur over historical periods and its temporal dimension should not be overlooked. (p. 331)

Sponsorship also occurs between professional organizations when a larger and more powerful organization permits a small, less powerful organization to use the resources of the more powerful organization to the advantage of the smaller one. Advantages may include publicity, recognition, joint conferences, use of physical faculties, use of expertise and technical skills, use of manpower, use of equipment and supplies, or any combination thereof.

Over the years, the profession of occupational therapy and its professional organization have experienced sponsorship with several professions and professional organizations. The various sponsorships may have occurred in part because of the diverse nature of the knowledge base in occupational therapy or because of sociocultural events occurring as the health care system developed in the United States. Sometimes the sponsorship was by mutual agreement, but other times the sponsorship happened without knowledge or consent. An example of the latter is the early courses developed and sponsored by nursing in what was called invalid occupation beginning in 1906 (Tracy, n.d.). The sponsorship by nursing was not by agreement or consent of the profession or professional organization because occupational therapy as a term did not exist until 1914, when Barton formally used it, and the Association was not formed until 1917. Occupational therapy, however, owes nurses and the nursing profession a debt of gratitude for developing the early courses in the application of occupations for therapeutic purposes, although the initial intent was largely for diversion of chronically ill patients.

On the other hand, the Association is totally responsible for agreeing to have its annual conference with the American Hospital Association (AHA) for several years during the early history of the Association. The rationale was to use the AHA conference as an opportunity to increase the visibility of occupational therapy to hospital administrators through exhibits of what occupational therapy could do and to encourage them to support the development of an occupational therapy service program in their hospitals and institutions. Although no record exists of how successful the joint venture was in increasing the number of occupational therapy service programs, the increased visibility appears to have been a good idea. The relationship with the AHA continued in the 1950s and 1960s with the joint development of 10 institutes for occupational therapists between 1954 and 1965.

Another example with more substantial results was the decision by the early leaders to require a medical prescription or referral by a physician to initiate services. The idea of a prescription was likely influenced by Dr. Dunton, but it was clearly evident in the definition of occupational therapy used by Dr. Pattison: "any activity, mental or physical, definitely prescribed...." (Pattison, 1922). The medical prescription bound occupational therapy to the medical profession until 1969, when the Statement on Referral (AOTA, 1969) allowed some referrals to be made by other professionals, especially when medical diagnoses or conditions were not the primary problem, such as educational problems or physical access in the home and safety in the workplace were the identified problems. Using the physician and practice of medicine as a sponsor gave occupational therapy an aura of scientific respectability that giving handicrafts to patients did not on the surface appear to have.

The professional organization further promoted sponsorship by the medical community when, in 1931, members of the Board of Management agreed with Kidner's suggestion to contact the American Medical Association (AMA) to request assistance in inspecting and accrediting educational programs. From 1935 to 1992, AOTA and the AMA jointly developed seven editions of the document entitled "Essentials of," followed by various wording related to occupational therapy or occupational therapists. Together, teams from the two organizations inspected and approved all occupational therapy educational programs. The support of the AMA increased the recognition and credibility of occupational therapy as a profession in a manner clearly visible for all to see.

Again, in contrast, the attempt by physical medicine in the late 1940s to sponsor occupational therapy by becoming directors of the education programs and service programs was not welcomed by the profession or professional organization. The idea that a physical medicine specialist would be in charge of the educational program and that all occupational therapy service programs would be administered under a physical medicine director was not acceptable to the profession. The idea that physical medicine physicians should direct both physical therapy and occupational therapy was outlined in Molander's (1931) article. Prior to his article, many occupational therapy service programs had functioned independently, often with the help of the Junior League and nurses serving as sources of referral to identify patients who could benefit from occupational therapy services. Physical medicine physicians, later physiatrists, went so far as to claim that occupational therapy was a form of physical medicine or that occupational therapy was a special type of physical therapy. Krusen (1934) stated that "the Council's definition of physical therapy is sufficiently broad so that it might include practically all occupational therapy" (p. 69). He was citing the Council on Physical Therapy definition that physical therapy is the treatment of disease by means of the "physical, chemical, and other properties of heat, light, water, electricity, massage, and exercise" (AMA, 1932).

Sponsorship can also result in a mixed outcome that includes both positive and negative results. Such is the case with allied health as an organizing strategy in institutions of higher education. The term allied health is an organizational concept formally adopted in 1966 with the passage of the Allied Health Professions Act (Maze, 1968) that included allied medical professions, associated health professions, allied health professions, and allied health sciences. All were designed to reorganize traditional academic structure to gather together paramedical disciplines that served the medical community and either required college-level course work or were being redesigned to move toward college-level education. Examples in addition to occupational therapy include medical technology, dieticians, radiological technology, cytotechnology, inhalation or respiratory therapy, hospital or health care administration, and physical therapy. The purpose of the reorganization was threefold: the lessening of course duplication, the implementation of an operational health team format, and the development of autonomous schools of allied health professions that could stand on par with schools of medicine, nursing, and dentistry (Meredith, 1971).

In the past, schools of occupational therapy had been integrated into the college and university system in a variety of departments. Some occupational therapy programs were a part of schools of art, home economics, education, nursing, or medicine. On the surface, location in a school of allied health seemed attractive because the occupational therapy program would be grouped with other similar health-focused programs as opposed to art, home economics, or education. The allied health unit would be on par with other units (departments, schools, or colleges) within the higher educational institution (college or university). The potential downside was the curriculum reorganization, which attempted to reduce perceived duplication of basic science courses such as anatomy, physiology, and other core courses. Content in the core courses may or may not address the need for knowledge in occupational therapy education. Loss of control over curriculum content is a major drawback to participation in an allied health school.

The relationship with allied health is unusual in terms of sponsorship. Usually the sponsoring group is older, more established, and more powerful than the group being sponsored. Such was not the case with allied health. The first use of the concept occurred in 1950, when the University of Pennsylvania established its School of Allied Medical Professions (Maze, 1968). The passage of the Allied Health Professions Act provided funds for rapid expansion of college- and university-based education for allied medical fields. However, occupational therapy was already well established as a profession and had been educating therapists in colleges and universities since 1949, so from a historical standpoint, it was the more established group. However, in the higher education system, it did not have a unique identity and thus could be reorganized by more a powerful but younger group with federal funds useful to both the allied health group and the occupational therapy education program.

The professional Association began to decrease the emphasis on medicine and medical subjects in the late 1950s and 1960s. The Board of Management discontinued inviting physicians to serve as Fellows on the Board in 1959. The minutes state the Association had outgrown the need for this kind of professional status (AOTA, 1959). Physicians had served on the Board as Fellows beginning in 1946. However, the Association severed ties completely. Instead, a Medical Advisory Committee was formed in 1954 and continued to meet and exist until at least 1968 (AOTA, 1968).

The 1965 Essentials of an Accredited Education Program for the Occupational Therapist does not list fieldwork assignments by diagnostic categories such as orthopedics or tuberculosis but instead use the general terms suggested by the recommendations from the Basic Approach Study: psychosocial dysfunction and physical dysfunction (AOTA, 1965). The Essentials do not specify medical lectures on certain diagnoses. In 1963, the new editor of the American Journal of Occupational Therapy (AJOT) dispensed with the Advisory Committee to the journal, which had been composed primarily of physicians representing areas of practice such as psychiatry, physical medicine, pediatrics, tuberculosis, and general medicine. These areas presented the categories of hospital affiliations under the Essentials adopted in 1949 (AMA, 1949; AOTA, 1950). Instead, the new editor invited occupational therapists to service as division editors and reviewers without any medical advisory oversight. The 1969 Statement on Referral does not require a prescription for all referrals to occupational therapy services, recognizing that occupational therapy may provide services in areas outside the purview of medical practice (AOTA, 1969).

In 1974, when the Delegate Assembly adopted the position to promote licensure, the Association formally began the process of declaring occupational therapy to be an independent profession (Johnson, 1975). If the profession wanted to be a subspecialty of medicine, it would have aligned with the state medical practice acts that cover medical specialties. However, occupational therapy personnel are educated as physicians, so they did not meet the qualifications. In addition, increasing numbers of practitioners were working in areas that did not require medical management, such as public schools, home medication, low vision, or health and wellness businesses. The time had come to make the break from medical sponsorship.

In summary, sponsorship is a double-edged sword, and the benefits must be measured against the drawbacks. Sponsorship always compromises the attainment of professional autonomy but may help build the framework or infrastructure that ultimately facilitates such attainment. Control over the standards for educational preparation (accreditation) and credentialing process (registration, certification, or licensure) at the initial and continuing levels are key elements in attaining professional autonomy. In addition, the profession must convince society that its services are of value, worthy of financial payment, and needed by citizens for some identified purpose or purposes. Occupational therapy has met the challenges over the years. Sponsorship, both solicited and unsolicited, has been part of the process.

Definition of Occupational Therapy

Occupational therapy has roots and shoots from many fields, but major influences come from social service (helping others), education (teaching and training), and maintenance of good health (wellness). Dr. Licht (1952) stated that "occupational therapy was originally supervised by craftsmen, then educators, still later by nurses, and now by occupational therapists" (p. 448). During the formative years, occupational therapy was reported to be a branch of social service (Hall, 1923). At the same time, an Association document stated that "treatment should be prescribed and administered under constant medical advice and supervision," suggesting that occupational therapy was considered a subspecialty or adjunct within the medical field (AOTA, 1923). Dunton (1928) may have been supporting the subspecialty status when he stated that "occupational therapy ... is an adjunct to other forms of treatment, supplementing them and increasing their value, so that from the combined treatment the duration of care is decreased or a better end result obtained" (p. 5). At the same time, he stated that "occupational therapy depends upon other branches, and especially upon psychology, for its own advancement" (p. 5).

On the other hand, Robinson (1919) supported the social science aspects, stating that:

> ...occupational therapy must take into consideration social as well as physical problems, and must have constantly as its aim the teaching of persons to fit better into their usual environment, as well as assisting them to return to their usual surroundings .... Occupational therapy should, therefore, be an adjunct to those forces of the hospital dealing with the social betterment as well as the physical betterment of the patient .... It is generally recognized that an important function of occupational therapy is to influence the mind as well as the body of those needing hospital care. (p. 524)

Rehfuss, Albrecht, and Price (1948) stated that:

> ...until modern psychology advances to the point where the physical and mental effects of emotions upon the individual can be accurately determine, occupational therapy must likewise lag as a science since it is believed that the creation of a pleasant mental attitude or emotion and the stimulation of interest are the bases for the successful employment of occupational therapy. (p. 766)

The profession of occupational therapy continues to develop as an autonomous profession focused on promoting life to the fullest and participation in all aspects of living. Sponsorship by medicine is no longer needed and tends to limit the scope of practice in a profession designed to maximize the use of occupation by, and the occupational performance of, persons in educational pursuits, living arrangements, vocational choices, qualify of life satisfaction, participation in activities of daily living, positive interpersonal relations, social inclusion, cultural diversity, community interaction, lifestyle decision making, and political involvement.

As the model definition for legislature and value statement imply, professionals with occupational therapy view the profession as a discipline separate from the medical profession that focuses on the use of occupation by humans to effect quality of life and participation. The study of occupation is part of the social science. However, aspects of occupational dysfunction will always have a relationship to body structure (anatomy) and function (physiology). Occupational therapy is a hybrid discipline, using knowledge from social, biological, and physical sciences.

Occupational therapy seems to best fit as a life and living science based on achieving occupational performance that has goal direction, meaning, and purpose to individuals, organizations, and communities and focuses on the structure and organization in time and space. Influencing factors include age, sex, health or disability status, socioeconomic status, cultural customs, family history and expectations, and past and present personal decision making. Many of these factors are beyond the scope of medicine and the influence of drugs and surgery. Sponsorship made sense when the profession was small and had few models of practice articulating its unique perspective of occupation as a life force capable of helping people develop habits and routines in their everyday life activities. In the past 100 years, occupational therapy has developed its own literature base and created its own body of research. Use of resources in medicine is no longer needed as a support tool.

The process of delivering therapy continues to need improvement and revision. Currently, the therapy process requires extensive clinical reasoning, which may be based largely on experience rather than on logical progression from assessment to planning to implementation to reevaluation. Too many assessments do not link to planning, implementation, and reevaluation. Too many practice models do not have identified assessment instruments. The Model of Human Occupation (MOHO) is an exception and is an example of what can be done in the occupational therapy

Table 11-1
OCCUPATIONAL THERAPY DEFINITIONS

2011	The practice of occupational therapy means the therapeutic use of occupations, including everyday life activities, with individuals, groups, populations, or organizations to support participation, performance, and function in roles and situations in home, school, workplace, community, and other settings. Occupational therapy services are provided for habilitation, rehabilitation, and the promotion of health and wellness to those who have or are at risk for developing an illness, injury, disease, disorders, condition, impairment, disability, activity limitation, or participation restriction. Occupational therapy addresses the physical, cognitive, psychosocial, sensory-perceptual, and other aspects of performance in a variety of contexts and environments, to support engagement in occupations that affect physical and mental health, well-being, and quality of life (RA 4/14/11 [Agenda A13 Charge 18] Policy 5.3.1.)
2013	Occupational therapy is a health, wellness, and rehabilitation profession that helps individuals maximize their performance and functioning throughout the lifespan (US, DHHS, Health Resources and Services Administration)
2015	Occupational therapy (OT) is a profession that seeks to help individuals to achieve their optimal level of independence and ultimately find satisfaction and meaning in their lives. The role of OT in health care enables people to live fuller lives by preventing or learning how to live with illness, injury, or disability. Through skilled activity analysis and purposeful activity, occupational therapists help individuals to achieve independence in performing activities of daily living, work, and leisure/play. (Lin, Zhang & Dixon, PM&R, 7, 945.)

Table 11-2
EXAMPLES OF OCCUPATION OVER THE LIFESPAN

- The occupation of infants is learning basic functions such as eating and responding to the environment around them
- The occupation of young children is mastering their developing bodies and performing the skills needed for learning
- The occupation of adolescents is learning social interaction behaviors and exploring career opportunities
- The occupation of young adults is developing a career and establishing a healthy and satisfying lifestyle of their own
- The occupation of adults is maintaining employment, fulfilling family responsibilities, and engaging in community activities
- The occupation of older adults is to maintain a healthy lifestyle in retirement and engage in satisfying activities

Adapted from the AOTA Calendar The World of Occupational Therapy 1990.

knowledge base. Linking assessment to planning, implementation, and reevaluation also facilitates research and, more importantly, the application of research back to improving practice. Presently, research studies often use a variety of assessment instruments in the methodology section and different intervention techniques to study the same or similar disorders. Different assessment instruments tend to measure different concepts and problems. Intervention techniques focus on different problems when the research studies are compared. More confusion than clarity may result within occupational therapy practice, making clear communication to other professionals nearly impossible. Examples of current definitions are presented in Table 11-1, and examples of occupation across the lifespan are listed in Table 11-2.

Challenges to Practice

Helping to make communities more livable can be a goal of future practitioners. Working with architects, engineers, and community planners, occupational therapists can evaluate how, when, and where occupations are best performed to provide maximum effectiveness and efficiency, giving meaning and purpose to individuals, organizations, and community members.

Occupational therapy personnel have an opportunity to be product evaluators, especially in the areas of safety and ease of use. Many products are recalled every year because of deficits and safety flaws not detected during prototype tryout. Basic safety in product use and potential problems of wear and tear could be observed by occupational therapy personnel, saving manufacturers money and loss of reputation. Better design and usability could increase revenue and improve manufacturers' reputations.

Occupational therapy personnel can increase their skills in working with people who have multisystem disorders. Multisystem disorders are often difficult to treat effectively because treatment of one system, such as the nervous system, may result in decreased effectiveness of another, such as the cognitive system. Examples of multisystem disorders are stroke, cancer, traumatic brain injury, and polytrauma from vehicle crashes or explosive devices. Finding ways to create a balancing act of effective treatment for one system while not seriously decreasing the effectiveness of another is the kind of challenge occupational therapy personnel can meet. Changes in the way occupations are performed and/or changes in the environmental demands may allow more aggressive treatment of one system, such as the nervous system, while supporting another system, such as the cognitive system, until the nervous system is better able to function with less therapy or adjustment to the therapy has been achieved.

LEGISLATION AND POLICY MAKING

Table 11-3 summarizes important legislation enacted from 2010 to 2015. The profession must continue its advocacy for legislation and policies that promote the profession and the consumers it services. Occupational therapy must be included in legislation that increases participation and inclusion of all individuals, organizations, and communities. Occupational therapy must be active in promoting and protecting civil rights. Occupational therapy personnel need to be included as qualified providers in all legislation and policy making that affects the ability of practitioners to provide services.

Table 11-3 LEGISLATION	
2010	Patient Protection and Affordable Care Act (ACA) (P.L.111-148) was enacted which reforms health care. All citizens are required to have or to purchase health insurance. Regulations for health insurance companies require increase consumer protection against loss of insurance eligibility due to pre-existing conditions or certain conditions previously considered uninsurable. To increase financial support for consumers, the ACA provide scholarships and loan repayments through National Health Service Corps (NHSC). Occupational therapy is classified within the rehabilitation habilitation required- benefit categories to cover services for a wide range of conditions (Brown, 2012)
2015	Every Student Succeeds Act (ESSA) (P.L. 114-95). Revises No Child Left Behind Act of 2001 . Preserves federal mandate for standardized testing but eliminates punitive consequences for states and districts that perform poorly.
2015	Medicare Access and CHIP Reauthorization Act (MACRA) (P.L. 114-10). Repeals the sustainable growth rate formula designed to control the rate of increase for physician services. Requires a review of documentation for outpatient occupational therapy services that exceed a threshold amount of $3,700 in 2016 (Snadhu, 2015)

Educational programs should be available in all 50 states at both the professional and technical levels in public and private institutions. Particular attention should be paid to the distribution of practitioners per 100,000 population. Shortages of practitioners continue to exist in certain areas of the country, whereas surpluses may exist in other areas. Research has shown that occupational therapy assistants tend to not be as mobile as occupational therapists. Therefore, availability of local education programs becomes more important. However, even at the professional level, the existence of an educational program increases the opportunity for awareness and education of the public sector about occupational therapy. The value of the physical location of the occupational therapy education program continues to be a significant factor in providing a supply of educated practitioners while also providing a physical presence of the profession in the sociocultural fabric of society and the health care system.

RESEARCH

The Research Advisory Panel (RAP) is a joint group formed by AOTA and the American Occupational Therapy Foundation (AOTF) to advise and inform on issues related to research (Rogers, 2010). A document titled the Occupational Therapy Research Agenda was created with an outline of activities considered relevant research topics for the profession. Five broad categories of research are listed: assessment/measurement, intervention, basic research, translational research,

Table 1. Occupational Therapy Research Agenda

Table 1 provides an overview of the research categories as well as an example of research goals and priorities. To see the complete research agenda, visit http://www.aota.org/DocumentVault/Research/45008.aspx or http://www.aotf.org/Portals/0/documents/Programs-Partnerships/AOTF-AOTA%20Joint/OT%20Research%20Agenda-FINAL.pdf.

Research Categories	Major Research Goals	Research Priorities
Assessment/ Measurement	Develop outcome instruments sufficiently responsive to measuring change in daily life activities, including activity and participation	Screening instruments to identify performance deficits in persons of all ages with chronic disorders and disability
Intervention— Preventive, Restorative, Compensatory	Evaluate the *efficacy* of occupational therapy interventions (in controlled conditions)	Application of interventions that: 1. Are client-centered 2. Manipulate an occupational therapy modality/method a. Occupation b. Cognitive, sensory, motor, and/or affective functions c. The environment
Translational Research	Evaluate the *effectiveness* of occupational therapy interventions (under conditions of usual care)	Examine the effects of stem cell transplantation, neural implants, and other novel and developing medical therapies on functional recovery (e.g., when is the best time to intervene to promote recovery of body structures/functions, activity, or participation?)
Basic Research	Delineate how productive occupation promotes life-long health and reduces the risk of chronic disease and disability, and maintains quality of life in people of all ages	Examine brain–behavior relationships in daily life activities
Health Services Research	Evaluate performance outcomes for diagnostic groups based on type of occupational therapy intervention, site of service delivery, professional training, and/or team composition	Design and implement studies comparing the effectiveness of different treatment options, including different occupational therapy approaches and different rehabilitation approaches
Research Training	Increase occupational therapy's research capacity	Prepare program directors in research universities to support early career (< 5 years postdoctoral degree) occupational therapist scientists

Figure 11-1. Occupational therapy research agenda. (Printed with permission from the Archive of the American Occupational Therapy Association, Inc.)

and health services research. The panel selected three of the five as most import to the Centennial Vision: intervention research, translational research, and health services research. Goals and priorities for each area of research are presented in Figure 11-1.

ASSOCIATION

State

State associations need to be strengthened so they can support members' needs for up-to-date information and can lobby on behalf of members and consumers for legislation to keep the occupational therapy practice act up-to-date and services to consumers in line with needs for services to which occupational therapy can contribute. In addition, state associations need to identify issues that should be referred to the national organization for action at the national level. The national association can address issues that are common to many states such as threats to scope of practice and lobbying for federal legislation.

National

Presidents, Executive Director, Board of Directors, and Representative Assembly

Three people have assumed the role of President of AOTA since 2010: Florence A. Clark, 2010-2013 (Figure 11-2); Virginia C. Stoffel, 2013-2016 (Figure 11-3); and Amy Lamb, 2015-2019 (Figure 11-4). Biographical sketches appear in Table 11-4. Frederick Somers continues to serve as Executive Director. The Association's Board of Directors set the Strategic Goals and Objectives for 2014 through 2017 (Table 11-5). The Centennial Vision Priorities for Fiscal Year 2015 are listed in Table 11-6. The Representative Assembly adopted the documents listed in Table 11-7. A major focus of the Association's activity has been on driving, especially older drivers, as the cover of a 2011 issue of *OT*

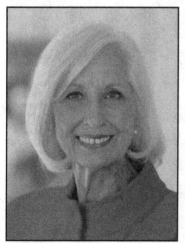

Figure 11-2. Florence A. Clark, PhD, OTR/L, FAOTA, President of AOTA, 2010-2013. (Printed with permission from the Archive of the American Occupational Therapy Association, Inc.)

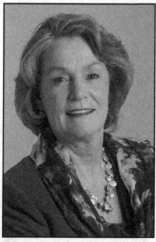

Figure 11-3. Virginia Stoffel, PhD, OT, BCMH, FAOTA, President of AOTA, 2013-2016. (Printed with permission from the Archive of the American Occupational Therapy Association, Inc.)

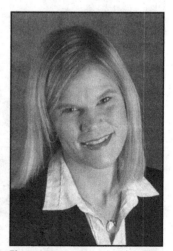

Figure 11-4. Amy Lamb, OTD, OTR/L, FAOTA, President of AOTA, 2016-2019. (Printed with permission from the Archive of the American Occupational Therapy Association, Inc.)

Table 11-4
BIOGRAPHICAL SKETCHES

FLORENCE ARCURI CLARK

Born September 8, 1946

Born in Brooklyn, New York. She received her Bachelor of Arts in English (major) and speech drama (minor from the State university of New York at Albany in 1968, her master of science in occupational therapy form the State university of New York at Buffalo in 1970 ad her Ph.D. in education with a dual major in educational psychology and special education from the University of Southern California in 1982. She was an instructor in occupational therapy at Suffolk State School in Melville, NY, from 1966-67, and a Trainee in occupational Therapy for the New York State Department of Mental Hygiene in Albany, NY, from 1968-70. She was the Coordinator of Rehabilitation and Education, Adolescent Unit, Buffalo State Hospital from 1970-72 From 1970-1973 she held positions as adjunction and clinical instructor in occupational therapy at the State University of New York at Buffalo and Elizabethtown College. From 1973-1976 she was Director of Occupational Therapy at Pennhurst State School and Hospital in Spring City, PA, and held an adjunct assistant professorship with the Department of occupational Therapy at Temple University. From 1976-1984 she was a faculty member at the Center for the Study of Sensory Integrative Dysfunction. She joined the faculty at the university of southern California in 1976, became professor and chair in 1989 and Associate Dean and professor of the Division of Occupational Science Occupational Therapy at the Ostrow School of Dentistry in 2006 . She was president from 2010-13. She received the Award of Merit in 1999, gave the Eleanor Clarke Slagle lectureship in 1993 and was named to roster of Fellows in 1981. She is also a charter member of the American Occupational Therapy Foundation Academy of Research She has authored and co-authored articles, chapters, and books.

VIRGINIA (GINNY) CARROLL STOFFEL

Born March 19, 1955

Born in Wisconsin. She has a bachelor's degree in occupational therapy from the College of St. Catherine in 1977, a master's of science in educational psychology from the University of Wisconsin-Milwaukee in 1983 and a doctorate in leadership for the advancement of learning and service from Cardinal Stritch University in 2007. She is board certified in mental health through the advanced certification program of the Association. She is chair and associate profession at the University of Wisconsin-Milwaukee, College of Health Sciences, Department of Occupational Therapy. Her research interests is on the strengths and needs of people with serious mental illness living in the community, the occupational nature of people with substance use disorders, and evidence based practice regarding behavior change. With Catana Brown, PhD, OTR, FAOTA, she has published the text book titled *Occupational Therapy in Mental Health: A Vision for Participation*, Philadelphia, F.A. Davis. She was named to Roster of Fellows in 1993.

AMY LAMB

Born December 16, 1975

She received her B.S. and OTD from Creighton University. She was chair of the Political Action Committee and Vice President before becoming President. She received the Lindy Boggs Advocacy Award in 2011 and was named to Roster of Fellows in 2012. She has worked as an occupational therapist at St. Joseph's Medical Center in Omaha, Nebraska from 1998-2000, Fairview Medical Center in St. Paul, Minnesota, in 2000, Monroe-Meyer Institute in Omaha from 2003-2005 and Brookdale Senior Living Center in Denver, Colorado from 2009-2010. She has been a faculty member at the College of Saint Mary's in Omaha, from 2001-2004, Creighton University form 2004-2005 and at Eastern Michigan University in Ann Arbor, Michigan from 2010 to the present. She is also the owner of AJLamb Consulting firm which she founded in 2000. In 2006 she was named Educator of the Year at Creighton University. Her areas of specialty are health policy and advocacy, management and leadership, and assessment and intervention with adults and older adults. She has published articles and chapters in textbooks. She is married and has two children.

Practice shows (Figure 11-5). Another focus has been on the military and wounded warriors. The 2014 annual conference opened with a program featuring three wounded warriors (Figure 11-6).

Leadership

Leadership continues to be a crucial need in the profession. The profession has multiple needs for leaders. Learning leadership skills is as important as learning practice skills. The format continues to be the same: leadership skills involve mentoring. Mentoring is most effective at the

Table 11-5
AOTA STRATEGIC GOALS AND OBJECTIVES 2014-2017
• Building the profession's capacity to fulfill its potential and mission • Demonstrating and articulating our value to individuals, organizations, and communities • Linking education, research, and practice • Creating an inclusive community of members • Securing the financial resources to invest in the profession's ability to respond to social needs
AOTA Board of Directors, Dated 3/1/2013

Table 11-6
CENTENNIAL VISION PRIORITIES FOR FISCAL YEAR 2015
• Boldly navigating a changing world • Enhance AOTA's role as an essential resource to the occupational therapy community in a changing world • Enhance the effectiveness of communications to members to help them message appropriately within their settings and in their decision makers • Engage in broad-based advocacy to ensure funding for occupational therapy in traditional and emerging areas • Identify and articulate occupational therapy's distinct value to individuals, organizations and communities • Promote occupational therapy's role in service delivery system redesign to assure fair payment and provision of quality care with particular emphasis on primary care, prevention and expansion of mental health • Provide strategic support for educators, practitioners, and researchers to meet rapidly changing social needs • Explore relationships with other global national and regional occupational therapy associations with similar levels of education/practice • Foster member cultural competence to meet changing demographics an societal needs • Define and promote quality occupational therapy • Collaborate with AOTF in support of research activities that build the occupational therapy knowledge base and support quality practice • Promote member awareness of AOTA PERFORM & National Outcomes Database • Promote evidence-based practice
Retrieved 8/21/2014 from www.aota.org/AboutAOTA/Get-InvolvedBOD/News/2014/FY14-CV-Iriorities.aspx

one-on-one level in which the mentor helps the mentee develop both skills and confidence to take on more difficult tasks in the practice arena and professional associations.

Public Relations

Occupational therapy must articulate the unique value of occupational therapy services to consumers in methods that reach target audiences. For many years, occupational therapy has been associated with medical disciples and medical rehabilitation services. The value of occupational therapy is not limited to serving those consumers with an identified medically diagnosed condition. Occupational therapy provides services to those who want to prevent or diminish the impact of changes in ability and skills due to aging or change the focus of their occupations in careers or from career to retirement. Occupational therapy in school systems promotes educational goals, not medical rehabilitation. The focus is on organizing the learning environment to enhance the student's learning potential, not on remediating dysfunction. Occupational therapy

Table 11-7
ASSOCIATION DOCUMENTS ADOPTED BY THE REPRESENTATIVE ASSEMBLY

2010	• Driving and Community Mobility • Enforcement Procedures for the Occupational Therapy Code of Ethics and Ethics Standards • Occupational Therapy Code of Ethics and Ethics Standards • Guidelines for Re-entry into the Field of Occupational Therapy • Occupational Therapy Services in the Promotion of Psychological and Social Aspects of Mental Health • The Scope of Occupational Therapy Services for Individuals with an Autism Spectrum Disorder Across the Life Course • Specialized Knowledge and Skills in Mental Health Promotion, Prevention, and Intervention in Occupational Therapy Practice • Specialized Knowledge and Skills in Technology and Environmental Interventions for Occupational Therapy Practice • Standards for Continuing Competence • Standards of Practice for Occupational Therapy • Telerehabilitation
2011	• Accreditation Council for Occupational Therapy Education Standards • AOTA's Societal Statement on Health Literacy • Complementary and Alternative Medicine • Occupational Therapy Services for Individuals who have Experienced Domestic Violence • Occupational Therapy Services in Early Childhood and School-based Settings • Occupational Therapy Services in Facilitating Work Performance • Philosophical Base of Occupational Therapy • The Role of Occupational Therapy in Disaster Preparedness, Response and Recovery: A Concept Paper • The Role of Occupational Therapy in End-of-Life Care (replaces document on hospice)
2012	• Fieldwork Level II and Occupational Therapy Students: Position Paper • Physical Agent Modalities replaces previous papers
2013	• AOTA' Societal Statement on Health Disparities • Cognition, Cognitive Rehabilitation and Occupational Performance • Guidelines for Documentation of Occupational Therapy • Obesity an Occupational Therapy • Occupational Therapy in the Promotion of Health and Well-being • The Role of Occupational Therapy in Wound Management • Telehealth
2014	• Guidelines for Supervision, Roles, and Responsibilities During the Delivery of Occupational Therapy Services (edited) • Occupational Therapy Practice Frame: Domain and Process, 3rd edition • Occupational Therapy's Commitment to Nondiscrimination and Inclusion (edited) • The Philosophical Base of Occupational Therapy Education • Scope of Practice • The Role of Occupational Therapy in Primary Care: Position Paper
2015	• Complex Environmental Modifications: Position Paper • Occupational Therapy for Children and Youth Using Sensory Integration Theory and Methods in School-based Practice • Occupational Therapy's Perspective on the Use of Environments and Contexts to Facilitate Health, Well-Being an Participation in Occupations

November-December issues of the American Journal of Occupational Therapy for each year.

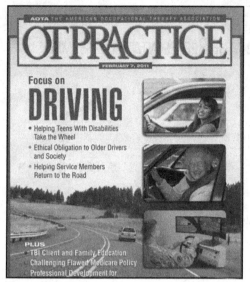

Figure 11-5. Driving project. (Printed with permission from the Archive of the American Occupational Therapy Association, Inc.)

in home modification promotes adapting space and technology to facilitate the occupations people want and/or need to perform in their daily lives. Creative use of available media is needed to promote the variety of occupational therapy services that occupational therapists and assistants can provide. Occupational therapy services should be available to all citizens and customers regardless of whether they live in rural or urban environments. As technology improves, telehealth and telemedicine communication systems (i.e., tele-occupational therapy) may provide answers to providing services to populations where geographic distances limit access.

Occupational therapists and assistants need to continue image building as a life science that helps people better organize their occupations to increase enjoyment, management, performance, and quality of life throughout the lifespan. Occupational therapy has a unique perspective, which is the ability to examine occupational performance from a variety of perspectives in time and space while taking into account personal likes and dislikes for doing occupations that must be done (obligatory) as well as those that are pleasurable but not required to maintain health and well-being but may enhance quality of life. The multidimensional perspective gives occupational therapy personnel an opportunity to help consumers make adjustments and adaptations in the performance of occupations that might not otherwise occur to the person, organization, population, or community.

Information Resources

The profession needs a worldwide accessible database that includes abstracts and access to all occupational therapy journals in all languages, as well as all textbooks, teaching manuals, and annual reports of occupational therapy organizations. Occupational therapy information and literature need to be stored to maximize distribution of knowledge

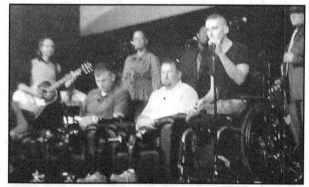

Figure 11-6. Wounded warriors at the 2014 AOTA annual conference opening ceremony. (Printed with permission from the Archive of the American Occupational Therapy Association, Inc.)

and promote resources for research activities to improve practice and promote the profession. A site that translates articles into several languages would further augment sharing of information and data.

Organizational Structure

The control of the professional Association has changed over the years. Some functions that the Association spent personal and financial capital to develop are no longer within the Association's domain of control, such as accreditation of educational programs and credentialing of personnel.

Both are now conducted independently of the professional organization. Continuing credentials or recertification is now primarily the responsibility of the state licensure boards. Even though the Association's financial management is now controlled largely by the requirements for incorporation under the District of Columbia code, members must maintain an active role in exercising their rights to determine how the money is spent. Whereas Association members used to determine the structure and organization of the Association, now the wishes of members are largely overshadowed by governmental controls. Those controls are designed to keep organizations financially viable and free of graft and corruption, but the same controls decrease the ability of members to determine how to run the organization. Power to control the organization rests with a small number of elected officers. Other members can advise but cannot override the elected officers and cannot change the organization structure without violating the incorporation requirements specified in the District of Columbia code. Membership in the professional organization may be voluntary, but the organization structure of the professional organization is not determined by the voluntary members. Instead, the membership is once again given only an advisory role through their state representative; the same role they once had under the old House of Delegates which functioned in the 1940s and 1950s before the 1964 bylaws gave the Delegate Assembly responsibility for policy making. The real power is held by the elected members of the Board of Directors.

Occupational Therapy Practice Framework, Third Edition

The Third Edition of the OTPF incorporates addition changes in the content, although the basic format of the document remains the same. Most of the changes were editorial or moving content from one section to another to better explain the purpose and clarify the process. Changes include removing the category "Therapeutic Use of Self" as an intervention technique because it is considered to be a general process. The category "Consultation Process" was removed as an intervention and is now described as a method of intervention in the process. The subtitle "Therapeutic Use of Occupations and Activities" was changed to "Occupations and Activities" because therapeutic use is supposedly implied. Feedback had suggested there was confusion regarding the use of interventions as hierarchical between occupation-based interventions and purposeful activities. "Preparatory Methods and Tasks" became a subcategory apart from "Occupations and Activities." Preparatory methods are not activities, so they are no longer grouped in the category considered with activities. Preparatory tasks are considered to be engagements (e.g., cones, clothespins) that are not a part of occupation but do address underlying client factors. The term task is used to distinguish these engagements from activities and occupations. The "Advocacy" section was expanded to include subsection "Self-Advocacy." Advocacy is seen as the manner or intervention that begins the process through which change occurs, as opposed to being the method. A "Preparatory Methods" subcategory was "Assistive Technology and Wheeled Mobility." "Education Process" was changed to "Education Training" with two subheadings: "Education" and "Training."

FOUNDATION

In 2014, the Annual Report stated that the Mission Statement was revised to read, "The mission of AOTF is to advance the science of occupational therapy to support people's full participation in meaningful life activities" (AOTF, 2014, p. 12). The Vision Statement reads, "We envision a vibrant science that builds knowledge to support effective evidence-based occupational therapy" (AOTF, 2014, p. 12). A new group called the AOTF Leaders & Legacies Society was started to honor

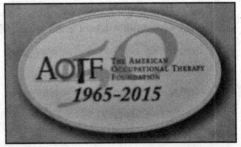

Figure 11-7. AOTF 50th anniversary symbol celebrating the Foundation. (Printed with permission from the Archive of the American Occupational Therapy Association, Inc.)

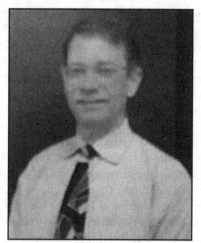

Figure 11-8. Scott Campbell, PhD, Chief Executive Officer, AOTF. (Printed with permission from the Archive of the American Occupational Therapy Association, Inc.)

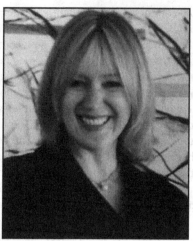

Figure 11-9. Diana L. Ramsay, Chair, Board of Directors of the AOTF, 2010-2015. (Printed with permission from the Archive of the American Occupational Therapy Association, Inc.)

occupational therapy professionals "who have demonstrate their leadership abilities and skills through service in a variety of civic and professional organizations" (AOTF, 2014, p. 9). In 2016, the Foundation celebrated its 50th year with a new logo (Figure 11-7). Scott Campbell (Figure 11-8) became the new Chief Executive Officer of the AOTF. Diana Ramsey (Figure 11-9) was Chair of the Board of Directors from 2000 to 2005. One of the fundraising activities was a "dancing with the stars" contest featuring couples who were leaders in the Association. Figure 11-10 shows the logo used for the contest. The Wilma L. West Library (Figure 11-11) has responded to requests for over 3,370 books; 36,476 journal and newspaper articles; 1,172 doctoral dissertations and master's theses; 1,000 audiovisual resources, including photos and videos; and 1,096 proceedings and other resources. The Annual Report also states that the Foundation had awarded 1,450 scholarships over the years, amounting to $1,316,646. The year 2015 was a pivotal year for the Foundation. Its second Executive Director, Charles H. Christiansen, retired, and its third Director, Scott Campbell, was hired (Figure 11-12).

LOOKING BACK AND LOOKING FORWARD

The Janus approach is one of looking forward and backward at the same time—how we did it and what is next.

The Vision

How Has the Vision Barton Had When He Created the Term *Occupational Therapy* Changed Over the Years?

Barton stated in 1914, "If there is an occupational disease, why not an occupational therapy?" (Barton, 1914). Barton further suggested that he believed that occupational

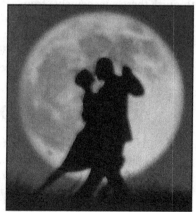

Figure 11-10. AOTF Event: "Dancing With the Stars" contest logo. (Printed with permission from the Archive of the American Occupational Therapy Association, Inc.)

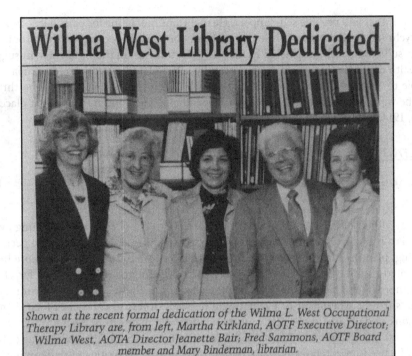

Wilma West Library Dedicated

Shown at the recent formal dedication of the Wilma L. West Occupational Therapy Library are, from left, Martha Kirkland, AOTF Executive Director; Wilma West, AOTA Director Jeanette Bair; Fred Sammons, AOTF Board member and Mary Binderman, librarian.

Figure 11-11. The Wilma L. West Library was formally dedicated in 1988. (Printed with permission from the Archive of the American Occupational Therapy Association, Inc.)

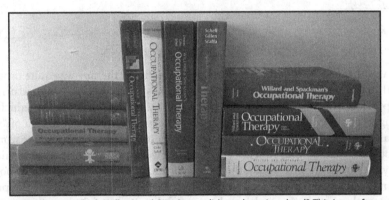

Figure 11-12. Which Willard and Spackman did you have in school? This is an often-asked question of occupational therapy practitioners. There have been 12 editions of Willard and Spackman published—the first in 1947 and the 12th in 2014. The other editions were published in 1954 (2nd), 1963 (3rd), 1970 (4th), 1978 (5th), 1983 (6th), 1988 (7th), 1993 (8th), 1998 (9th), 2003 (10th), and 2009 (11th). Pictured on the left from top to bottom in order are the first through fourth editions. Pictured on the right from top to bottom in order are the fifth through eighth editions. Pictured in the center from left to right are the nineth through 12th editions. (Copyright © Dr. Lori T. Andersen. Reprinted with permission.)

therapy could provide an occupation that would produce "a similar therapeutic effect to that of every drug in material medico" (italics in original), the original name of the Physician's Desk Reference (PDR) (Barton, 1914, p. 139). In other words, he suggested that a doctor's prescription could be filled by the right occupation and dosage just as well as a pharmaceutical drug. He also suggested that there is an occupation that will provide "exercise for each separate organ, joint, and muscle of the human body" (Barton, 1914, p. 139). What is more, the occupation will be "a useful occupation" that will provide self-support. He mentions morphine for pain, a leucotoxin for leuke-mia, strychnine, and digitalis. While there may not be specific occupation that produces equal (or better) results than each drug listed in the PDR, Barton was on the right track in suggesting that good health could be obtained through carefully selected and administered occupation. We have been able to "use the hospital (and other settings) as a re-educational institution through which to put the waste products of society (social dependents) back and into the right place" in society (Barton, 1914, p. 140).

The Image

How Has the Image of Occupational Therapy Changed Over the Years Since the Practice of Occupational Therapy Formally Began?

One early image is that of a basket lady carrying craft supplies in a basket hung over her arm. Another is a room in a hospital or institution in which crafts activities are being performing such as weaving, printing, or woodworking. Both are rather rare today. A clinic is more likely to have items related to self-care for adults and selected sensorimotor play activities for children. The image is more likely that of a therapist helping a person with dressing or performing kitchen and work tasks from a wheelchair or evaluating a person's fitness to drive. The focus is more on the occupations of daily life in the 21st century. Handcrafts may still be seen as tasks to teach skills such as hand manipulation and following directions but are rarely the main focus of intervention which is focused on activities of daily living, instrumental activities of daily living, work, play, leisure, rest and sleep, and social participation.

The Message

How Has the Public Message (Definitions and Descriptions) About Occupational Therapy Changed Over the Years?

Originally, the definition and description of occupational therapy was quite broad: "any activity, mental or physical, definitely prescribed ... to hasten recovery...." and return to roles and activities previously pursued and enjoyed (Pattison, 1922). The focus was on reducing, curing, or eliminating, if possible, the effects of illness and disease. At the time, the idea of "working one's way to health" was radial. The prevailing view was resting and avoiding active work. Preventing health problems, maintaining function, and saying well and safe in the home and community were rarely, if ever, mentioned. Today, the focus is on enabling participation in the home, at school, at work, and in the community. However, occupation continues to be art of the process toward achieving a goal, whether the goal is reduction of the effects of disease, increased community participation, or both.

The Public "Face"

How Have We Changed Our Approach to Identifying and Interacting With Other Stakeholders (Professional Organization, Consumer Coalitions/Groups, Policy Makers, Service Recipients)?

Initially, interaction was primarily with physicians and hospital administrator groups such as the AHA, AMA, American Psychiatric Association, and American Tuberculosis Association. In the 1960s, the Association officers became more involved with other groups, such as the Coalition of Independent Professions, Society of Allied Health Professions, and American Public Health Association. Today, interaction with occupational therapy associations in other countries has been useful, such as the joint annual conference with Canada in 1994. Establishing and maintaining contact with legislators at both the state and national levels has become essential to provide an "occupational therapy face" for legislation and policy making.

Education

How Has Our System of Education and Training Approach Changed in Preparing Our Practitioners, Educators, and Researchers?

The original 6-week (or fewer) courses focused on how to perform craft activities, follow hospital etiquette, and interact with patients. The length and content of the curriculum have both increased. The course of study for occupational therapists has increased from 6 weeks to about 6 years of university- or college-level education. The content now includes biological and behavioral sciences, training in multiple media and modalities, theory and application of occupational therapy, management techniques, and supervised practice training. In addition, a certification examination is required before a person is recognized as qualified to practice and become licensed. Formal educational criteria and practice guidelines for occupational therapy assistant did not exist in the early days of the profession and were not formalized until 1958; they have also expanded from short courses of several weeks to several months of formal course work.

Standards and Standard Setting

How Has Our System of Quality Controls or Standards Setting (Accreditation and Credentialing) Changed?

From 1917 to 1922, there was no generally accepted and published quality control. Starting in 1923, the Association developed and published minimum standards for educational programs in the Archives of Occupational Therapy. In 1932, the first directory of recognized credentialing (registered occupational therapist) was published based on standards developed in 1928 and finalized in 1931, including formal training in a recognized occupational therapy training school and/or experience practicing in an occupational therapy service program. Formal recognition of accredited education programs began in 1938 based on a set of essential factors first published in the Journal of the American Medical Association in 1935. One examination for persons not previously recognized in the National Register of qualified occupational therapists was administered in 1939. Admission to the directory of registered occupational therapists by examination for new graduates began in 1944 based on essay and short-answer questions and by multiple-choice questions beginning in 1947. Cooperation with the AMA in developing and implementing accreditation procedures occurred from 1933 to 1992. The ACOTE took over formal accreditation of occupational therapy education programs at both the professional and assistant levels in 1992. Registration was changed to certification in 1986 with the formation of the American Board for Certification of Occupational Therapy (ABCOT) when membership in the Association was formally separated from the process of certification. The name of the certifying organization was changed in 1996 to the National Board for Certification of Occupational Therapy (NBCOT), and it became an independent organization. The requirements to sit for an initial certification examination continue, and the results are accepted by all 50 states and three jurisdictions (Guam, Puerto Rico, and the District of Columbia). States started to require licenses to practice in 1975. All states and the three jurisdictions required a license to practice as an occupational therapist as of 2014. Licensure for occupational therapy assistants was achieved in 2015.

Defense Against Encroachment

How Have We Changed Our Defense of Our Curriculum of Study (Pedagogy) and Scope of Practice From Encroachment Over the Years?

In 1948/1949, we defended occupational therapy education and practice from a takeover bid by the Council of Physical Medicine of the AMA through a series of meetings pointing out that the practice of occupational therapy was broader than the content or service programs provided by physical medicine alone. In 1979, the Association began a series of meetings with the American Physical Therapy Association (APTA) regarding the broadening of scope of physical therapy to include self-care in home, school, and community. The Association's Government and Legislative Affairs Department has reported threats to occupational therapy practice from physical therapists, art therapists, music therapists, recreational specialists, optometrists, orthotics and prosthetics practitioners, speech-language pathologists, naturopathic physicians, orientation and mobility specialists, polysomnographic technologists (sleep specialists), exercise physiologists, and massage therapists (2014 National Office report, p. 30). Others have included psychologists, physicians, nurses, and kinesiotherapists. These threats most often occur today through attempts to revise, update, or expand the scope of practice outlined in a licensure law. However, threats can also occur from language written into a federal or state law.

Practice

How Have We Changed (Contracted and Expanded) Our Practice Arena or Sphere of Influence (Illness to Wellness and Promotion, Rehabilitation of Disability to Prevention of Disability)?

Two of the original areas of practice have decreased, and two others have increased. Tuberculosis is no longer listed as a separate area of practice in occupational therapy data collection statistics and mental illness, originally the largest area of practice, has decreased significantly in numbers of practitioners over the years. In contrast, orthopedics was originally a minor area of practice but is now a major area, along with physical disabilities and rehabilitation. The other major practice area that has increased is pediatrics, which was a minor area in the 1930s and is now a major area of practice in early intervention and school-based practice. Other diagnoses rarely seen today are poliomyelitis, post-polio syndrome, and rheumatic fever as a cause of a person being labeled a "cardiac cripple." Increased diagnoses seen today include Alzheimer's disease, spinal cord injury, and head (traumatic brain) injury.

Legislation and Policy Making

How Have We Changed Our Approach to Achieving Legislation Favorable to Occupational Therapy Education, Practice, and Research?

The Association had no lobbyist or department addressing legislation prior to the 1950s. The Association was not involved in writing the original Medicare and Medicare legislation as physical therapy was. Although occupational therapy was included in the 1943 Vocational Rehabilitation Act, the inclusion was not a result of Association actions. Beginning in the 1970s, the Association began increased involvement in federal legislation. In 1974, the Association formally agreed to support state licensure. In 1980, efforts by the Association resulted in the inclusion of occupational therapy in Medicare Part B. The Association began publishing the Legislative Alert in 1973 (changed to the Federal Report in 1977) to inform members about the status of pending or adopted federal legislation. In 1999, the Association began published the State Policy Department News to cover state news regarding licensure law development, passage, and sunset review. The title was changed to State Policy Update in 2007, and it was discontinued in 2011. The Government Affairs Office of the Association publishes an occasional column in *OT Practice* regarding legislative issues.

How Have We Changed Our Approach to Achieving Policy Regulations Favorable to Occupational Therapy (Salary Schedules, Inclusion of Occupational Therapy in Legislation for Evaluation and Intervention, and Reimbursement for Services)?

The Association developed a Civil Service Committee to keep track of state salaries beginning in the 1940s. Later, the Civil Service Committee became the Legislative and Civil Service Committee. The Legislative Committee was formed under the Developmental Council in 1964. In 1968, the Association hired its first lobbyist, Russell J. N. Dean, Director of the Washington Consulting Service. Early interaction with Congress related to hearings on the amendments to the Vocational Rehabilitation Act. Early interactions with federal agencies were with the Division of Allied Health Manpower and Division of Medical Care Administration of the U.S. Public Health Services, Department of Health Education and Welfare (HEW). One request was to explore grant and contract possibilities for recruitment and refresher courses. A second was a recommendation that independent occupational therapy practitioners be allowed direct payment under supplementary medical insurance part of the Medicare Program (Tiebel, 1968). The national office first listed governmental affairs in 1973 under the Public Affairs Department. The Legislative Alert was published from 1973 to 1975. The Federal Report was published by the Government and Legal Affairs Department from 1977 to 1987 as a separate publication and was included in *OT Week* for 2 more years. The Government and Legal Affairs Department was formed in 1976.

Research

How Have We Changed Our Approach to Facilitate Research on the Effectiveness and Efficiency of Practice, Education, and Research Methodology?

Research has been a focus since the founding of the Association. Dunton was the first chair of the Research Committee. The primary focus was on collecting information about research publications rather than supporting research through education of how to conduct research or through grants or contracts. However, both Dunton and Louis Haas conducted studies related to the practice of occupational therapy in psychiatry and mental illness. A series of studies appears in Occupational Therapy and Rehabilitation on types of arts and crafts and their effect on mood or emotion. Haas reported on the organization and administration of occupational therapy. Support for education and research and financial grants became available with the formation of the AOTF in 1965. Research activities has increased in the Association as more people have applied for and received funding through the National Institutes of Health and other funding organizations.

Association Finances, Grants, and Outside Funding

How Has the Association Attracted Outside Funds (Non-Membership Dues) Over the Years, Including Scholarships, Traineeships, Grants, and Contracts?

Over the years, many source of outside funds have been sought by the Association. However, as Executive Director Marjorie Fish pointed out, grants provide money and cost money (Annual Report, 1961/1962). The financial hazards are that the more grants, the more personnel, the more activities that cannot be suddenly cut off at termination (of grant funding) but require some

Table 11-8
PARTIAL LIST OF EARLY ASSOCIATION GRANTS AND CONTRACTS

- Kellogg grants (scholarships, traineeships, grants, contracts), 1946-1969
- United Cerebral Palsy 1951-67 (undergraduate scholarships) Note: UCP took over awarding scholarships after 1967. 1955-56, $10,000; 1950, $10,000; 1963, $1500
- National Institute of Mental health, NIH, PHS, DHEW 3M-9083 1955-59, Allenberry Conference held in 1956. Proceedings published in 1959.
- Office of Vocational Rehabilitation, DHEW, 1955 Institute held in New York, June 20-25, 1955. Proceedings published
- National Foundation for Infantile Paralysis: recruitment 1955-56 $23,850, 1957-58, 1959-62
- Office of Vocational Rehabilitation, DHEW, 4 Regional Institutes, 1955-1956, $10,000. Proceedings published
- Office of Vocational Rehabilitation, Institute held October 2-25, 1957 Proceedings published
- Office of Vocational Rehabilitation, Grant 123-T-1957-61
- Office of Vocational Rehabilitation, Field Consultant, Rehabilitation of the Physically Disabled (Irene Hollis), 1958-1962
- Office of Vocational Rehabilitation, Field Consultant in Psychiatry (Mary Alice Combs, 1961-1964; June Mazer, 1964-69)
- National Foundation for Infantile Paralysis. Curriculum Study grant 1950-1958
- Office of Vocational Rehabilitation 1952. Traineeships for 1 person from each OT educational program to attend WFOT conference in Philadelphia, PA
- OVR/VRA/SRA graduate education traineeships, 1960-1972
- Vocational Rehabilitation Administration 123-T-1962-1969 (Curriculum Study)
- Vocational Rehabilitation Administration (VRA 367-T-66 1966-69 Recruitment)
- National Institutes of Health (Training Institutes for OT educators), 1973-74
- Public Health Services (Educator Training workshops, 1974-76)

provision of an ongoing character (Fish, 1961-1962, p. 9). Major grant funds have been included scholarships and traineeships, professional development, curriculum review, and student recruitment (Table 11-8).

The National Office

How Has the Role of the National Office Changed Over the Years?

The first "offices" were in Consolation House (Barton's home) and Mrs. Slagle's kitchen. The focus was on membership, educational standards, job placement, finances, and qualifications/registration. In the 1950s, grant development and administration and the publication of conference proceedings and practice manuals was added. In the 1960s, legal consultation and lobbying at the federal level was added. In the 1970s, legal consultation for states seeking licensure was added, and the office was move from New York City to the Washington, DC, area. The Government and Legal Affairs Department was added first to deal with federal legislation and then with state licensure. Reimbursement demands and coding for insurance claims was also added to meet membership demands. The office staff grew from one person and a secretary to multiple people occupying a variety of positions as the needs and expectations of the Association grew to encompass accreditation, registration, scholarships, continuing education and competency, recruitment, public information, practice standards and guidelines, research, documentation and reimbursement, state licensure, federal legislation, and legal affairs. Some of the activities would later become parts of separate organizations, such as registration/certification (NBCOT), scholarships, and research (AOTF). However, the initial organizing efforts were accomplished in the national office.

Workforce Demographics

How Has the Change in Location and Number of Practitioners Occurred Over the Years?

The first membership list in 1917 was represented primarily by three states: Illinois, Massachusetts, and New York, plus Canada. In the first National Registry of qualified practitioners published in 1932, 80 of the 318 names are of therapists living in New York State. Membership remains predominately from the North Central (12) and Northeast (9) states. California, Texas, and Florida are the only states to be included in the top states reporting a significant number of therapists that are not from the North Central or Northeast states. In 1997, the regional breakdown of therapists showed that 53.9% of therapists responding to the survey lived in North Central or Northeast areas of the country, comprising 21 states (AOTA, 1998a). In the 2010 Compensation Survey, 52.4% of therapists responding to the survey lived in the North Central or Northeast areas. Student enrollment from the two regions was 60.2% (AOTA, 2010, pp. 11, 62). In the 2015 Salary and Workforce Survey, 51% of practitioners live in the North Central or Northeast states, and 56.4% of students attend occupational therapy educational programs located in the North Central or Northeast states (AOTA, 2015a, pp. 12, 42). There is slight decreasing trend, but the influence of the North Central and Northeast states will remain for many years to come.

Specialization Versus Generalist

What Is the Argument for and Against Specialization in Occupational Therapy?

The argument has two aspects: one related to education and the other to practice. In education, the argument concerns whether practitioners should be educated as generalists or should select a field of specialization during their educational preparation. Over the years, the generalist approach has dominated in educational preparation. The Essentials and Standards documents have uniformly supported the generalist view. Not everyone agreed. In 1953, Dr. Dunton wrote an editorial in support of permitting shorted periods of education "with more emphasis on specialties for which pupils seem best adapted" (Dunton, 1953, p. 215). His rationale was that allowing specialization during educational preparation permitted students to finish their education quicker and thus join the workforce sooner to alleviate the manpower shortage. Welles (1958) makes the point that registration (certification) may imply that the person is qualified "for any type of position on any level" in the practice of occupational therapy (p. 289). She states further that there is no defined body of knowledge in occupational therapy that when mastered will automatically qualify a person for a particular position. Nevertheless, she recommends that the concept of specialization be accepted in the field of occupational therapy and that the profession should continue to define function with greater precision. Hirama (1982) also supports specialization. She suggests that the profession needs to define what advanced occupational therapy knowledge is and establish criteria for the status of "specialist." Dunn and Rask (1989) also support specialization and outline additional steps needed to develop specialty areas of practice. Later, the recommendations of all the authors would be adopted in the specialty certification program as advanced practice concepts. In the final analysis, both concepts have been accepted. Initial education and certification are at the generalist level, but postgraduate education (degree or non-degree) is available to support specialization in many aspects and areas of practice.

Definition of Core Concept

Is Occupation or Activity the Common Core of Occupational Therapy?

Barton chose the word *occupation* when he created the term *occupational therapy* in 1914. However, Pattison used the word *activity* in the definition he created, which was widely used in the profession for many years. The definition begins "any activity." Thus, the profession has used the two words interchangeably for many years. Dictionaries are of limited help because both words have the additional meaning of an implied health benefit or therapeutic potential attached, which dictionaries do not address. For many years, the term *purposeful activity* was suggested, but the nature of purpose was likewise difficult to fully define or describe.

Looking Forward: Workforce Trends

The National Center for Health Workforce Analysis (NCHWA) under the Health Resources and Services Administration of the U.S. Department of Health and Human Services conducted an analysis of the projected workforce needs for occupational therapy and physical therapy using the Health Workforce Simulation Model (HWSM) (NCHWA, 2013). The HWSM assumes that demand equals supply in the base year. Major components include characteristics of the existing workforce, newly trained workers entering the workforce, and workforce decisions such as retirement and pattern of work hours. For demand modeling, the major components include population demographics, health care use patterns, and demand for health care services. Based on the HWSM, three statements were made that between 2012 and 2025:

- Supply is estimated to grow by 46% for occupational therapists and 33% for physical therapists.
- Demand is estimated to grow by 20% for occupational therapists and 23% for physical therapists.
- The projected supply of individuals in each occupation exceeds the projected growth in service demand for occupational therapists and physical therapists.

According to these findings, there should be a more-than-sufficient supply of occupational therapists and physical therapists to meet the project growth in demand for services by 2025. A surplus of 22,300 occupational therapists and 19,100 physical therapists is projected. The calculations do not include numbers for occupational therapy or physical therapy assistants.

However, the estimated supply in 2012 is stated as 86,300. The source of the number is not stated. According to the 2010 survey of state occupational therapy regulatory boards, the workforce of occupational therapists was approximately 102,500 occupational therapists and 34,500 occupational therapy assistants (AOTA, 2010). The source of entrants (58,200) and projected supply (126,200) by 2025 is not provided.

On the other hand, a study by Lin, Zhang, and Dixon (2015) suggests that a shortage of occupational therapists exists now and will increase in the future. Their model included both a demand and supply concept and is based on the difference between the national mean of available practitioners for currently available positions as determined by the Bureau of Labor (given a grade of C) and each state's shortage (or overage) ratio using a fixed standard deviation. Grades A and F were ±2.50, grades B and D grades were ±1.50, and grades C+ and C- were ±0.5 standard deviations from the mean. Their findings suggest that a shortage is expected to increase in all 50 states through the year 2030, the final year calculated. Using the grading system of A through F, they report that the number of states with a grade of D or below will increase from three in 2010 to 18 in 2020 and 37 in 2030. The three states with the greatest shortage ratio are projected to be Arizona, Hawaii, and Utah. The three states with the largest shortages (the number of practitioners available for jobs) are projected to be California, Florida, and Texas. States in the Northeast region as a whole are projected to have the smallest shortages of practitioners, whereas states in the South and West regions are projected to have the largest shortages.

Projecting future needs is always risky. Events such as political and legislative changes can quickly change the outlook for occupational therapy practitioners, as the Balanced Budget Act of 1997 showed. As of 2014, the Bureau of Labor projects an increased need for occupational therapists of 29% and for occupational therapy assistants of 41% through to 2025. Throughout our history, shortages have been the rule. Time will tell if the trend continues.

Changing Work Settings

Where or in What Settings Will Occupational Therapy Personnel Be Employed in the Future?

Changes in work settings appear to be occurring. In 2007, the primary work settings of new graduates were rehabilitation (24%), schools (23%), skilled nursing facilities (21%), and acute care facilities (14%) (NBCOT, 2008). In 2012, the primary work settings were skilled nursing facilities (20%), rehabilitation (17%), acute care (13%), and school systems (13%). However, in the same 2012 survey, the percentage of practitioners working in pediatrics is listed at 19%, whereas the number working in geriatrics is listed at 8% (NBCOT, 2012a). The primary work setting for new occupational therapy assistants is also skilled nursing facilities, followed by rehabilitation and school systems (NBCOT, 2012b). However, data from AOTA (2015a) show a different pattern for occupational therapists, without regard for number of years in practice. Overall, hospitals are the major employers (26.6%), followed by schools (19.9%), long-term care/skilled nursing facilities (12.2%), and freestanding outpatient facilities (10.8%). The data for occupational therapy assistants have remained consistent since 2000: long-term care/skilled nursing facilities followed by schools and hospitals (AOTA, 2015a). If the trends hold, nursing homes will be the primary employers of both occupational therapists and occupational therapy assistants, although hospitals will continue to employ a substantial percentage of occupational therapists, along with schools.

What Kinds of Conditions or Diagnoses Will Be Seen by Occupational Therapy Practitioners?

If past is prologue, the conditions or diagnoses seen by occupational therapy practitioners can be organized into six major groups: neurological, developmental, musculoskeletal/orthopedic, cardiopulmonary, psychosocial dysfunction disorders, and general medical/systemic disorders (NBCOT, 2012a, 2012b. For occupational therapists, the top three disorders in each group are:

- Neurological: cerebral vascular accident, dementia, traumatic brain injury
- Developmental: developmental delay, sensory integrative disorder, intellectual disability
- Musculoskeletal/orthopedic: fractures, joint replacement, osteoarthritis
- Cardiopulmonary: chronic obstructive pulmonary disease, congestive heart failure, myocardial infarction
- Psychosocial: anxiety disorders, autism spectrum disorders, behavior disorders
- General medical/systemic: general deconditioning/debilitation, cancer, diabetes

For occupational therapy assistants, the top three diagnoses in each category are:

- Neurological: dementia, cerebral vascular accident, Parkinson's disease
- Development: developmental delay, sensory integrative disorder, visual processing deficit
- Musculoskeletal/orthopedic: fracture, joint replacement, osteoarthritis
- Cardiopulmonary: congestive heart failure, chronic obstructive pulmonary disease, myocardial infarction
- Psychosocial dysfunction: anxiety disorders, behavior disorders, mood disorders
- General medical/systemic: diabetes, general deconditioning/debilitation, rheumatoid arthritis

What Do We Really Know About the Process of Occupational Therapy Practice?

There have been five analyses of practice conducted to develop rationale for questions on the initial certification examinations. The first analysis of occupational therapy practice was conducted in 1991 by the Educational Testing Service for the ABCOT and was based on a survey from approximately 1,400 therapists and assistances practitioners and educators. The goal was to establish the importance of knowledge of certain tasks for entry-level clinicians (Lang, 1994). The results were organized into seven categories: assess occupational performance, develop treatment plan, implement treatment plan, evaluate treatment plan, develop discharge plan, organization and management of services, and promote professional practice.

The second practice analysis was completed in 1997 (Dunn & Cada, 1998; NBCOT, 1998). The survey included 4,000 occupational therapists and 3,000 occupational therapy assistants. The sample was designed to represent all geographical areas, experience levels, and practice areas. The results were organized into four domains:

1. Provide occupational therapy services for person within the performance contexts of their lives

2. Provide occupational therapy services that address the occupational needs of populations with the context of their physical, social, temporal, and cultural environments

3. Manage the delivery of occupational therapy services

4. Advance the effectiveness of the occupational therapy profession

A third practice analysis was conducted in 2003 (Bent, Crist, Florey, & Strickland, 2005; NBCOT, 2004a, 2004b). The format was similar to the 1991 study. Results were organized in five domains:

1. Evaluate the individual/group to determine needs and priorities for occupation-based intervention

2. Develop intervention plan that addresses the occupational needs of individuals/groups

3. Implement occupationally meaningful interventions with individuals/groups that support participation in relevant environments

4. Provide occupational therapy services that address the occupational performance needs of populations

5. Manage, organize, and promote occupational therapy services

The fourth practice analysis was conducted in 2008. A total of 1,282 occupational therapists were requested to participate, and 1,156 completed the survey. Participations had to be working 36 months or less. Thus the study sample was different from the previous practice analysis studies, which included practitioners with a variety of years of work experience. Four domains were created:

1. Gather information regarding factors that influence occupational performance

2. Formulate conclusions regarding the client's needs and priorities to develop a client-centered intervention plan

3. Select and implement evidence-based interventions to support participation in areas of occupation (activities of daily living, education, work, play, leisure, social participation) throughout the continuum of care

4. Uphold professional standards and responsibilities to promote quality in practice

The fifth practice analysis was conducted in 2012. The sample included 2,826 occupational therapists who had been certified for less than 3 years. Response rate was 79% (2,235). Again, four domains were established:

1. Acquire information regarding factors that influence occupational performance throughout the occupational therapy process

2. Formulate conclusions regarding client needs and priorities to develop and monitor an intervention plan throughout the occupational therapy process

3. Select interventions for managing a client-centered plan throughout the occupational therapy process

4. Manage and direct occupational therapy services to promote quality in practice

An analysis of the five analyses shows the changing terminology in the occupational therapy literature, such as meaningful intervention, performance contexts, areas of occupation, and client-centered. However, the basic process is evident: gathering and evaluating information, developing and implementing a plan of care, and managing and directing occupational therapy services. What is missing from the 2012 domains (and was included in the 2008 domains) for the occupational therapist is a domain concerned with upholding ethical and professional standards. Why the domain was dropped is not clear. Such a domain is included for the occupational therapy assistant in addition to assisting occupational therapists to acquire information that influences occupational performance and implementing interventions in accordance with the intervention plan and under the supervision of the occupational therapist (NBCOT, 2012b). In summary, the process of delivering occupational therapy services remains consistent, although the descriptions of the process change to reflect current terminology.

Will the Profession of Occupational Therapy Support Licensure Portability?

Now that licensure has been achieved in all states for both the occupational therapist and the assistant, the next question concerns portability of the license across state lines. Initial certification is uniform because all states use the examination results from the examinations administered by the NBCOT. However, license renewal can vary depending on the frequency of renewal, the cost, the number of continuing educational units required, and the type or category of continuing education. Therapists and assistants who work in more than one state or jurisdiction or those who move from one state or jurisdiction are most affected. The Association can help by providing model legislation, just as it did for licensure laws, but state associations will need to step in to make the portability happen. State licensure laws, the rules and regulations, or both may need to be modified to permit portability to occur. The result may save practitioners money and time in renewing licensures, but the greater payoff may occur in facilitating movement of practitioners across state lines, especially during times of natural or manmade disasters.

What Is the Continuing Role of the National Association?

In 1997, Steib wrote in OT Week that the role of the Association was to help practitioners create and grow a strong, viable, and relevance profession; gain and maintain the respect and recognition they deserved; and maintain acceptable salary and reimbursement levels (Steib, 1997). Professional growth included "maintaining competency, gaining new skills, taking advantage of increased educational opportunities, and accessing new technologies and research" and the Association was actively involved in all of these (Steib, 1997, p. 19).

REFLECTION

This period of AOTA history includes the implementation of the Centennial Vision in AOTA operations, beginning with intensified continual education of the public about the profession's progress and accomplishments. Initiatives toward the critical appraisal of existing related literature on specific areas of occupational therapy provide validation and documentation for practitioners. Demand for evidence-based practice adds impetus for increased research. Revision of ACOTE standards reflected realignment to current practice and graduate level of education.

This period also revealed increased vigilance for protecting the profession's scope of practice. Consistent with the Centennial Vision of a global practice, there was increased recognition of the value of international and interprofessional education in the curriculum. Conversations stemmed from intensified awareness of the need for and a move toward higher degrees for entry into the profession: doctoral degrees for occupational therapists and bachelor's degrees for assistants, with the number of applicant entry-level doctoral programs continuing to increase.

REFERENCES

Accreditation Council for Occupational Therapy Education. (2011). Standards and interpretive guide. Bethesda, MD: Author

Allied Health Professions Personnel Training Act (P.L. 89-751)

American Medical Association. (1932). *Handbook of physical therapy*. Chicago, IL: AMA Press.

American Medical Association. (1949). Essentials of an acceptable school of occupational therapy. *Journal of the American Medical Association, 141*(16), 1167.

American Occupational Therapy Association. (1923). *Bulletin No. 1*. New York, NY: Author.

American Occupational Therapy Association. (1950). Essentials of an acceptable school of occupational therapy. *American Journal of Occupational Therapy, 4*(3), 125-128.

American Occupational Therapy Association. (1959). Board of Management minutes. New York, NY: Author.

American Occupational Therapy Association. (1965). *Guidebook for an accredited curriculum in occupational therapy*. New York, NY: Author.

American Occupational Therapy Association. (1968). *Roster: Medical Advisory Committee*. New York, NY: Author.

American Occupational Therapy Association. (1969). Statement on referral. *American Journal of Occupational Therapy, 23*(6), 530-531.

American Occupational Therapy Association. (1998a). *1997 member compensation survey: Summary report and tables*. Bethesda, MD: Author.

American Occupational Therapy Association. (2010). *2010 occupational therapy compensation and workforce study*. Bethesda, MD: Author.

American Occupational Therapy Association. (2014). FAQs: AOTA Board of Directors position statement on doctoral level single point of entry for occupational therapists. Retrieved from www.aota.org/AboutAOTA/Get-Involved/BOD/OTD-FAQs.aspx

American Occupational Therapy Association. (2015a). *2015 AOTA salary & workforce survey*. Bethesda, MD: Author.

American Occupational Therapy Association. (2015b). Statement on occupational therapy's distinct value. *OT Practice, 20*(11), 3.

American Occupational Therapy Association. (2016). Annual Meeting (Verbal Report with Slides). Bethesda, MD: Author.

American Occupational Therapy Foundation. (2014). *Celebrating 60 years of advancing the science of occupational therapy*. Bethesda, MD: Author.

Barton, G. Occupational therapy. *Trained Nurse and Hospital Review, 54*, 138-140.

Bent, M. A., Crist, P. A., Florey, L., & Strickland, L. R. (2005). A practice analysis of occupational therapy and impact on certification examination. *OTJR: Occupation, Participation and Health, 25*(3), 105-118.

Brandenburg, E. (1963). Building toward professionalism. In *Vocational Rehabilitation Administration/American Occupational Therapy Association workshop on graduate education in occupational therapy* (pp. 4-20). St. Louis, MO: Washington University.

Brown, E. J. (2012a). Mapping out the new ACOTE standards. *Advance for Occupational Therapy Practitioners, 28*(17), 13-30.

Dunn, W., & Cada, E. (1998). The national occupational therapy practice analysis: findings and implications for competence. *American Journal of Occupational Therapy, 52*(9), 721-728.

Dunn, W., & Rask, S. (1989). Entry level and specialized practice: A professional encounter. *American Journal of Occupational Therapy, 43*(1), 709.

Dunton, W.R., Jr. (1928). Prescribing occupational therapy. Springfield, IL: Charles C Thomas.

Dunton, W. R., Jr. (1953). Specialization. *American Journal of Occupational Therapy, 6*(5), 214-216.

Evans, K. A. (1987). Nationally speaking: Definition of occupation as the core concept of occupational therapy. *American Journal of Occupational Therapy, 41*(10), 637-628.

Fish, M. (1961/1962). Annual report of the executive director. New York, NY: American Occupational Therapy Association.

Hall, H.J. (1923). *OT – A new profession.* Concord, NH: Rumford Press.

Hirama, H. (1982). Toward specialization. *American Journal of Occupational Therapy, 36*(9), 601-602.

Johnson, J. (1975). Nationally speaking: Licensure. *American Journal of Occupational Therapy, 29*(2), 73.

Krusen, F. H. (1934). The relationship of physical therapy and occupational therapy. *Occupational Therapy and Rehabilitation, 13*(2), 69-77.

Lang, S. M. (Ed.). (1994). *AOTCB study guide for the OTR certification examination.* Rockville, MD: National Board for Certification in Occupational Therapy.

Licht, S. (1952). Occupational therapy. In W. Bierman & S. Licht (Eds.), *Physical medicine in general practice* (3rd ed., pp. 448-471). New York, NY: Paul B. Hoeber.

Lin, V., Zhang, X., & Dixon, P. (2015). Occupational therapy workforce in the United States: Forecasting nationwide shortages. *Physical Medicine & Rehabilitation, 7,* 946-954.

Maxwell, J. D., & Maxwell, M. P. (1984). Inner fraternity and outer sorority: Social structure and the professionalization of occupational therapy. In A. Wipper (Ed.), *The sociology of work: Papers in honour of Oswald Hall* (pp. 330-357). Ottawa, Canada: Carleton University Press.

Maze, D. J. (1968). The growth and development of the allied health schools. *Journal of the American Medical Association, 206*(7), 1548-1550.

Meredith, G. (1971). Schools of allied health professions. *American Journal of Occupational Therapy, 25*(1), 29-31.

Molander, C. O. (1931). An experiment in the combining of occupational therapy and physical therapy under single management. *Archives of Physical Therapy, X-Ray, and Radium, 12,* 279-286.

National Board for Certification in Occupational Therapy. (1998). *National study of occupational therapy practice: final report.* New York, NY: Professional Examination Service.

National Board for Certification in Occupational Therapy. (2004a). *OTR certification examination blueprint.* Gaithersburg, MD: Author.

National Board for Certification in Occupational Therapy. (2004b). *COTA certification examination blueprint.* Gaithersburg, MD: Author.

National Board for Certification in Occupational Therapy. (2008). *NBCOT 2008 practice analysis: Executive summary for the practice analysis study.* Gaithersburg, MD: Author.

National Board for Certification in Occupational Therapy. (2012a). *2012 practice analysis of the occupational therapist registered: Executive summary.* Gaithersburg, MD: Author.

National Board for Certification in Occupational Therapy. (2012b). *2012 practice analysis of the certified occupational therapy assistant: Executive summary.* Gaithersburg, MD: Author.

National Center for Health Workforce Analysis. (2012). Health workforce projections: Occupational therapy and physical therapy. Retrieved from bhw.hrsa.gov/healthworkforce/index.html

Pattison, H. A. (1922). The trend of occupational therapy for the tuberculous. *Archives of Occupational Therapy, 1*(1), 19-24.

Rehfuss, M. E., Albrecht, F. J. K., & Price, A. H. (1948). *A course in practical therapeutics.* Baltimore, MD: Williams & Wilkins.

Robinson, C. (1919). *Occupational therapy in the general hospital. Modern Hospital, 13,* 524-527.

Rogers, J. C. (2010). AOTA and AOTF announce new research agenda. *OT Practice, 15*(1), 11-12.

Steib, P. A. (1997). AOTA: Shaping the future. *OT Week, 11*(15), 18-20.

Tiebel, H. (1968). Annual report to the membership of the executive director. New York, NY: American Occupational Therapy Association.

Tracy, S. (n.d.). [Letter to Dr. Dunton]. Bethesda, MD: AOTA/AOTF Archives.

Welles, C. (1958). Da Vinci is dead: The case for specialization. *American Journal of Occupational Therapy, 12*(6), 289-290.

BIBLIOGRAPHY

American Occupational Therapy Association. (1998). *1997 member compensation survey: Final report.* Bethesda, MD: Author.

Brown, E. J. (2012). Health reform and occupational therapy. *Advance for Occupational Therapy Practitioners, 28*(15), 12-15.

Evans, K. A. (1987). Nationally speaking: Definition of occupation as the core concept of occupational therapy. *American Journal of Occupational Therapy, 41*(10), 637-628.

Hanft, B. E. (1989). Early intervention: Issues in specialization. *American Journal of Occupational Therapy, 43*(7), 431-432.

Sandhu, S. (2015). Medicare Part B policy changes coming in 2016. *OT Practice, 20*(22), 7.

Appendix A

Presidents of NSPOT and AOTA

Term	President
1917 (NSPOT)	George Edward Barton
1918–1919 (NSPOT)	William Rush Dunton, MD (NSPOT)
1919–1920 (NSPOT)	Eleanor Clarke Slagle (NSPOT)
1920–1923 (NSPOT/AOTA)	Herbert J. Hall, MD (NSPOT/AOTA)
1923–1928 (AOTA)	Thomas B. Kidner
1928–1930 (AOTA)	C. Floyd Haviland, MD
1930–1938 (AOTA)	Joseph C. Doane, MD
1938–1947 (AOTA)	Everett D. Elwood
1947–1952 (AOTA)	Winifred Conrick Kahmann, OTR
1952–1955 (AOTA)	Henrietta W. McNary, OTR
1955–1958 (AOTA)	Colonel Ruth A. Robinson, OTR, FAOTA
1958–1961 (AOTA)	Helen S. Willard, OTR, FAOTA
1961–1964 (AOTA)	Wilma L. West, OTR, FAOTA
1964–1967 (AOTA)	Ruth W. Brunyate Wiemer, MEd, OTR, FAOTA
1967–1973 (AOTA)	Florence S. Cromwell, MA, OTR, FAOTA
1973–1978 (AOTA)	Jerry A. Johnson, EdD, MBA, OTR, FAOTA
1978–1982 (AOTA)	Mae D. Hightower-Vandamm, OTR, FAOTA
1982–1983 (AOTA)	Caroline M. Baum, PhD, OTR/C, FAOTA
1983–1986 (AOTA)	Robert Bing, EdD, OTR, FAOTA
1986–1989 (AOTA)	Elnora M. Gilfoyle, ScD (Hon), OTR, FAOTA
1989–1992 (AOTA)	Ann P. Grady, PhD, OTR, FAOTA
1992–1995 (AOTA)	Mary M. Evert, MBA, OTR, FAOTA
	(continued)

Andersen, L. T., & Reed, K. L.
The History of Occupational Therapy: The First Century (pp. 359-360).
© 2017 Taylor & Francis Group.

Term	President
1995–1998 (AOTA)	Mary Foto, OTR, FAOTA
1998–2001 (AOTA)	Karen Jacobs, EdD, OTR/L, CPE, FAOTA
2001–2004 (AOTA)	Barbara L. Kornblau, JD, OT/L, FAOTA
2004–2007 (AOTA)	Carolyn Baum, PhD, OTR/L, FAOTA
2007–2010 (AOTA)	Penelope (Penny) Moyers-Cleveland, PhD, OTR/L, BCMH, FAOTA
2010–2013 (AOTA)	Florence Clark, PhD, OTR, FAOTA
2013–2016 (AOTA)	Virginia (Ginny) Stoffel, PhD, OT, BCMH, FAOTA
2016–2018 (AOTA)	Amy Jo Lamb, OTD, OTR/L, FAOTA

Appendix B

Executive Officers of NSPOT and AOTA

TERM	OFFICER	POSITION
1921–1937	Eleanor Clarke Slagle	Secretary-Treasurer
1937–1938	Maud Plummer	Executive Secretary
1938–1947	Meta R. Cobb	Executive Secretary
1948–1951	Wilma L. West	Executive Director
1951–1963	Marjorie Fish	Executive Director
1964–1968	Frances Helmig	Executive Director
1968–1971	Harriet Tiebel	Executive Director
1972–1974	Leo Fanning	Executive Director
1975–1987	James J. Garibaldi	Executive Director
1987–1999	Jeanette Bair	Executive Director
2000–2003	Joseph Isaacs	Executive Director
2004–present	Frederick P. Somers	Executive Director

Andersen, L. T., & Reed, K. L.
The History of Occupational Therapy: The First Century (p. 361).
© 2017 Taylor & Francis Group.

Appendix C

Locations of Headquarters for NSPOT and AOTA

Years	Location
1917	Consolation House (Home of George Edward Barton) A School Workshop and Vocational Bureau for Convalescents 16 Broad Street, Clifton Springs, NY
1921–1922	Home of Mrs. Eleanor Clarke Slagle 541 Madison Avenue, New York, NY
1922–1925	American Occupational Therapy Association, Inc. 370 Seventh Avenue, New York, NY
1925–1945	American Occupational Therapy Association Fuller Building (called Flatiron Building) 175 Fifth Avenue, New York, NY
1945–1955	American Occupational Therapy Association 33 West 42nd Street (Aeolian Building), New York, NY
1955–1967	American Occupational Therapy Association 250 West 57th Street (Fiske Building), New York, NY
1967–1972	American Occupational Therapy Association 251 Park Avenue South, New York, NY
1972–1980	American Occupational Therapy Association 6000 Executive Boulevard, Suite 200 (Wilco Building), Rockville, MD
1980–1994	American Occupational Therapy Association, Inc. 1383 Piccard Drive, Rockville, MD
1994–present	American Occupational Therapy Association, Inc. 4720 Montgomery Lane, Bethesda, MD

Andersen, L. T., & Reed, K. L.
The History of Occupational Therapy: The First Century (p. 363).
© 2017 Taylor & Francis Group.

Appendix D

Official Organ/Journal of NSPOT and AOTA

Publication Dates	Organ/Journal
1911–1921	*Maryland Psychiatric Quarterly*
1922–1924	*Archives of Occupational Therapy*
1925–1946	*Occupational Therapy & Rehabilitation*
1937	*Journal of Occupational Therapy* (only one edition published)
1947–present	*American Journal of Occupational Therapy*

Andersen, L. T., & Reed, K. L.
The History of Occupational Therapy: The First Century (p. 365).
© 2017 Taylor & Francis Group.

Appendix E

Annual Meetings of NSPOT and AOTA

DATE	LOCATION
September 3, 1917	New York, New York
September 2-4, 1918	New York, New York
September 8-11, 1919	Chicago, Illinois
September 13-14, 1920	Philadelphia, Pennsylvania
October 20-22, 1921	Baltimore, Maryland
September 25-29, 1922	Atlantic City, New Jersey
October 30–November 1, 1923	Milwaukee, Wisconsin
October 7-9, 1924	Buffalo, New York
October 19-22, 1925	Louisville, Kentucky
September 26-29, 1926	Atlantic City, New Jersey
October 10-13, 1927	Minneapolis, Minnesota
August 6-10, 1928	San Francisco, California
June 16-19, 1929	Atlantic City, New Jersey
October 20-24, 1930	New Orleans, Louisiana
September 28-30, 1931	Toronto, Canada
September 12-14, 1932	Detroit, Michigan
September 12-13, 1933	Milwaukee, Wisconsin
September 25-27, 1934	Philadelphia, Pennsylvania
September 30–October 1, 1935	St. Louis, Missouri
September 28–October 1, 1936	Cleveland, Ohio
September 14-17, 1937	Atlantic City, New Jersey
September 11-15, 1938	Chicago, Illinois
	(continued)

Andersen, L. T., & Reed, K. L.
The History of Occupational Therapy: The First Century (pp. 367-370).
© 2017 Taylor & Francis Group.

Date	Location
October 15-16, 1939*	New York, New York
September 15-19, 1940	Boston, Massachusetts
August 31–September 5, 1941	Washington, DC
October 8-9, 1942*	New York, New York
October 12-15, 1943*	Indianapolis, Indiana
November 12-15, 1944*	New York, New York
June 26-27, 1945*	Detroit, Michigan
August 10-15, 1946	Chicago, Illinois
November 2-7, 1947	Coronado, California
September 4-11, 1948	New York, New York
August 23-25, 1949	Detroit, Michigan
October 14-21, 1950	Glenwood Springs, Colorado
September 8-15, 1951	Portsmouth, New Hampshire
August 9-16, 1952	Milwaukee, Wisconsin
November 13-20, 1953	Houston, Texas
October 16-22, 1954	Washington, DC
October 21-28, 1955	San Francisco, California
September 29–October 5, 1956	Minneapolis, Minnesota
October 17-25, 1957	Cleveland, Ohio
October 17-23, 1958	New York, New York
October 19-23, 1959	Chicago, Illinois
November 13-17, 1960	Los Angeles, California
November 6-8, 1961	Detroit, Michigan
October 22-25, 1962	Philadelphia, Pennsylvania
September 29–October 3, 1963	St. Louis, Missouri
October 26-29, 1964	Denver, Colorado
October 31–November 4, 1965	Miami Beach, Florida
October 11-14, 1966	Minneapolis, Minnesota
October 11-14, 1967	Boston, Massachusetts
October 20-26, 1968	Portland, Oregon
November 3-7, 1969*	Dallas, Texas
November 20-24, 1970	New York, New York
October 31–November 5, 1971	Cleveland, Ohio
October 23-27, 1972	Los Angeles, California
October 29–November 2, 1973	Chicago, Illinois
October 21-25, 1974	Washington, DC
October 14-18, 1975	Milwaukee, Wisconsin
	(continued)

Date	Location
October 11-15, 1976	San Francisco, California
October 16-20, 1977	San Juan, Puerto Rico
May 7-13, 1978	San Diego, California
April 23-27, 1979	Detroit, Michigan
April 15-18, 1980	Denver, Colorado
March 9-13, 1981	San Antonio, Texas
May 10-14, 1982	Philadelphia, Pennsylvania
April 18-22, 1983	Portland, Oregon
May 7-11, 1984	Kansas City, Missouri
April 15-19, 1985	Atlanta, Georgia
April 20-23, 1986	Minneapolis, Minnesota
April 5-8, 1987	Indianapolis, Indiana
April 17-20, 1988	Phoenix, Arizona
April 15-19, 1989	Baltimore, Maryland
April 28–May 2, 1990	New Orleans, Louisiana
June 1-5, 1991	Cincinnati, Ohio
March 28–April 1, 1992	Houston, Texas
June 19-23, 1993	Seattle, Washington
July 9-13, 1994	Boston, Massachusetts (Can-Am Conference)
April 8-12, 1995	Denver, Colorado
April 19-23, 1996	Chicago, Illinois
April 11-15, 1997	Orlando, Florida
April 3-7, 1998	Baltimore, Maryland
April 16-20, 1999	Indianapolis, Indiana
March 31–April 4, 2000	Seattle, Washington
April 19-23, 2001	Philadelphia, Pennsylvania
May 2-5, 2002	Miami Beach, Florida
June 6-9, 2003	Washington, DC
May 20-23, 2004	Minneapolis, Minnesota
May 12-15, 2005	Long Beach, California
April 27-30, 2006	Charlotte, North Carolina
April 20-23, 2007	St. Louis, Missouri
April 9-13, 2008	Long Beach, California
April 23-26, 2009	Houston, Texas
April 29–May 2, 2010	Orlando, Florida
April 14-17, 2011	Philadelphia, Pennsylvania
April 26-29, 2012	Indianapolis, Indiana

(continued)

Date	Location
April 25-28, 2013	San Diego, California
April 2-6, 2014	Baltimore, Maryland
April 16-19, 2015	Nashville, Tennessee
April 7-10, 2016	Chicago, Illinois
March 30–April 2, 2017	Philadelphia, Pennsylvania

*No National meeting held because of war emergency.

Annual Meetings from 1922 to 1937 were held in conjunction with the American Hospital Association.

Adapted from:

AOTA. (1967). *50th Anniversary: Then...1917 and Now...1967.* New York, NY: American Occupational Therapy Association.

AOTA. (2014). Annual Meetings and Conferences of The National Society for the Promotion of Occupational Therapy and The American Occupational Therapy Association. Received from Mindy Hecker, May 21, 2014.

Appendix F

Eleanor Clarke Slagle Lecturers and Lectures

Year	Lecturer	Title of Lecture
1955	Florence M. Stattel	Equipment Designed for Occupational Therapy
1956	June Sokolov	Therapist Into Administrator: Ten Inspiring Years
1957	Ruth W. Brunyate	Powerful Levers in Common Things
1958	Margaret S. Rood	Every One Counts
1959	Lillian S. Wegg	The Essentials of Work Evaluation
1960	Muriel E. Zimmerman	Devices: Development and Direction
1961	Mary Reilly	Occupational Therapy Can Be One of the Great Ideas of 20th Century Medicine
1962	Naida Ackley	The Challenge of the Sixties
1963	A. Jean Ayres	The Development of Perceptual-Motor Abilities: A Theoretical Basis for Treatment of Dysfunction
1965	Gail S. Fidler	Learning as a Growth Process: A Conceptual Framework
1966	Elizabeth June Yerxa	Authentic Occupational Therapy
1967	Wilma L. West	Professional Responsibility in Times of Change
1969	Lela A. Lorens	Facilitating Growth and Development: The Promise of Occupational Therapy
1971	Geraldine L. Finn	The Occupational Therapist in Prevention Programs
1972	Jerry A. Johnson	Occupational Therapy: A Model for the Future
1973	Alice C. Jantzen	Academic Occupational Therapy: A Career Specialty
1974	Mary R. Fiorentino	Occupational Therapy: Realization to Activation
		(continued)

Andersen, L. T., & Reed, K. L.
The History of Occupational Therapy: The First Century (pp. 371-373).
© 2017 Taylor & Francis Group.

Year	Lecturer	Title of Lecture
1975	Josephine C. Moore	Behavior, Bias, and the Limbic System
1976	A. Joy Huss	Touch with Care or Caring Touch?
1978	Lorna Jean King	Toward a Science of Adaptive Responses
1979	L. Irene Hollis	Remember?
1980	Carolyn Manville Baum	Occupational Therapists Put Care in the Health System
1981	Robert K. Bing	Occupational Therapy Revisited: A Paraphrastic Journey
1983	Joan C. Rogers	Clinical Reasoning: The Ethics, Science, and Art
1984	Elnora M. Gilfoyle	Transformation of a Profession
1985	Anne Cronin Mosey	A Monistic or a Pluralistic Approach to Professional Identity?
1986	Kathlyn L. Reed	Tools of Practice: Heritage or Baggage
1987	Claudia Kay Allen	Activity: Occupational Therapy's Treatment Method
1988	Anne Henderson	Occupational Therapy Knowledge: From Practice to Theory
1989	Shereen D. Farber	Neuroscience and Occupational Therapy: Vital Connections
1990	Susan B. Fine	Resilience and Human Adaptability: Who Rises Above Adversity?
1993	Florence Clark	Occupation Embedded in Real Life: Interweaving Occupational Science and Occupational Therapy
1994	Ann P. Grady	Building Inclusive Community: A Challenge for Occupational Therapy
1995	Catherine A. Trombly	Occupation: Purposefulness and Meaningfulness
1996	David L. Nelson	Why the Profession of Occupational Therapy Will Flourish in the 21st Century
1998	Anne G. Fisher	Uniting Practice and Theory in an Occupational Framework
1999	Charles H. Christiansen	Defining Lives: Occupation as Identity: An Essay on Competence, Coherence, and the Creation of Meaning
2000	Margo B. Holm	Our Mandate for the New Millennium: Evidence-based Practice
2001	Winnie Dunn	The Sensation of Everyday Life: empirical, Theoretical, and Pragmatic Considerations
2003	Charlotte Brasic Royeen	Chaotic Occupational Therapy: Collective Wisdom for a Complex Profession
2004	Ruth Zemke	Time, Space, and the Kaleidoscopes of Occupation
2005	Suzanne M. Peloquin	Embracing Our Ethos, Reclaiming Our Heart
2006	Betty Risteen Hasselkus	The World of Everyday Occupation: Real People, Real Lives
2007	Jim Hinojosa	Becoming Innovators in a Era of Hyperchange
2008	Wendy J. Coster	Embracing Ambiguity: Facing the Challenge of Measurement
2009	Kathleen Barker Schwartz	Reclaiming Our Heritage: Connecting the Founding Vision to the Centennial Vision

(continued)

YEAR	LECTURER	TITLE OF LECTURE
2010	Janice Posatery Burke	What's Going on Here? Deconstructing the Interactive Encounter
2011	Beatriz C. Abreu	Accentuate the Positive: Reflections on Empathetic Interpersonal Interactions
2012	Karen Jacobs	PromOTing Occupational Therapy: Words, Images, and Actions
2013	Glen Gillen	A Fork in the Road
2014	Maralynne D. Mitcham	Education as Engine
2015	Helen S. Cohen	A Career in Inquiry
2016	Susan L. Garber	The Prepared Mind
2017	Roger O. Smith	Technology and Occupation: Past 100, Present and Next 100 Years

Note: Eleanor Clarke Slagle lectureship is not awarded every year.

Appendix G

AOTA Award of Merit Recipients

Year	Recipient(s)	Year	Recipient(s)
1950	Munzesheimer, Eva Otto	1968	McDaniel, Myra L. Wiemer, Ruth Brunyate
1951	Greene, Marjorie B. West, Wilma L.	1971	Spelbring, Lyla M.
1952	Kahmann, Winifred C.	1972	Crampton, Marion W.
1954	Taylor, Marjorie M. Willard, Helen S.	1973	Hollis, L. Irene
1955	McNary, Henrietta	1974	Cromwell, Florence S.
1956	Rouse, Dorothy D. Spackmann, Clare S.	1975	Welles, Carlotta
1957	Dunton, William Rush	1976	Hopkins, Helen L. Kilburn, Virginia T. Schwagmeyer, Mildred
1959	Robinson, Ruth A.	1977	Matthews, Martha E.
1960	Spear, Marion R.	1978	Moersch, Martha T.
1962	Wade, Beatrice D.	1979	Jantzen, Alice C. Johnson, Jerry A.
1964	Fish, Marjorie	1980	Fidler, Gail S.
1965	Ayres, A. Jean Jeffers, Lucie Spence	1982	Butz, Clyde W.
1967	Gleave, G. Margaret	1983	Hightower-VanDamm, May D. Reed, Kathlyn L. (continued)

Andersen, L. T., & Reed, K. L.
The History of Occupational Therapy: The First Century (pp. 375-376).
© 2017 Taylor & Francis Group.

Year	Recipient(s)	Year	Recipient(s)
1984	Baum, Carolyn Manville Devereaux, Elizabeth B. Hamant, Celestine Sammons, Fred	2000	Evert, Mary Margaret Grady, Ann P.
1985	Jaffe, Evelyn Grossman	2001	Anderson, Reba Fine, Susan B. Rourk, Jane Davis
1986	Llorens, Lela A. Slominski, Anita H.	2003	Jacobs, Karen Ottenbacher, Kenneth J.
1987	Bing, Robert Kendall Yerxa, Elizabeth J.	2004	Miller, Lucy Jane
1988	Tyndall, Dean R.	2006	Gillette, Nedra
1989	Hays, Carole Ann	2007	Clark, David D.
1990	Rogers, Joan C.	2008	Foto, Mary Elizabeth Smith
1991	Dunn, Winifred W. Gilfoyle, Elnora M.	2009	Kornblau, Barbara L.
1992	Gilkeson, Grace E. Mitchell, Marlys	2010	Carrasco, Ricardo C.
1993	Henderson, Anne	2011	Kielhofner, Gary (Posthumous)
1994	Hinojosa, Jim	2012	Kramer, Paula
1995	Prendergast, Nancy D.	2013	Moyers Cleveland, Penelope
1996	Hansen, Ruth Izutsu, Satoru	2014	Holm, Margo
1997	Kolodner, Ellen L.	2015	Mitcham, Maralynne D. (Posthumous)
1998	Stattel, Florence	2016	Fisher, Thomas F.
1999	Clark, Florence A.	2017	Christiansen, Charles

Note: Award of Merit is not given every year.

Appendix H

AOTA Membership Summary

Year	No. of Members		Year	No. of Members
1917	40		1970	9,348
1920	190		1975	20,120
1925	749		1980	30,616
1930	883		1985	40,941
1935	831		1990	44,792
1940	1,207		1995	54, 884
1945	2,177		2000	46,093
1950	2,967		2005	34,368
1955	3,896		2010	49.226
1960	4,938		2015	53,203
1965	5,350			

Notes: Based on unpublished membership numbers supplied by the Association. Two external events slowed the growth of the Association's membership. One was the Great Depression of the 1930s and the other was the introduction of the managed care payment system and therapy cap imposed by the Balanced Budget Act of 1997.

Andersen, L. T., & Reed, K. L.
The History of Occupational Therapy: The First Century (p. 377).
© 2017 Taylor & Francis Group.

INDEX